Cancer biotherapy

Cancer biotherapy
An introductory guide

Edited by

Annie Young
Three Counties Cancer Network,
Cheltenham, UK

Lewis Rowett
Annals of Oncology,
ESMO Head Office,
Viganello-Lugano,
Switzerland

David Kerr
Department of Clinical Pharmacology,
Radcliffe Infirmary,
Oxford, UK

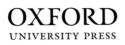

OXFORD
UNIVERSITY PRESS

*This book has been printed digitally and produced in a standard specification
in order to ensure its continuing availability*

OXFORD
UNIVERSITY PRESS

Great Clarendon Street, Oxford OX2 6DP

Oxford University Press is a department of the University of Oxford.
It furthers the University's objective of excellence in research, scholarship,
and education by publishing worldwide in

Oxford New York

Auckland   Cape Town Dar es Salaam   Hong Kong   Karachi
Kuala Lumpur Madrid Melbourne Mexico City   Nairobi
New Delhi Shanghai Taipei Toronto
With offices in
Argentina Austria Brazil Chile Czech Republic France Greece
Guatemala Hungary Italy Japan South Korea Poland Portugal
Singapore Switzerland Thailand Turkey Ukraine Vietnam

Oxford is a registered trade mark of Oxford University Press
in the UK and in certain other countries

Published in the United States
by Oxford University Press Inc., New York

ISBN 978-0-19-856631-1

Acknowledgements

Thanks go to all those who contributed time and effort to getting this book written and published. In addition to all authors we would want to thank in particular Savita Anderson, Katharine Clayden, and the ever-patient editorial staff of Oxford University Press.

AY
LR
DK
2006

Contents

Contributors

Kenneth D. Bagshawe
Department of Oncology
Hampstead Campus
Royal Free and University College
Medical School
University College London
Rowland Hill Street
London
UK

Richard H. J. Begent
Royal Free and University College
London Medical School
Department of Oncology
Rowland Hill Street
London
UK

Deborah Beirne
CRUK Clinical Cancer Centre
St. James Hospital
Leeds
UK

Peter Borchmann
Medizinische Einrichtungen der
Universität zu Köln
Klinik I für Innere Medizin
Kerpener Straße 62
D - 50924 Köln
Germany

Aniruddha Choudhury
Immune and Gene Therapy
Laboratory
Cancer Center Karolinska
Karolinska University Hospital
Stockholm
Sweden

Andreas Engert
Medizinische Einrichtungen der
Universität zu Köln
Klinik I für Innere Medizin
Joseph-Stelzmann-Strasse 9
Köln, D - 50924
Germany

Dirk Laurent
Schering AG
Global Medical Development
Oncology
D-13342 Berlin
Germany

Wan-Teck Lim
National Cancer Centre Singapore
Republic of Singapore

Howard L. McLeod
Washington University School of
Medicine
Division of Oncology
Campus Box 8069
660 South Euclid Avenue
St. Louis, MO 63110
USA

Håkan Mellstedt
Managing Director
Cancer Centre Karolinska
Department of Oncology
Karolinska University
Hospital Solna
SE-171 76 Stockholm
Sweden

Rachel Midgley
Department of Clinical
Pharmacology and Cancer
Therapeutics
University of Oxford
Radcliffe Hospital
Oxford
UK

Monica M. Mita
Institute for Drug Development
Cancer Therapy and Research Center
7979 Wurzbach Rd., 4th Floor, Rm
#Z414
San Antonio, TX 78229
USA

Kees Nooter
Department of Medical Oncology
Erasmus University Medical Center
Daniel den Hoed Cancer Center
Rotterdam
The Netherlands

Cornelis J. A. Punt
University Hospital Nijmegen St.
Radboud
Department of Medical Oncology
NL - 6500 HB Nijmegen
The Netherlands

Eric K. Rowinsky
Imclone Systems
33, Imclone Drive
Branchburg, NJ 08876
USA

Gary K. Schwartz
Memorial Sloan Kettering Cancer
Center
Gastrointestinal Oncology Research
Laboratory
1275 York Avenue
New York, NY 10021
USA

Leonard Seymour
University of Oxford
Radcliffe Infirmary
Dept. of Clinical Pharmacology
Oxford
UK

Manish A. Shah
Department of Medicine
Division of Solid Tumour Oncology,
and Laboratory of New Drug
Development
Memorial Sloan-Kettering Cancer
Center
New York
USA

Surinder K. Sharma
CRUK Targeting and Imaging Group
Department of Oncology
Hampstead Campus
Royal Free and University College
Medical School
University College London
Rowland Hill Street
London
UK

Stefan Sleijfer
Department of Medical Oncology
Erasmus University Medical Center
Daniel den Hoed Cancer Center
Rotterdam
The Netherlands

Neil Steven
CRC Institute for Cancer Studies
Clinical Research Block
The Medical School
Edgbaston
Birmingham
UK

Archie Tse
Department of Medicine
Division of Solid Tumour Oncology,
and Laboratory of New Drug
Development

Memorial Sloan-Kettering Cancer
Center
New York
USA

Carla M. L. van Herpen
Department of Medical Oncology
Radboud University Medical Centre
Nijmegen
The Netherlands

Jaap Verweij
Erasmus University Medical Centre
Department of Medical Oncology
Groene Hilledijk 301
NL - 3075 EA Rotterdam
The Netherlands

Cancer biotherapy—an introduction

David Kerr, Lewis Rowett, and Annie Young

1 Gotta dance!

An introduction of this kind, in this kind of book, is where the editors get to claim that the book you have in your hands is the book they set out to produce. Through a winning combination of intelligent choices, hard work, and thoughtful editing, the goals they set for themselves at the outset have all been reached, if not surpassed. Perhaps we will get to that introduction shortly, but first let's talk about *Singin' in the rain* (bear with us, we hope to make a serious point).

Made in 1951, *Singin' in the rain* is arguably the greatest musical ever written directly for the screen, and we would like to contend here that it is one of the great collaborative works of art of the twentieth century. Conceived by the producer Arthur Freed as an opportunity to use songs from his own back catalogue, co-written with Nacio Herb Brown, the film uses only two specially written songs, and one of those, *Make 'em laugh*, is widely considered to plagiarise Cole Porter's *Be a clown*. The song *Singin' in the rain* had been used repeatedly in films since the late 1920s and had already been memorably performed on film by both Jimmy Durante and Judy Garland. Taking the songs as their starting point, screenwriters Betty Comden and Adolph Green initially imagined an *Oklahoma*-style western musical, which finally became the story of a stuntman turned actor during the days of silent films and the emergence of the talkies. Stanley Donen, the director, had directed Fred Astaire a year before in *Royal Wedding*, had worked on numerous films through the 1940s as a choreographer, and had demonstrated a rare gift for filming dancing as director of the film version of *On the town*, where he had worked with Frank Sinatra and Gene Kelly.

It is Gene Kelly that most of us immediately think of at the mention of *Singin' in the rain*: Kelly the star singing and dancing in the rain, Kelly the uncompromising, pushing the young Debbie Reynolds to a career-best performance, Kelly the perfectionist redubbing the sounds of tap dancing that did not meet his exacting standards. But the performances of the entire cast are quite wonderful, from Jean Hagen's shrill, and Oscar-nominated, embodiment of Lina Lamont, to Donald O'Connor's buoyant sidekick, Cosmo, and Cyd Charisse's nameless dancer during the memorable *Broadway melody* ballet.

Suffice to say *Singin' in the rain* represents an extraordinary coming together of extraordinary talents. There is a strong element of that in this book—a world-class team of cancer researchers and clinicians, who have the ability to make the complex comprehensible. The second element that is celebrated in *Singin' in the rain,* is the emergence of new technology, i.e. talking pictures, and how such new technology can best be used to increase the sum of human well-being, a recurrent theme of this book.

Indeed the extraordinary technological insights that the last decade has given to the molecular mechanisms underpinning transformation of normal to cancer cells and development of new cancer therapies, offers an extraordinary potential to increase the sum of associated human well-being. The three key technological breakthroughs used to manufacture large quantities of biological molecules, are: (1) the discovery of the hybridoma technique in 1975 to produce monoclonal antibodies (Chapter 7) and for which Kohler and Milstein were awarded a Nobel prize; (2) the discovery of restriction enzymes, which permit isolation of genes that can be manipulated in another setting, again to produce amounts needed for clinical application; and (3) the discovery of growth factors, proteins that bind to cell surfaces promoting cellular differentiation and growth, for which Cohen and Levi-Montalcini were awarded a Nobel prize. However, despite some significant successes in more recent years, the problem of cancer remains great.

2 The problem of cancer

Cancer incidence, the number of new cancer cases occurring, has, with a few notable specific cancer exceptions, been increasing continuously since the time that reliable cancer statistics became available. It has been estimated that in 2002 there were 10.9 million new cases of cancer globally, with 6.7 million deaths, and 24.6 million persons living with cancer (Parkin *et al.* 2005). Over the last 20 years, increasing life expectancy has become a major determinant of increasing cancer incidence, and the World Health Organization has estimated that with this ageing of populations there could, by 2020, be 16 million new cases per year and around 10 million deaths. In Europe, where primary prevention, i.e. lifestyle changes that can reduce cancer incidence, screening, and application of modern cancer therapies, has led in recent years to generally decreasing trends in age-standardized rates, it has nevertheless been estimated that there will be around 1.25 million cancer deaths in 2015, almost 130 000 (11%) more deaths than in 2000 (Quinn *et al.* 2003).

Lung cancer has been the most common cause of cancer death since the mid-1980s, and in 2002, there were 1.35 million new cases, with 1.18 million deaths, 17.6% of the global total. Significantly, almost half of the cases occur in developing countries (Parkin *et al.* 2005). The largest part of this is due to tobacco smoking. Indeed, in the developed world, it is estimated that 25–30% of all, not just lung, cancer deaths are tobacco-related (Boyle *et al.* 2003). Adequate intervention, however, has been shown by the Nordic countries, which, since the early 1970s, have adopted integrated programmes against smoking that have significantly reduce lung cancer rates. In the UK, tobacco consumption has declined by 46% since 1970 and lung cancer mortality among men has been decreasing since 1980, although the rate still remains high (Peto *et al.* 2000).

Similarly, screening and early diagnosis can play a major role in reducing cancer mortality. Cervical cancer, although only the seventh most frequent cancer overall, is the second most common cancer among women globally, with an estimated 493 000 new cases and 274 000 deaths in 2002. Some 83% of these cases occurred in developing countries, where cervical cancer accounts for 15% of female cancers. By contrast, in developed countries where cervical screening using the Papanicolaou (Pap) test is commonplace, cervical cancer accounts for only 3.6% of new cancers (Parkin *et al.* 2005).

If, however, we consider those reductions in age-standardised cancer mortality, it is hard to establish what role therapy (chemotherapy, radiotherapy, or surgery, alone or in combination) has played, since improvements in diagnostics may have allowed earlier diagnosis and so increased survival (Garattini and La Vecchia 2001). There are, however, a few selected cancers or groups of cancers that have shown clear therapy-related improvements in mortality over recent decades. These are essentially the lymphoreticular and germ cell tumours.

For example, despite an increase in the incidence of testicular cancer since the 1970s, mortality rates have fallen in North America and Western Europe (Levi *et al.* 2001). In the USA and the EU countries, testicular cancer mortality has fallen by around 70% since their peaks in the late 1960s and early 1970s.

This fall can in the largest part be attributed to developments in cancer therapeutics, significant among them being platinum-based chemotherapeutics. This can be demonstrated by mortality data from Eastern Europe, where access to newer therapies has been limited or delayed, and mortality rates rose on average by approximately 60% over the same period; indeed, they have only started to decline in the last few years (Levi *et al.* 2001).

In short, cancer incidence is increasing globally, and while primary prevention and screening can be effective, new therapies are urgently needed. Where a new therapy becomes available it can have a dramatic effect on mortality.

3   Chemotherapy and biotherapy

At this stage it may be useful if we define what we mean by cancer biotherapy and explain how we see it as being different from chemotherapy.

3.1   Cytotoxic chemotherapy

The origins of modern cancer chemotherapy date back to World War I when mustard gas (sulphur mustard) was used as a weapon with cytotoxic, i.e. cell killing, effects. During World War II, Gilman and Philips, working for the Medical Division of the Chemical Warfare Service of the US Army investigated the cytotoxic effects of analogues of the sulphur mustards and noted that the cytotoxicity was related to the extent that the cells were proliferating (Gilman and Philips 1946). They suggested that such cytotoxic chemicals had potential in the treatment of cancer.

Cytotoxic chemotherapy, as we know it today, has the potential to kill proliferating cells. Since, as we will see in subsequent chapters (see Chapter 1), uncontrolled cell growth and proliferation are characteristic of cancer cells, cytotoxic chemotherapy can kill cancer cells. Unfortunately, chemotherapy is a systemic therapy, it enters the bloodstream and is distributed throughout the body; and the body contains many types of cell that are proliferating but are not cancer cells, e.g. bone marrow cells developing red and white blood cells, cells of mucosal linings, and skin cells.

The fluoropyrimidine drug 5-fluorouracil (5-FU) is a well-established example of a cytotoxic cancer chemotherapeutic and has been used in the treatment of a variety of cancers, including breast cancer, head and neck cancer, and most significantly in colorectal cancer (IMPACT 1995). The fluoropyrimidine drugs were developed during the 1950s following the finding that rat hepatomas used the pyrimidine uracil, one of the four bases found in RNA, at a higher rate than did normal tissues. 5-FU is an antimetabolite, it acts to inhibit an essential biosynthetic process and so promote cell death.

Essentially, 5-FU is an analogue of uracil with a fluorine atom replacing one of the hydrogen atoms; it enters the cell via the same pathways as uracil but is then metabolised to a variety of active products that can disrupt RNA synthesis by insertion into RNA instead of uracil. These active 5-FU metabolites can also disrupt DNA synthesis and inhibit the nucleotide-synthesising enzyme thymidylate synthase (Longley *et al.* 2003). However, the cytotoxic effects of 5-FU are indiscriminate, leading to cell death in bone marrow, skin, and mucosae, and so producing some of the typical side-effects of chemotherapy, e.g. mouth ulcers, rashes, diarrhea, fatigue due to anaemia, and susceptibility to infection.

3.2 Biotherapy

Biotherapy is now regarded as the fourth treatment modality for patients with cancer. Biotherapy encompasses the use of agents derived from biological sources or of agents that affect biological responses (Oldham 1998).

Biotherapy, or biological therapy, attempts to use the great increases in our knowledge of molecular biology, cell biology, and immunology (Chapter 2) that have arisen since World War II, and in particular since Richard Nixon passed the National Cancer Act in 1971, so declaring the War on Cancer, to achieve tumour control. Cell death remains a fundamental part of what biotherapy aims for, but another key feature is that through increased understanding of cancer biology, the therapies may be targeted to act specifically on cancer cells. Biotherapy may also be characterised by the use of naturally occurring biological molecules, such as cytokines and antibodies, or by the manipulation of normal biological mechanisms to control or inhibit tumour growth.

This is not to say that biotherapies are without side-effects. Indeed significant side-effects of biotherapies have been reported (see, for example: Bendell *et al.* 2003; Hurwitz *et al.* 2004), but these effects occur, not as a result of the indiscriminate killing of proliferating cells, rather as a consequence of the complexity of the biological systems the therapies are intended to interact with or manipulate.

4 The future is now...

We are in the midst of a revolution in the treatment of cancer. Speaking to the Royal College of Physicians in March 2002, Karel Sikora, former head of the World Health Organization Cancer Programme, noted that there were over 500 anticancer drugs in clinical development. He predicted that that number might exceed 1000 by 2005. Analysing the possible development pathways of a variety of new anticancer technologies, predominantly biotherapies, e.g. monoclonal antibodies (Chapter 7), cancer vaccines (Chapter 12), and kinase inhibitors (Chapter 4), he identified the years 2005 to 2010 as potentially critical (Sikora 2002).

In mid-1980, the US Food and Drug Administration (FDA) approved interferon alpha, soon followed by the approval of granulocyte colony stimulating factor (GCSF) and granulocyte macrophage colony stimulating factor (GMCSF). As of writing, twenty years on in early 2005, the US FDA's Center for Drug Evaluation and Research website lists some 120 drugs approved for use in oncology (*http://www.fda.gov/cder/cancer/druglistframe.htm*). Of these, 12 have been approved for the first time since January 2000; but of these 12, four are preparations of antibodies, two are enzymes, one is a modified growth factor, one is the endocrine therapy fulvestrant developed as a consequence of our increased knowledge of, and targeted to, the oestrogen receptor, and one is the biologically active small molecule imatinib, which has specific enzyme inhibitory activities. And this is to ignore the approvals in the late 1990s of the monoclonal antibodies rituximab and trastuzumab (Chapter 7), and the cytokine interferon-α2b (Chapter 9).

At the turn of the new millennium, it was certainly possible to argue that anticancer drug development was going through a transition. That remains true today. What we want to make clear here, and what we believe this whole book demonstrates, is that this transition is now passing into clinical practice.

5 So what do we do now?

The other thing we hope this book can do is provide some pointers as to what we can expect from this transition and what we might do next.

5.1 Don't believe the hype

The emergence of talking pictures, the technological transition that *Singin' in the rain* deals with, had a profound effect on films and film production. Critics have argued that it inhibited diversity in films and set back film aesthetics, making film makers lazy and over-reliant on expositionary dialogue and narration (Crafton 1999). Indeed, Alfred Hitchcock, who had directed the first British talkie, famously said that American films were mostly pictures of actors talking. Herein lies an important lesson for those us working to develop cancer biotherapeutics and bring them to the clinic: we should not forget what we already know, either about drug development or clinical practice. The issue is not simply how we use the knowledge base, although that must necessarily be part of it, but how we ensure that patients benefit.

Despite the acknowledged successes of the last 30 or so years, it is probably not unfair to characterise the history of the War on Cancer as a series of false dawns. Few military metaphors can have become quite so hackneyed in that time as the 'breakthrough', with the hype too frequently being succeeded by public disappointment, disenchantment, and backlash (Sporn 1996; Daugherty 2002). And it is impossible to argue with Christopher Daugherty (Daugherty 2002) when he writes:

> Can the media report the hope without the hype? Well, they should. Their ability to do so would be increased if the oncology research community recognised its own potential role in contributing to the kind of hype that can never be lived up to. When we contribute to the hype, knowingly or ignorantly, we then fail to stand firm in protecting the primary interests of our patients. In so doing, we put ourselves at risk of further losing our patients' trust in our abilities both to care for them and to improve the future care of patients with cancer.

What can we do now? Ask how the new biotherapeutics can improve patient benefit and work towards those answers.

5.2 Cure or care?

It has been suggested that attempts to incorporate our enhanced biological knowledge into new clinical protocols will favour trials of targeted biotherapies, of the kind this book is focused on, while limiting the funds available for testing genetic findings that may offer more immediate benefits to patients (Anonymous 2003). The potential of genetic information to benefit patients is outlined in Chapter 14. It is becoming increasingly apparent that the collecting and testing of genetic data will contribute to our understanding of the effectiveness of those targeted biotherapies, as many may work best, or work only, in distinct genetically defined patient populations (for review see Rothenberg *et al.* 2003). It is, consequently, beholden on us to use our existing knowledge of clinical research to design the most appropriate studies and ensure that relevant data for identification of patient populations is collected. Certainly infrastructure for this kind of research has been lacking but developments such as the National Cancer Tissue Resource in the UK (Knox and Kerr 2004) are helping to fill these gaps.

6 Caveat lector

Cancer drug development and cancer clinical practice are now going through important transitions. This is not hype but a reality, which all of us working to improve cancer patient care must now face. This book is an attempt to bring some of the elements of these transitions into focus. The field of biotherapy is moving rapidly, and we must admit that this book is, at least in part, merely a snapshot of that field as it was at the end of 2004 and the beginning of 2005. Our understanding of individual therapies may have changed since then.

Nevertheless, we have tried to promote an understanding of the underlying biological principles. Cancer remains a vast global problem; biotherapeutics are potentially valuable additions to our armamentarium against that problem.

References

Anonymous (2003) Acceleration of cure or optimisation of care? *Lancet*; 4: 261.

Bendell JC, Domchek SM, Burstein HJ *et al.* (2003) Central nervous system metastases in women who receive trastuzumab-based therapy for metastatic breast carcinoma. *Cancer*; 97: 2972–77.

Boyle P, Autier P, Bartelink H *et al.* (2003) European Code Against Cancer and scientific justification: third version (2003). *Ann Oncol*; 14: 973–1005.

Crafton D (1999) *The Talkies: American Cinema's Transition to Sound, 1926–31*. University of California Press. Berkeley, CA.

Daugherty CK (2002) The 'cure' for cancer: can the media report the hope without the hype? *J Clin Oncol*; 20: 3761–4.

Garattini S, La Vecchia C. (2001) Perspectives in cancer chemotherapy. *Eur J Cancer*; 37 Suppl 8: S128–47.

Gilman A, Philips FS (1946) The biological actions and therapeutic applications of the B-chloroethyl amines and sulfides. *Science*; 103: 409–15.

Hurwitz H, Fehrenbacher L, Novotny W *et al.* (2004) Bevacizumab plus irinotecan, fluorouracil, and leucovorin for metastatic colorectal cancer. *N Engl J Med*; 350: 2335–42.

IMPACT (1995) Efficacy of adjuvant fluorouracil and folinic acid in colon cancer. International Multicentre Pooled Analysis of Colon Cancer Trials (IMPACT) investigators. *Lancet*; 345: 939–44.

Knox K, Kerr DJ (2004) Establishing a national tissue bank for surgically harvested cancer tissue. *Br J Surg*; 91: 134–6.

Levi F, La Vecchia C, Boyle P, Lucchini F, Negri E (2001) Western and eastern European trends in testicular cancer mortality. *Lancet*; 357: 1853–4.

Longley DB, Harkin DP, Johnston PG (2003) 5-fluorouracil: mechanisms of action and clinical strategies. *Nat Rev Cancer*; 3: 330–8.

Oldham R (ed.). (1998) *Principles of cancer biotherapy* (3rd edn). Kluwer Academic Publishers, Boston MA.

Parkin DM, Bray F, Ferlay J, Pisani P (2005) Global Cancer Statistics, 2002. *CA Cancer J Clin*; 55: 74–108.

Peto R, Darby S, Deo H, Silcocks P, Whitley E, Doll R (2000) Smoking, smoking cessation, and lung cancer in the UK since 1950: combination of national statistics with two case-control studies. *BMJ*; 321: 323–9.

Quinn MJ, d'Onofrio A, Moller B *et al.* (2003) Cancer mortality trends in the EU and acceding countries up to 2015. *Ann Oncol*; 14: 1148–52.

Rothenberg ML, Carbone DP, Johnson DH (2003) Improving the evaluation of new cancer treatments: challenges and opportunities. *Nat Rev Cancer*; 3: 303–9.

Sikora K (2002) The impact of future technology on cancer care. Clin Med; 2: 560–8.

Sporn MB (1996) The war on cancer. *Lancet*; 347: 1377–81.

Chapter 1

An introduction to the cell biology of cancer

Lewis Rowett and Annie Young

1 Introduction

As you certainly know, and if not it will become apparent from a reading of the subsequent chapters of this book, cancer is a genetic disease and a disease of cells. Commonly, cancer is described as a disease of unregulated, or dysregulated, cell growth. Significantly, we will see that cancer is a disease of cellular control systems. Before we look at these systems in more detail, it may be useful to consider what cells are.

All living things are composed of at least one cell. Many are composed of no more than one cell, e.g. bacteria, amoebae, but the human body is composed of billions of cells. The exact number is unclear and varies, of course, with the body in question, but estimates of cell numbers in the human body go as high as 100 trillion, i.e. 10^{14}. Similarly, the exact number of types of cells in the human body is not known. Nevertheless, all the cells in the human body, with a few important exceptions, have an underlying structural similarity.

2 Cell structure

The cells of the human body are described as being **eukaryotic**: the contents of the cell are separated from the outside world by a lipid bilayer membrane, the various biological processes conducted by the cell, e.g. respiration, protein synthesis, digestion of cellular debris and ingested materials, are compartmentalised into separate intracellular bodies called **organelles**, and, fundamentally, the great majority of the cell's genetic material, its **DNA**, is separated from the rest of the cell within a **nucleus**. Within the DNA's, now famous, double-helical structure, is encoded the cell's genetic information. This is achieved through the order, or sequence, of the **nucleotide** bases, adenine (A), thymine (T), guanine (G), and cytosine (C) along each strand. Each base may thus be considered as a letter in a four-letter alphabet spelling out biological messages in the chemical sequence of the DNA.

Generally, the nucleus occupies about 10% of the total cell volume, with the separation from the rest of the cell being effected by the nuclear envelope, two further concentric lipid bilayer membranes. This nuclear envelope is perforated at intervals by large nuclear pores, which allow transport of molecules between the nucleus and the rest of the cell contained within the cell membrane, the **cytosol**. Embedded within the cytosol, which is predominantly water, is a meshwork of tubules, the cytoskeleton, which gives the cell shape, effects intracellular transport, and can bring about cell movement. It is the tubules of the cytoskeleton that pull the DNA-containing **chromosomes** apart during **mitosis** and subsequently splits the dividing cell in two. Most human cells are between 10 μm and 100 μm in diameter.

2.1 The cell membrane and membrane proteins

The bilayer structure of the cell membrane is formed as a result of the properties of the lipid, i.e. fatty, molecules. The lipid molecules of cell

Table 1.1 Cell structures and their functions

Structure	Function
Cell membrane	Forms boundary of the cell, maintaining integrity while allow control of molecules crossing the membrane.
Nucleus	Houses the majority of the cells DNA and so controls protein synthesis.
Endoplasmic reticulum (ER)	Membranous structures involved in lipid (smooth ER) and protein synthesis (rough ER).
Ribosomes	Attached to the rough ER, the sites RNA translation leading to protein synthesis.
Golgi apparatus	Carbohydrate synthesis, site of covalent modification of products of the rough and smooth ER prior to their despatch to cellular locations.
Mitochondria	Oxidation to produce the cell's ATP.
Lysosomes	Digestion, has a relatively high pH and contains digestive enzymes that break down cellular and ingested materials.
Peroxisomes	Detoxification, contains the enzyme catalase which converts hydrogen peroxide to water and oxygen.
Cytoskeleton	Confers shape on the cell and provides a mechanism for cell movement and intracellular transport.

membranes are amphipathic, i.e. they contain a hydrophilic 'water-loving' and a hydrophobic 'water-fearing' end. In aqueous environments, such as the cytosol, these amphipathic lipids naturally organise themselves into double layers, with the hydrophobic ends facing inwards towards each other and the hydrophilic ends facing outwards towards the aqueous environment. While this bilayer structure is common to cell membranes, it is the proteins within them that achieve most of the specific functions of membranes, serving as specific receptors for certain hormones, enzymes, transport proteins, and so on. It is the proteins, therefore, that give each type of membrane in the cell its characteristic functional properties. Some of these membrane proteins are structurally linked to the cytoskeleton.

2.2 Organelles

All eukaryotic cells contain essentially the same basic set of organelles, literally little organs, suspended within the cytosol. These organelles are themselves delimited from the rest of the cytosol by lipid bilayer membranes and, since the lipid bilayer of organelle membranes is impermeable to most hydrophilic molecules, the membrane of each organelle contains membrane transport proteins that are responsible for passage of specific metabolites through the organelle membrane. Similarly, each organelle membrane holds mechanisms for importing and incorporating into the organelle, the specific proteins that make the organelle unique. Again, we see that it is the proteins that give each type of organelle in the cell its characteristic functional properties.

Approximately half of the membrane area in a eukaryotic cell encloses a network of interconnected tubules, vesicles, and sacs that constitutes the organelle called the **endoplasmic reticulum** (ER). Membrane-bound **ribosomes** coating the cytosolic surface of the ER, create regions termed rough endoplasmic reticulum, or rough ER. The ribosome is a complex of more than 50 different proteins and several RNA molecules and is, when bound to the ER, the site of protein synthesis within the cell. The ER is also the site of most of the lipid production for the rest of the cell and serves as a store for calcium ions.

Many of the proteins and lipids produced in the ER are passed to the **Golgi apparatus**. The Golgi apparatus is a major site of carbohydrate synthesis within the cell, and it also serves as a sorting and despatching point for the products of the ER, usually modifying those products covalently before despatching them to various cellular destinations.

Mitochondria occupy a substantial part of the eukaryotic cytosol and are the site of most cellular oxidations, producing most of the cell's **ATP**, the basic energy molecule of the cell. Each mitochondrion has a double-membrane structure, an outer membrane and a highly convoluted inner membrane. The inner membrane is folded into structures called cristae that project into the central mitochondrial matrix. These cristae greatly increase the available surface area of the inner membrane and it is in this membrane that the enzymes of the respiratory chain, those responsible for the production of ATP, are embedded. The mitochondrial matrix contains, among other things, mitochondrial DNA, which is inherited exclusively from the maternal line. In human cells, mitochondrial DNA represents less than 1% of the total cellular DNA.

A further significant membrane-enclosed organelle is the **lysosome**. The internal space of the lysosome is maintained at an acidic pH of around pH 5.0, and it contains digestive enzymes, proteases, lipases, phosphatases, etc., that degrade ingested macromolecules and particles drawn into the cell by the process of **endocytosis**. Lysosomes also play a part in breaking down other organelles trafficked to them from within the cell itself.

Although each organelle performs an essentially similar set of basic functions in all cell types, and while all cells do contain an essentially similar set of organelles, variations in the functions of cells can lead to variations in the abundance of the various organelles and can result in further organelle specialisations.

2.3 The nucleus

The cell nucleus is a particularly specialised organelle and the defining characteristic of eukaryotic cells. The nucleus contains the DNA of the cell's **genome**, and it is the site of DNA replication, transcription of DNA to **RNA**, and post-transcriptional processing of RNA. Indeed it is only the final step in gene expression, the **translation** of RNA to protein, occurring in the ribosomes of the rough ER, that takes place outside the nucleus. This separation of **transcription** and translation affords the eukaryotic cell further levels at which gene expression can be regulated.

The nucleus is contained within a double-membrane structure called the nuclear envelope composed of inner and outer nuclear membranes. The outer nuclear membrane is connected to, and continuous with, the endoplasmic reticulum. Moreover, the cytosol-facing surface of the outer nuclear membrane has ribosomes bound to it. The inner nuclear membrane, by contrast, holds proteins that are specific to the nucleus. Beneath the inner nuclear membrane is the nuclear lamina, a meshwork of interconnected protein subunits called nuclear lamins that provides structural support to the nucleus. These nuclear lamins are a specialised class of intermediate filament proteins, one of the three classes of protein otherwise found in the cytoskeleton. The nuclear envelope is perforated by pore complexes which together with other membrane bound proteins anchor it to the nuclear lamin.

Internally, the nucleus appears to mirror the cell itself in localising particular functions to particular regions. Most obvious among these internal regions of the nucleus is the nucleolus, which is the site of ribosomal (r)RNA gene transcription and ribosomal subunit assembly. Other regions of localised function giving rising to the internal organisation of the nucleus include the organisation of DNA into chromosomes, the localisation of DNA replication, and post-transcriptional processing of pre-mRNA molecules.

3 Cell growth

So there we have our cell, one of billions in the human body. What happens to turn this one cell into what Robert Weinberg (Weinberg 1998) has called the one renegade cell, the cell that leads to cancer?

We said at the outset that cancer is a disease of unregulated cell growth, more specifically unregulated cell proliferation by cell division. Yet cell proliferation is a natural and necessary multistep process. Typically, human cells proliferate, grow to a preprogrammed size and extent, become mature, and eventually die. The single fertilised ovum must divide and proliferate to make the billions of cells that make up the body; skin cells and cells of mucosal epithelia are constantly being worn away and must be replaced. Clearly, it is not the proliferation itself that makes cells cancerous, rather it is the loss of regulation leading to continual proliferation that is the defining characteristic of cancer cells. These cells do not respond to the various signals and controlling systems that regulate normal cell behaviour. Consequently, cancer cells grow and divide continuously, invading normal tissues and organs and ultimately, if unchecked by medical intervention, spreading throughout the body. It is important to understand that this loss of cell growth regulation is the result of accumulated malfunctions, occurring as genetic mutations, in multiple cell regulatory systems.

4 Cell division and the cell cycle

The term **mitosis** was first used to describe **somatic**, i.e. non-reproductive, cell division in the 1880s by the German anatomist Walther Flemming (Flemming 1882), and the essential mechanics of this process by which daughter chromosomes are separated, the nucleus divided, and daughter cells formed (**cytokinesis**) were established over the following 50 years. How this process is controlled has, however, only begun to be elucidated over the last 20 years or so with our growing understanding of the cell cycle. The cell cycle is a key regulator of the processes of cell proliferation and growth. The molecular machinery of the cell cycle and its potential to provide targets for cancer therapy are discussed in some detail elsewhere in this book (see Chapter 6).

Nevertheless, we should understand that irrespective of the specific genetic damage leading to cancer or the type of cancer, the common feature is disruption of the cell cycle (Sherr 1996).

Mitosis (see Table 1.2) and cytokinesis only occupy about 5% of the cell cycle, the remaining time being spent in interphase, during which actual cell growth and DNA replication occur in preparation for cell division. The cell cycle (Fig. 1.1) is divided into four distinct phases—G_1, S, G_2 and M—with quality-control checkpoints switching the cell from one phase to the next, ensuring accurate time and order of the molecular events (Sherr 1996). The essential role of each phase is as follows:

G_1 The interval (gap) between the end of mitosis and the beginning of DNA replication. The cell grows and prepares metabolically for DNA replication.

S   The phase of DNA synthesis and replication.

G_2 The interval (gap 2) between the end of DNA synthesis and the beginning of mitosis. The cell continues to grow and proteins are synthesised in preparation for mitosis.

M   Mitosis.

The duration of these phases may vary considerably depending upon the cell type. Typically, a rapidly proliferating human cell in culture will have a total cycle time of 24 h, of this the G_1 phase might last about 11 h, S phase about 8 h, G_2 about 4 h, and M about 1 h.

Often after mitosis the cell may exit completely, either temporarily or permanently, from the cell cycle and enter what is called G_0. It is in G_0 that the cell performs its routine functions. Entry from G_0 into the cell cycle (G_1) is governed by a restriction point, a transition point beyond which the cell progresses into S phase and through the cell cycle, independent of external stimuli such as exposure to nutrients or **mitogen** activation (Pardee 1974).

The regulatory mechanisms controlling the switching between the various phases of the cell cycle fall into two main classes: intrinsic mechanisms, which occur routinely in every cell cycle and form part of the driving mechanism of the cycle; and extrinsic mechanisms, which operate quality control when defects are detected (Ekholm & Reed 2000).

4.1 Cyclins, cyclin-dependent kinases, and cyclin-dependent kinase inhibitors

In human cells, the principle intrinsic control system is a family of **protein kinases** known as **cyclin-dependent kinases (Cdks)**. These Cdks, when complexed with specific regulatory proteins called cyclins, drive the cell

Table 1.2 The phases of mitosis. Mitosis is usually followed by cytokinesis, i.e. division of cytoplasm and formation of daughter cells

Phase	Events
Prophase	DNA contained in chromatin condenses into chromosomes composed of two chromatids and a centromere. Centrioles, microtubule organising centres, move to opposite poles of the cell and begin forming the mitotic spindle between them.
	The nuclear membrane breaks down.
Metaphase	Chromosomes attach to the centre of the mitotic spindle at their centromeres.
Anaphase	Each centromere splits and the daughter chromatids are drawn apart to opposite poles of the cell by the spindle.
Telophase	The daughter chromatids, now chromosomes, begin to decondense. The spindle breaks down and the nuclear membrane reappears.

forward through the cell cycle. The Cdk/cyclin complex is itself subject to both positive and negative regulation, such that the activity of the Cdks fluctuates as the cell progresses through the cell cycle. These variations can lead to cyclical changes in the phosphorylation of intracellular proteins that initiate or regulate the major events of the cell cycleDNA replication, mitosis, and cytokinesis (Morgan 1995).

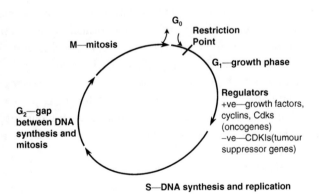

Fig. 1.1 The phases of the cell cycle. Note that not all cells enter G_0, the post-mitotic state, on passing through the cycle. Cdk, cyclin-dependent kinases; CDKI, cyclin-dependent kinase inhibitors. (See also Chapter 6.)

The cyclins themselves, as mediators of Cdk activities, represent a further intrinsic control mechanism, with cyclin levels also fluctuating through the various phases of the cycle. A large number of different cyclins have been identified (A to T) but generally they can be divided into four main classes: G_1 cyclins, e.g. the cyclin D isoforms that drive the cell through the G_1 phase; G_1/S cyclins, e.g. cyclin E isoforms that direct entry of the cell into S phase; S cyclins, e.g. cyclin A isoforms that drive the cell through S phase; and M cyclins, e.g. cyclin B isoforms that are necessary for mitosis (Sherr 1996, 2000). Cyclin levels are controlled primarily by gene expression and protein degradation, and unscheduled expression of cyclin genes has been implicated in several human cancers (Sherr 2000; Sutherland & Musgrove 2004; Tetsu & McCormick 1999; Yu *et al.* 2000).

Negative regulation of Cdk activities is achieved by a class of proteins called the **Cdk inhibitors** (CDKIs), which can serve to stop cell progression through the cell cycle. There are mainly two families of CDKI: the INK4 (inhibitors of Cdk4) family, including $p16^{ink4a}$, $p15^{ink4b}$, $p18^{ink4c}$, and $p19^{ink4d}$, which bind and inhibit cyclin D-bound Cdks; and the KIP family, including $p21^{waf1}$, $p27^{kip1}$ and $p57^{kip2}$, which negatively regulate cyclin E-bound and cyclin A-bound CDK2 (Sherr & Roberts 1999). Disruption of CDKI activities has been identified in a variety of different human cancers, and the CDKIs are believed to play a role in preventing uncontrolled cell proliferation and tumour formation, such that several of the genes encoding CDKIs are considered as **tumour suppressor genes** (Reed *et al.* 1996; Solomon & Kaldis 1998; Talve *et al.* 1999).

4.2 Tumour suppressors

Genes in which a mutation can lead to loss of protein function that may result in uncontrolled cell proliferation and tumour formation have been called tumour suppressor genes, and their products are considered tumour suppressors, i.e. they negatively regulate cell proliferation by encoding proteins that block the action of growth promoting proteins. Tumour suppressor genes are recessive in that both **alleles** of a pair must mutate for the gene to be inactivated. Within the cell cycle, the two best-characterised tumour suppressors are the retinoblastoma (Rb) protein and the transcription factor **p53** (see Chapter 6 for details).

Retinoblastoma is a childhood cancer of the eye occurring in about one child in 20 000 as a result of mutation of the *Rb* gene located on human chromosome 13. This gene was the first human tumour suppressor gene to be isolated. The

Rb protein encoded by the gene is normally expressed in almost all the cells of the body and serves to regulate the cell cycle by communicating between the cell cycle and the machinery of transcription, in particular Rb regulates the G_1/S transition. In its active state, Rb is hypophosphorylated and forms an inhibitory complex with a group of nuclear transcription factors, known as E2F-DP (E2F-1, -2, and -3), which are involved in cellular replication during S phase. In its hyperphosphorylated state, however, the Rb protein does not bind to this transcription factor; this phosphorylation is achieved by CDKs. Mutations in the *Rb* gene can lead to Rb becoming constitutively phosphorylated and so permanently unable to bind and inhibit the transcription factors leading to uncontrolled entry of cells in the S phase (reviewed by: Malumbres & Barbacid 2001; Weinberg 1995). Dysregulation of the cell cycle by mutation of *Rb* has now been implicated in several common types of cancer, including lung, breast and bladder cancer (Hickman *et al.* 2002). Indeed it seems that mutation of *Rb* or the *p53* gene may occur in most human cancers.

p53 is a DNA-binding protein that regulates the expression of genes involved in cell cycle arrest. Normal cellular levels of p53 are low, largely due to the short half-life of the protein; however, both intracellular and extracellular stress signals, e.g. DNA damage, can lead to rapid induction of p53. This activates transcription of the p21 CDKI, which inhibits cell cycle progression by general inhibition of CDK/cyclin complex formation and by inhibiting DNA replication. The resulting cell cycle arrest allows time for DNA damage to be repaired before it is replicated or for the cell to enter programmed cell death—apoptosis (reviewed by: Hickman *et al.* 2002; Sandal 2002). Mutation of the *p53* gene may lead to failure of the damage-induced cell cycle arrest, resulting in increased mutation rates and a general instability of the cell genome. Such genetic instability is a common property of cancer cells, and indeed *p53* is the most commonly disrupted gene in human cancers, with more than 50% of human cancers showing *p53* mutations. It is important to note, however, that activation of the p21 CDKI is not itself necessary for p53-mediated apoptosis. p53 transcriptionally activates many other genes including the gene encoding Mdm2, its own inhibitor, so providing a negative feedback mechanism, and a number of genes involved in apoptosis (reviewed by Sherr 2004).

5 Programmed cell death—apopotosis

Programmed cell death is a normal physiological process that plays a crucial role both in embryonic development and the maintenance of adult tissues (see Chapter 6). In adults, programmed cell death is responsible for balancing cell proliferation and maintaining constant cell numbers in tissues undergoing cell turnover; it is estimated that each year, a mass of cells almost equal to the weight of the body is lost as a result of programmed cell death (Reed 1999a). As we have seen with p53, programmed cell death also provides a defence mechanism that can eliminate damaged and potentially dangerous cells. The underlying morphological process of programmed cell death is called apoptosis and is characterised morphologically by shrinking of the **cytoplasm**, membrane blebbing, condensation of nuclear chromatin, and fragmentation into membrane-enclosed vesicles (Reed 1999b). These changes are accompanied by biochemical changes, including the release of mitochondrial cytochrome C, the degradation of the genomic DNA into high-molecular mass and oligonucleosomal fragments by endoncleases, activation of apoptotic protease activating factor (Apaf-1), and the cleavage of a specific subset of cellular polypeptides by **caspases**, a family of intracellular proteases (Kerr *et al.* 1972; Martin & Green 1995). These caspases are synthesised as inactive precursors that can be converted to the active form by proteolytic cleavage, catalysed by other caspases. So the initial activation of a caspase begins a cascade leading to activation of additional caspases and, ultimately to cell death.

This biochemical cascade of apoptosis is subject to regulation at multiple levels. Proteins of the Bcl-2 family may either inhibit apoptosis, e.g. Bcl-2, Bcl-XL, Bcl-W, Mcl-1, A1/Bfi-1, or act to enhance apoptosis, e.g. BAD, Bak, Bax, Bid, Bik, Bcl-2, and Bcl-XL both act by binding and inhibiting Apaf-1 and so prevent caspase activation. However, Bax, when present in excess, can displace Bcl-2 from Apaf-1 allowing caspase cleavage and activation. Bax also promotes apoptosis by mediating the release of cytochrome C from the mitochondria. In addition, the caspases are themselves subject to regulation through the action of a number of caspase inhibitors (Reed 1999b).

With an increased understanding of the nature and role of apoptosis has come the recognition that, while cancer is certainly a disease of dysregulated cellular proliferation, abnormal proliferative capacity is only one side of the story. Abnormal cellular survival, as a consequence of a failure to induce apoptosis, also plays a major part in tumorigenesis. For example, loss of Bax function has been implicated in the pathogenesis of colorectal cancers (Rampino *et al.* 1997). Moreover, the failure of many chemotherapeutic agents is now thought to reflect the inability of these drugs to induce **apoptosis**.

6 Oncogenes

Although mutation of the *Rb* or *p53* gene may occur in most human cancers, no mutation of a single gene has been identified, which alone can cause cancer. Multiple mutations must occur causing dysregulation of multiple systems before a cancer cell can arise. Rb and p53 are tumour suppressors: their normal functions are as safeguard systems preventing loss of growth control and it is loss of this inhibitory effect through gene mutation that leads to their role in oncogenesis. **Proto-oncogenes**, by contrast, are genes that by mutation to **oncogenes** encode proteins that can play an active role in disrupting cell growth.

6.1 Ras

The first human oncogene to be identified and sequenced was a mutation of the *ras* proto-oncogene. Significantly, a mutated *ras* gene had been previously identified as the tumour-causing gene in a **retrovirus** that causes sarcomas in mice. The *ras* proto-oncogene was subsequently shown to be mutated in up to 30% of human cancers (reviewed in Malumbres & Barbacid 2003). The structure and function of Ras and its potential as a target for cancer therapy are discussed in detail in Chapter 5; we should nevertheless understand here that normal Ras proteins are GTPases that cycle between inactive guanosine diphosphate (GDP)-bound and active guanosine triphosphate (GTP)-bound states. The Ras protein is anchored in the cell membrane and is activated either by cell stimulation by growth factors such as erbB or insulin-like growth factor (IGF), or by intracellular signalling proteins such as oestrogen receptor-a and, subsequently, transient conversion of Ras proteins to the active GTP-bound form. Ras occupies a key position helping to transmit signals from these growth factor receptors on the cell surface to downstream targets regulating cell growth. The mutations in *Ras* genes have been shown to be point mutations, i.e. single DNA base changes resulting in conversion of single amino acids in the Ras protein sequence, but these mutations generate a hyperactive Ras that persists in its active GTP-bound state, so causing persistent and inappropriate transmission of signals via protein kinases promoting cell growth and proliferation (Bogusky & McCormick 1993). Importantly, a mutation of this kind need only affect one of the cell's two gene copies to achieve an effect, since the mutant protein is hyperactive. The Ras proteins are, in fact, a family of related proteins each encoded by a separate proto-oncogene and playing roles in several different growth factor pathways through the regulation of protein kinases.

6.2 BCR-ABL

While formation of the mutant *ras* oncogene is caused by a single base change in the DNA sequence of the *ras* proto-oncogene, oncogenes can also be formed by much larger mutational events.

The **Philadelphia chromosome** was the first consistently found chromosomal abnormality identified as being associated with human cancer. The chromosome is a shortened chromosome 22 resulting from the reciprocal **translocation**, i.e. exchange, of DNA between the long arms of chromosomes 9 and 22 (reviewed Kurzrock *et al.* 2003). The Philadelphia chromosome is found in more than 90% of patients with chronic myelogenous leukaemia (CML), a cancer that accounts for about 15% of adult leukaemia cases.

Underlying the Philadelphia chromosome's involvement in the development of CML is the exchange of DNA that comes with translocation. As a result of the translocation, the 3' part of the *ABL* gene (the end of the gene where transcription stops) is moved from its normal position on chromosome 9 to chromosome 22 and is brought adjacent to the proximal end of the *BCR* gene, which is itself disrupted. The product of this fusion is a **chimeric *BCR-ABL* gene**, an oncogene. The normal *ABL* gene found on chromosome 9 encodes Abl, a ubiquitously expressed 145-kDa protein, which can act as a protein kinase, a tyrosine kinase, and plays a role in cellular signalling and cytoskeletal molding in response to growth factor receptor signals. Moreover, unlike the BCR-ABL oncoprotein, normal Abl is able to pass into the cell nucleus and has been implicated in regulation of the cell cycle (Van Etten 1999) and in monitoring DNA damage (Wang 1998).

The formation of the BCR-ABL oncoprotein results in a change from the structure of the normal ABL protein such that regulation of its tyrosine kinase function is lost. This results in constitutive expression of the ABL tyrosine kinase function and disruption/dysregulation of those growth factor receptor signalling pathways in which ABL normally functions.

7 Receptors and cellular signalling

Cell surface receptors involving kinase functions have themselves been implicated in the development of cancer cells (see Chapter 4). The epidermal growth factor receptor (EGFR) family, also called the ErbB family, consisting of EGFR (HER1), HER2 (Neu), HER3, and HER4, has been widely studied. These receptors are critical for regulating the proliferation and **differentiation** of normal cells, and dysregulation of their signalling, particularly of EGFR and HER2, is commonly seen in human cancers. Over-expression of EGFR has been demonstrated in several human tumour types including breast, ovarian cervical, colorectal, bladder, gastric, non-small cell lung, head and neck, and oesophageal cancer (reviewed in: Gelmon *et al.* 1999; Rowinsky 2003). The HER2 receptor has been associated with 20–30% of invasive breast cancers and its expression is an indicator of poor prognosis.

The EGFR proteins are composed of three structural domains: an extracellular domain that binds the appropriate **ligand**; a transmembrane domain; and an intracellular domain with a tyrosine kinase function. Ligand binding to the extracellular domain leads to dimerisation, which can be between two identical receptors (homodimerisation) or between different EGFR species (heterodimerisation), depending upon the ligand bound. The dimerisation process activates the tyrosine kinase function of the receptor leading to phosphorylation of intracellular proteins that activate downstream signalling processes, so ultimately controlling physiological events through a signal **transduction** cascade (reviewed in Olayioye *et al.* 2000). A number of different mechanisms have been identified as involved in increased EGFR activation in cancer including over-expression of the receptor protein, mutation leading to constitutive expression of the tyrosine kinase function, mutation leading to ligand-independent signalling, phosphatase deficiencies resulting in decreased receptor degradation (reviewed in Rowinsky 2003). Other tyrosine kinase-containing receptor families implicated in the development of human cancers include platelet-derived growth factor receptor (PDGFR), vascular endothelial growth factor receptor (VEGFR), fibroblast growth factor receptor (FGFR), and the insulin receptor families (Madhusudan & Ganeson 2004). An acquired self-sufficiency in growth signals is now considered to be one of the hallmarks of cancer cells (Hanahan & Weinberg 2000).

8 Cell adhesion, migration, and metastases

The expression of molecules at the cell's surface also plays a significant role in the latter stages of tumour development, which are characterised by the invasion of the cells into surrounding tissues and their dissemination to form metastases in distant organs. Indeed, it is estimated that around 90% of all cancer deaths arise from the formation of such metastases. These events are accompanied by changes in cell-to-cell and cell-to-substrate interactions, which are mediated by families of structurally related molecules. These include the cadherins and the **immunoglobulin** superfamily cell adhesion molecules (Ig-CAMs), both of which effect cell–cell adhesion, and the **integrins**, which bind predominantly to the intracellular matrix. Recently it has been suggested that these molecules can also interact with and modulate the signalling functions of receptor tyrosine kinases (Cavallaro & Christofori 2004).

8.1 Cadherins and E-cadherin

The cadherin superfamily consists of classical cadherins, the main mediators of calcium-dependent cell–cell adhesion, and non-classical cadherins, which includes desmosomal cadherins and the protocadherins, but whose role in tumour progression is unclear. Structurally, the classical cadherins are glyco-proteins composed of an extracellular region with multiple cadherin sequence repeats of about 110 amino acids, a single-span transmembrane-domain, and an intracellular domain that effects attachment to the cytoskeleton via inter-actions with various catenin proteins forming the cytoplasmic cell-adhesion complex. The connections between successive extracellular domains are main-tained by conserved calcium-binding sites, which are the most notable feature of these repeat sequences. Cadherin-mediated cell–cell adhesion is achieved through protein–protein interactions between two cadherin molecules of the same class, i.e. homophilic binding, on the surface of the respective cells (reviewed in Patel *et al.* 2003).

The majority of human cancers arise from epithelial tissues in which E-cadherin is the predominant cell–cell adhesion molecule. A number of studies have suggested that in cancers of epithelial origin, E-cadherin cell–cell adhesion is lost with tumour progression. Moreover, while E-cadherin can still be found in differentiated tumours, E-cadherin expression shows an inverse correlation with tumour grade and patient mortality (Birchmeier & Behrens 1994; Hiroshi 1998). Tyrosine kinases, such as the receptor tyrosine kinases of EGFR and FGFR, and non-receptor tyrosine kinase of c-Src can phosphorylate E-cadherin, N-cadherin, β-catenin, and γ-catenin and so promote the disas-sembly of the cytoplasmic adhesion complex, disrupting cadherin-mediated cell–cell adhesion (reviewed in Cavallaro & Christofori 2004). These observa-tions have led to the proposal that the loss of E-cadherin mediated cell–cell adhesion is a prerequisite for tumour cell invasion and metastasis.

8.2 Ig-CAMs and N-CAM

While the cadherins exhibit calcium-dependent cell–cell adhesion, most cal-cium-independent adhesion is mediated by the Ig superfamily CAMs. These CAMs contain one or more Ig domains. Each Ig domain is composed of around 110 amino acids and has a three-dimensional structure based on the immuno-globulin fold, consisting of two β-sheets held together by a disulfide bond.

One of the best-studied of the Ig-CAMs is the neural cell adhesion molecule (N-CAM), which is widely expressed in a variety of cell types, including most nerve cells. N-CAM is the most prevalent calcium-independent cell–cell adhesion molecule, and its role in neuronal development has been investigated extensively (Kiss & Muller 2001). There are at least 20 forms of N-CAM, all generated from a single gene by alternative splicing of the RNA transcript, but all feature a large extracellular region folded into five Ig domains. Some forms of N-CAM have transmembrane and intracellular domains, while others are anchored to the cell membrane via glycosylphosphatidylinositol (GPI). Like the cadherins, N-CAM is thought to achieve cell–cell adhesion by means of a homophilic mechanism, between N-CAM molecules on adjacent cells. In various tumour types, the pattern of N-CAM expression shifts from the adult, GPI-linked, 120-kDa isoform to the embryonic 140-kDa and 180-kDa transmembrane isoforms (reviewed in Cavallaro & Christofori 2004). In addition, an overall down-regulation of N-CAM expression has been shown to correlate with malignancy in certain tumour types, such as colon cancer, pancreatic cancer and astrocytoma. These changes in patterns of N-CAM expression and the role they play in tumour progression are not fully understood; however, the differential levels of polysialylation of the various N-CAM isoforms have been shown to modulate the adhesive functions of N-CAMs, with heavily polysialylated molecules actually limiting adhesion by virtue of the negative charge of the sialic acid (Kiss & Muller 2001).

As with E-cadherin, N-CAM may also play a role in signal transduction associated with tumour transformation: N-CAM has been found in a signalling complex associated with N-cadherin and FGFR-4, and in β tumour cells, the association of N-CAM and N-cadherin with FGFR-4 triggers FGFR signalling, leading to increased cell–extracellular matrix (ECM) adhesion (Cavallero et al. 2001).

Other members of the Ig-CAMs have also been implicated in tumour progression. The expression of carcinoembryonic antigen (CEA) has been found to be up-regulated in a number epithelial tumours, including colon, stomach, lung, pancreas, bladder, and ovarian carcinoma (reviewed in Hammarstrom 1999). CEA, which features a single Ig domain, is involved in mediating both homotypic and heterotypic cell–cell adhesion, but the role it plays in tumour progression is unclear.

9 Multi-drug resistance and ATP-binding cassette (ABC) transporters

An aspect of cancer cell biology that frequently becomes apparent during therapy is drug resistance, which remains a primary cause of suboptimal therapeutic outcomes. There are generally two forms of drug resistance in cancer cells: those that impair delivery of drugs to tumour cells, and those that occur within the cell and affect its sensitivity to the drugs. Impairment of drug delivery may involve reduced absorption in the gut, for orally administered drugs, or reduced drug levels in the blood due to increased metabolism; the role and development of tumour vasculature has also been held to be important (Jain 2001).

Drug resistance resulting from changes in cellular sensitivity to a drug may occur by alterations in the drug's cellular target, activation of repair mechanisms to increase repair of drug-induced damage, frequently DNA damage, reduction in drug influx, activation of detoxification mechanisms, e.g. cytochrome P450, blocking of apoptosis, or active removal of the drug from the cell by transmembrane pumping molecules (reviewed by Gottesman *et al.* 2002). Significantly, cells grown in culture and selected for resistance to a single drug or class of drugs, frequently show cross-resistance to other unrelated drugs. This phenomenon is multi-drug resistance, and its development is indicative of, and a consequence of, ongoing cellular mutations.

9.1 ABC transporters

Classical multi-drug resistance, the resistance to natural-product hydrophobic drugs, e.g. anthracyclines, etoposides, and the vinca alkaloids, generally arises from the expression of ATP-dependent efflux pumps. These pumps belong to the ATP-binding cassette (ABC) transporter family that share sequence similarity and structural homology. Over 40 human ABC genes have so far been identified and these have been divided into seven subfamilies (ABCA–ABCG) on the basis of sequence and domain organisation (reviewed by Gottesman *et al.* 2002). However, most of our knowledge of these molecules comes from study of the 170-kDa cell membrane protein P-glycoprotein, which is encoded by the gene *MDR1* (ABCB1). P-glycoprotein has 12 transmembrane regions and two ATP-binding sites, and in cancer multi-drug resistance it has been shown to be involved in mediating resistance to anthracyclines, vinca alkaloids, colchicines, epipodophyllotoxins, and paclitaxel (Avendano & Menendez 2002). The transmembrane regions bind hydrophobic drugs and then two ATP hydrolysis events are required to achieve the removal of one drug molecule from the cell. First, binding of the drug to the transmembrane regions stimulates the ATPase activity of P-glycoprotein; this leads to an ATP hydrolysis event and a conformational change that releases the drug to the outside of the cell. Hydrolysis of ATP at the second ATP-binding site then occurs to restore the original conformation and complete the catalytic cycle (reviewed by Gottesman *et al.* 2002). Expression of P-glycoprotein has been demonstrated in a variety of multi-drug-resistant tumour types, e.g. renal cell, colon, and hepatocellular cancers (Fojo *et al.* 1987).

10 The hallmarks of cancer

We have said that the loss of cell growth regulation seen in cancer is the result of accumulated genetic mutations in multiple cell regulatory systems. Although some mutations, e.g. p53 mutations, are extremely common in cancer cells, no one mutation can make a cell cancerous. Mathematical modelling of tumorigenesis has suggested that the number of rate-limiting mutations for a given adult tumour is probably of the order of five to eight (Renan 1993).

In addition, we have seen how the biology of cancer cells involves changes in cell adhesion molecule expression and the development of multi-drug resistance. With more than 100 distinct types of human cancer, the potential complexity of cancer has seemed to place tumorigenesis beyond the reach of explanation by an underlying set of biological principles. Recently, however, Hanahan and Weinberg have proposed that the great variety in cancer cell **genotypes** can be seen as giving rise to six essential alterations in cellular physiology (Hanahan & Weinberg 2000). These hallmarks of cancer are as follows:

> self-sufficiency in growth signals;
> insensitivity to growth-inhibitory signals;
> evasion of programmed cell death (apoptosis);
> limitless replicative potential;
> sustained **angiogenesis**;
> tumour invasion and metastasis.

Hanahan and Weinberg have suggested that these characteristics are shared by most, if not all, human tumours. The genetic mechanisms by which these characteristics are acquired may vary from tumour to tumour, but the end result will be the expression of these capabilities.

Considering the previous sections of this chapter we have seen, for example, how mutation of the *ras* proto-oncogene can lead to sustained growth signals, how mutations in the *Rb* gene lead to Rb becoming unable to inhibit the entry of cells into the S phase of the cell cycle, and how mutation of the *BAX* gene may lead to failure of apoptosis.

10.1 Limitless replicative potential

The capacity for limitless replication, immortalisation, rather than the 60–70 doublings displayed by normal human cells in culture, appears to be based, at least in part, on **telomere** maintenance and on the avoidance of cellular senescence.

Telomeres, the ends of chromosomes, are composed of thousands of repeats of a six-base pair sequence element, which are eroded by 50–100 base pairs during each cell cycle. As such, the telomeres represent a cellular counter of successive generations, with the progressive depletion of the telomeres through the cell cycles ultimately leading to exposure of chromosomal DNA, chromosome fusion, and cell death (Counter *et al.* 1992). Telomere mainten-ance has been shown to occur in almost all tumour types primarily by up-regulation of the enzyme **telomerase**, which adds further six base pair repeats to the telomere ends (reviewed in: Bryan & Cech 1999; Shay & Bacchetti 1997).

10.2 Sustained angiogenesis

It is now generally accepted that in order for solid tumours to grow beyond microscopic dimensions they require angiogenesis, the formation of new blood vessels able to supply the tumour with critical nutrients and oxygen from the peripheral blood supply (Folkman 1971). Tumour cells appear to activate angiogenesis by changes in the pattern of expression of angiogenesis inducers and inhibitors, e.g. increases in levels of VEGF an angiogenesis inducer, and decreases in levels of the inhibitor thrombospondin-1 (reviewed by Hanahan & Weinberg 2000). Tumour angiogenesis and its potential as a therapeutic target are considered in detail in Chapter 10.

10.3 Tumour invasion and metastasis

The capacity of tumour cells to invade adjacent tissues, travel to distant sites, and form metastases, represents the ultimate cause of some 90% of human cancer deaths (Sporn 1996). We have discussed above how changes in the pattern of expression of cell surface molecules that anchor the cells into their environment, e.g. Ig-CAMs, cadherins, and integrins, may play a part in the process of metastasis. Importantly, all of these molecule types also seem to play a role in cellular signalling.

A second component of the invasive and metastatic capacity of tumour cells involves extracellular proteases that can degrade the ECM. These enzymes involved in remodelling the ECM are known as **matrix metalloproteinases** (**MMPs**), and their activities, regulation and potential as therapeutic targets are also considered further in Chapter 10.

11 Conclusion

Our knowledge of cancer cell biology has advanced hugely over the last 30 years, with the development of new techniques initially offering hope-inspiring insights that have often subsequently revealed bewildering complexities. With this knowledge, and from these complexities, however, an understanding of underlying principles has now begun to emerge. Cancer is a disease of cells: we are only just beginning to explore the therapeutic potential of this know-ledge and understanding. Both the lay and the scientific communities are continually bombarded with media releases, covering exciting breakthroughs in genetic discoveries that enhance our understanding of cancer. It is incumbent upon us all to competently guide our patients through each one of these discoveries.

References

Alberts B, Johnson A, Lewis J, Raff M, Roberts K, Walter P (2002) *Molecular biology of the cell* (4th edn). Garland Science, New York.

Avendano C, Menendez JC (2002) Inhibitors of multi-drug resistance to antitumor agents (MDR). *Curr Med Chem*; 9:159–93.

Birchmeier W, Behrens J (1994) Cadherin expression in carcinomas: role in the formation of cell junctions and the prevention of invasiveness. *Biochim Biophys Acta*; **1198**: 11–26.

Bogusky MS, McCormick F (1993) Function and regulation of Ras and its relatives. *Nature*; **366**: 643–54.

Bryan TM, Cech TR (1999) Telomerase and the maintenance of chromosome ends. *Curr Opin Cell Biol*; **11**: 318–24.

Cavallaro U, Niedermeyer J, Fuxa M, Christofori G (2001) N-CAM modulates tumour-cell adhesion to matrix by inducing FGF-receptor signalling. *Nat Cell Biol*; **3**: 650–7.

Cavallaro U, Christofori G (2004) Cell adhesion and signalling by cadherins and Ig-CAMs in cancer. *Nat Rev Cancer*; **4**: 118–32.

Counter CM, Avilion AA, LeFeuvre *et al.* (1992) Telomere shortening associated with chromosome instability is arrested in immortal cells which express telomerase activity. *EMBO J*; **11**: 1921–9.

Ekholm SV, Reed SI (2000) Regulation of G (1) cyclin-dependent kinases in the mammalian cell cycle. *Curr Opin Cell Biol*; **12**: 676–84.

Flemming W (1882) *Zellsubstanz, kern und zelltheilung*. FCW Vogel, Leipzig.

Fojo AT, Ueda K, Slamon DJ, Poplackt DG, Gottesman MM, Pastan I (1987) Expression of a multi-drug-resistance gene in human tumors and tissues. *Proc Natl Acad Sci USA*; **84**: 265–9.

Folkman J (1971) Tumor angiogenesis: therapeutic implications. *N Engl J Med*; **285**: 1182–6.

Gelmon KA, Eisenhauer EA, Harris AL, Ratain MJ, Workman P (1999) Anticancer agents targeting signaling molecules and cancer cell environment: challenges for drug development? *J Natl Cancer Inst*; **91**: 1281–7.

Gottesman MM, Fojo T, Bates SE (2002) Multi-drug resistance in cancer: role of ATP-dependent transporters. *Nat Rev Cancer*; **2**: 48–58.

Hammarstrom S (1999) The carcinoembryonic antigen (CEA) family: structures, suggested functions and expression in normal and malignant tissues. *Semin Cancer Biol*; **9**: 67–81.

Hanahan D, Weinberg RA (2000) The hallmarks of cancer. *Cell*; **100**: 57–70.

Hickman ES, Moroni MC, Helin K (2002)The role of p53 and pRB in apoptosis and cancer. *Curr Opin Genetics Dev*; **12**: 60–6.

Hirohashi S (1998) Inactivation of the E-cadherin-mediated cell adhesion system in human cancers. *Am J Pathol*; **153**: 333–9.

Jain RK (2001) Normalizing tumor vasculature with anti-angiogenic therapy: a new paradigm for combination therapy. *Nat Med*; **7**: 987–9.

Kerr JFR, Wyllie AH, Currie AR (1972) Apoptosis: a basic biological phenomenon with wide ranging implications in tissue kinetics. *Brit J Cancer*; **26**: 239–57.

Kiss JZ, Muller D (2001) Contribution of the neural cell adhesion molecule to neuronal and synaptic plasticity. *Rev Neurosci*; 12: 297–310.

Kurzrock R, Kantarjian HM, Druker BJ, Talpaz M (2003) Philadelphia chromosome-positive leukemias: from basic mechanisms to molecular therapeutics. *Ann Intern Med*; 138: 819–30.

Madhusudan S, Ganesan TS (2004) Tyrosine kinase inhibitors in cancer therapy. *Clin Biochem*; 37: 618–35.

Malumbres M, Barbacid M (2001) To cycle or not to cycle: a critical decision in cancer. *Nat Cancer Rev*; 1: 222–31.

Malumbres M, Barbacid M (2003) *Ras* oncogenes: the first 30 years. *Nat Cancer Rev*; 3: 459–65.

Martin SJ, Green DR (1995) Protease activation during apoptosis. Death by a thousand cuts? *Cell*; 82: 349–52.

Morgan DO (1995) Principle of CDK regulation. *Nature*; 374: 131–4.

Olayioye MA, Neve RM, Lane HA, Hynes NE (2000) The ErbB signaling network: receptor heterodimerization in development and cancer. *EMBO J*; 19: 3159–67.

Pardee AB (1972) A restriction point control for normal animal cell proliferation. *Proc Natl Acad Sci USA*; 71: 1286–90.

Patel SD, Chen CP, Bahna F, Honig B, Shapiro L (2003) Cadherin-mediated cell–cell adhesion: sticking together as a family. *Curr Opin Struct Biol*; 13: 690–8.

Rampino N, Yamamoto H, Ionov Y *et al.* (1997) Somatic frameshift mutations in the BAX gene in colon cancers of the microsatellite mutator phenotype. *Science*; 275: 967–9.

Reed AL, Califano J, Cairns P *et al.* (1996) High frequency of p16 (CDKN2/MTS-1/INK4a) inactivation in head and neck squamous cell carcinoma. *Cancer Res*; 56: 3630–3.

Reed JC (1999a) Mechanisms of apoptosis avoidance in cancer. *Curr Opin Oncol*; 11: 68–75.

Reed JC (1999b) Dysregulation of apoptosis in cancer. *J Clin Oncol*; 117: 2941–53.

Renan MJ (1993) How many mutations are required for tumorigenesis? Implications from human cancer data. *Mol Carcinogenesis*; 7: 139–46.

Rowinsky EK (2003) Signal events: Cell signal transduction and its inhibition in cancer. *Oncologist*; 8 Suppl 3: 5–17.

Sandal T (2002) Molecular aspects of the mammalian cell cycle and cancer. *Oncologist*; 7: 73–81.

Shay JW, Bacchetti S (1997) A survey of telomerase activity in human cancer. *Eur J Cancer*; 33: 787–91.

Sherr CJ (1996) Cancer cell cycles. *Science*; 274: 1672–7.

Sherr CJ (2000) The Pezcoller lecture: cancer cell cycles revisited. *Cancer Res*; 60: 3689–95.

Sherr CJ (2004) Principles of tumor suppression. *Cell*; 116: 235–46.

Sherr CJ, Roberts JM (1999) CDK inhibitors: positive and negative regulators of G1 phase progression. *Genes & Dev*; 13: 1501–12.

Solomon MJ, Kaldis P (1998) Regulation of CDKs by phosphorylation. *Results Probl Cell Differ*; 22: 79–109.

Sporn MB (1996) The war on cancer. *Lancet*; 347: 1377–81.

Sutherland RL, Musgrove EA (2004) Cyclins and breast cancer. *J Mammary Gland Biol Neoplasia*; 9: 95–104.

Talve L, Sauroja I, Collan Y, Punnonen K, Ekfors T (1999) Loss of expression of p16INK4/ CDKN2 gene in cutaneous malignant melanoma correlates with tumor cell proliferation and invasive stage. *Int J Cancer*; 74: 255–9.

Tetsu O, McCormick F (1999) Beta-catenin regulates expression of cyclin D1 in colon carcinoma cells. *Nature*; 398: 422–6.

Van Etten RA (1999) Cycling, stressed-out and nervous: cellular functions of c-Abl. *Trends Cell Biol*; 9: 179–86.

Wang JY (1998) Cellular responses to DNA damage. *Curr Opin Cell Biol*; 10: 240–7.

Weinberg RA (1995) The retinoblastoma protein and cell cycle control. *Cell*; 81: 323–30.

Weinberg RA (1998) *One renegade cell: the quest for the origins of cancer.* Basic Books, New York.

Yu Q, Geng Y, Sicinski P (2001) Specific protection against breast cancers by cyclin D1 ablation. *Nature*; 411: 1017–21.

Chapter 2

An introduction to the immune system and cancer

Rachel Midgley

1 Introduction

Immunology as a science celebrated its bicentenary just before the dawn of the new millennium. In 1796 Jenner reported his finding that inoculation of a young man, James Phipps, with pus obtained from a cowpox lesion (or vaccinia from the latin term '*vacca*' meaning cow) resulted in protection against human smallpox, a frequently fatal disease. This was the first documented evidence for the effectiveness of 'vaccination'. Despite Jenner's firm evidence, the resistance of the Church to his methods meant that smallpox vaccination did not become routine until the twentieth century.

Even before the coining of the term 'vaccination', the importance of prior exposure to, and recovery from, a disease in order to confer resistance had been recognised. Indeed 2500 years ago, during the ravaging of Athens by the plague, Thucydides noted that those who were able safely to tend to the sick had previously contracted the disease but recovered; essentially they were now 'immunised'.

However, the birth of modern immunology came only with Louis Pasteur and the discovery of the 'Germ Theory of Disease'. At this time (mid-1800s), it was known that chicken cholera bacillus was the causative agent for chicken cholera, a disease devastating fowl farms. Pasteur inadvertently created the tools for the first non-randomised two-armed trial of vaccination, when one summer he accidentally left a flask of cholera bacillus out on his bench. Returning after his summer break he decided to use the old culture to infect a group of chickens. To his surprise, despite the culture looking essentially normal, the chickens did not display the normal physical manifestations of the disease and all remained alive. Pasteur then prepared a new stock of the bacteria, and inoculated the original group of eight plus ten more chickens. The new group of ten, with no prior exposure to the bacteria, quickly became ill and died, while the original group again survived with no detrimental effects. Pasteur concluded that exposure of the original group of eight chickens to the old culture had somehow altered their susceptibility to the second fresh batch of bugs. Indeed he invented the phrase 'attenuation' to describe the effect that sitting on the bench had had upon the virulence of the old culture. This culture was no longer capable of inducing clinical disease but had created an 'immune response' that protected inoculated chicken from later more potent bacterial insult. Later in the same century, Theobold Smith demonstrated that the chicken cholera bacteria could also be harnessed as a protective agent by heat-killing and then injecting the resultant dead culture into the recipient, showing that the bugs did not need to be alive to confer immunity.

The discovery of the rabies vaccine highlighted yet another way of attenuating organisms, by passage in an unnatural host. Pasteur isolated the rabies **virus** from a fox and passaged it through a series of rabbits; that is inoculated the first rabbit, waited for it to become clinically unwell and then re-isolated the virus and injected the next rabbit and so on. By doing this it was postulated that he would select for strains possibly pathogenic to the rabbit but decreasingly pathogenic to the fox. Eventually he prepared a vaccine from the nervous system of the final rabbit. On 4 July 1885, Joseph Meister, a 9-year-old boy, was severely bitten by a rabid dog. His desperate parents hearing of Pasteur's work travelled to Paris in the hope of a cure. Pasteur injected the boy with his vaccine and waited. The boy did not contract rabies and became the first survivor of an otherwise certain rabid death.

By the beginning of the twentieth century, immunologists had split into two camps: the humoralists believing that immunity was based upon a non-cellular transferable factor in the serum; and cellularists who suggested that dedicated immune effector cells were responsible for **immune surveillance**. This was really the birth of modern immunology as we know it. Although the two factions were diametrically opposed in their views of the immune system, it is now clear that both theories are correct and the immune system comprises a highly orchestrated interaction between cellular and **humoral** components.

1.1 Modern understanding of the immune system

Modern immunologists separate the immune system into two major strategies: **innate** and **adaptive immunity**. Innate immunity refers to the broad but non-specific immediate response that occurs irrespective of the nature of the invader. For example, as demonstrated later, **natural killer (NK) cells** circulate round the body and engulf and digest foreign cells they encounter. The innate response provides the initial anti-microbial battle, and prevents overwhelming spread of the infection throughout the body while the adaptive immune response, which is slower but more specific and sophisticated, is being raised. This adaptive response provides long-term protection or immunity from subsequent exposure to the same invaders.

As hypothesised 100 years ago, the adaptive immune system can be divided into two main branches: the cellular or **cell–mediated** immune response, sometimes known as the Th1-type response; and the humoral immune response, known as the Th2-type response. These two immune functions are inextricably intertwined and the fine balance between them, in an immune response against a specific organism, depends on the nature of the organism, the route of infection, and the general health of the immune system as a whole. It has largely been accepted that, in response to infection with bacteria (which generally remain in the extracellular compartment), it is largely the **B cells** (**B lymphocytes**) of the humoral arm (Th2 response) that proliferate and produce large amounts of specific antibodies that mark out the invading organisms as foreign and dictate their eventual elimination from the body. In contrast, the cellular (Th1) immune response uses specialised **T cells** (T lymphocytes) to recognise and destroy host cells infected by viruses or parasites.

However, it has become increasingly evident that this traditional separation is incompletely borne out in practice, with recognition now that antibody responses are very important in the clearance of viruses and the raising of anti-viral immunity through vaccination; and the acknowledgement of the role of **helper T cells** in coordinating anti-bacterial responses.

We will now review in more detail the specifics of the main effectors of the immune system, antibodies (humoral system), and T and B lymphocytes (the cellular immune system).

2 The humoral immune system

Antibodies were the first specific component of the immune system to be delineated and they are the cornerstone of humoral immunity. Antibodies are sometimes termed **immunoglobulins** and they are produced and secreted by B lymphocytes that have differentiated into plasma cells, in response to infection. They are Y-shaped molecules (Fig. 2.1) whose arms form the antigen-binding sites—the parts of the molecule that bind and recognise specific parts (**epitopes**) of invaders proteins. Antibodies tend to recognise non-contiguous amino acids of a particular protein while it is *in situ* within the pathogens structure, with the amino acid residues in between the recognition points being hidden in the complex folding of the protein structure (Fig. 2.2). This is in contrast to T cells (see below).

Variable regions = antigen-binding sites

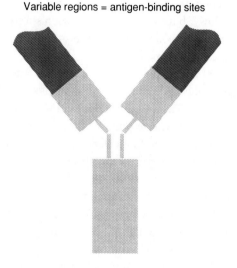

Constant region = effector function

Fig. 2.1 Basic structure of an antibody.

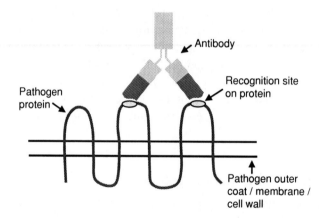

Fig. 2.2 Antibodies recognise non-contiguous *amino acids* of a protein while it is *in situ*.

The single stem of the Y of the antibody determines its 'class', which defines its functional capabilities and downstream effector mechanisms. The classes are also known as **isotypes** and are named G, A, M, D, and E. In humans, IgG immunoglobulins (antibodies) are further separated into four classes (Ig G1 to IgG4 with IgG1 being the most abundant) and IgA immunoglobulins are divided into IgA1 and IgA2. Table 2.1 outlines the defining characteristics of each of the immuoglobulin isotypes. The importance of each isotype relative to one another within a particular response depends upon the infective agent, the stage of infection (first encounter or re-challenge), and the site of infection.

Table 2.1 Immunoglobulin isotypes

Isotype	Characteristics
IgG	Classical pathway of complement activation. Placental transfer (IgG1 and IgG3 particularly). Some binding to macrophages and other phagocytes. Clearance bacterial, viral, and other infection (e.g. Candida, Toxoplasma).
IgM	Classical pathway of complement activation. Clearance of some bacterial and viral infections (particularly streptococcus and staphylococcus).
IgA	Alternative pathway of complement activation. Binds to macrophages and other phagocytes. Usually mucosal secretion. Clearance of influenza infections.
IgD	Probably important for cell signalling. May substitute for some of functions of IgM if that isotype is low.
IgE	High-affinity binding to mast cells. Implicated in immediate-type hypersensitivity.

2.1 The humoral immune response and mechanisms of action of antibodies

The extracellular spaces of the body are generally guarded by the humoral immune response, in which antibodies produced by B cells bring about the destruction or neutralisation of invading organisms. Resting B cells circulating in the body are stimulated to differentiate into mature antibody-secreting plasma cells in the presence of foreign antigen and with the help of so-called helper T cells (usually Th2). This is a subset of **CD4+** T cells, which will be discussed in more detail later.

The first and simplest process of anti-microbial action by antibodies is neutralisation, which is a 'soaking up' mechanism. In order to gain a foothold in infection, viruses and intracellular bacteria need to bind to specific target molecules on the host cells to be internalised. Antibodies can bind the pathogen in order to prevent this process. Antibodies can also neutralise the specific toxins of pathogens prohibiting their internalisation, which would result in cell death.

A slightly more complicated process involves opsonisation. Here antibodies coat extracellular bacteria and the stem region of the bound antibodies (the so-called 'constant' region) is recognised by the **Fc receptor** of phagocytic cells, priming the latter for their consumptive action (Fig. 2.3).

Antibody binding to antigen expressed on pathogens can also activate **complement**. The complement system is a large series of plasma proteins that react with one another in a cascade, with the final consequence of bacterial

Antibodies coating pathogen

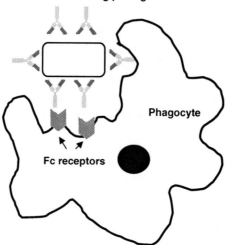

Fig. 2.3 Opsonisation. Antibodies coat the bacteria and then the constant region of the antibodies are recognised by the Fc receptor on the phagocyte, inducing phagocytosis.

opsonisation, chemo-attraction for phagocytes, and activation of recruited phagocytes. There are two major activation routes for complement, the classical and the alternative pathways, but the details of these are not appropriate for this text.

A final method of antibody action requires the integrated action of the other division of the immune system—the cellular arm. In this process, virus-infected human host cells signal the presence of intracellular infection by expressing non-native viral proteins on their cell surfaces. The proteins are then recognised and bound by antibody, and subsequently the infected cell is killed by natural killer (NK) cells. This process is called **antibody-dependent cell-mediated cytotoxicity** (ADCC). It is thought to be particularly important in the destruction of cells bearing cancer-related proteins and is therefore particularly pertinent for this book.

2.2 Genetic recombination and the generation of antigen-specific antibodies

Figure 2.4 shows a more detailed structure of an antibody, comprising two identical heavy chains and two identical light chains. Each chain has a constant region and a variable region. The face presented by the four variable regions (two heavy, two light) constitutes the antigen-binding site. In order to recognise the huge spectrum of pathogens that the human host may encounter, each individual human being harbours a plethora of B cells that, in total, are capable of producing antibodies of almost limitless antigen-binding capacity. For many years there was confusion as to how such a range of antigen specificities could be encoded by a small number of genes. In 1976, Susumu Tonegawa discovered that the genes determining the antibody variable regions were not inherited as whole genes but rather as gene segments, each segment encoding a portion of the variable region for one of the antibody polypeptide chains. During the development of B cells in the foetal bone marrow, these gene segments are joined by a process of genetic recombination to form a complete stretch of DNA, which encodes a single whole variable region. There are many gene segments in each set; different segments are joined in different cells; the recombination is not precise and random additional **nucleotides** are often inserted at the joins; and different light and heavy chains come together in different cells. Thus, a large spectrum of potential antigen-binding sites is generated in each individual, but each B cell has the capability of producing antibody with only one specific binding capacity. When this cell divides in response to infection, because of the irreversibility of the genetic rearrangement, all progeny cells will generate antibodies with the same parental antigen-binding specificity.

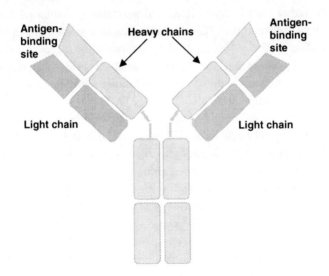

Fig. 2.4 Detailed structure of an antibody. There are four chains: two heavy (light grey) and two light (dark grey). Each chain has a constant region and a variable region. The distal portions of the four chains make up the variable antigen-binding region (see Fig. 2.1).

3 The cellular immune system

3.1 Cytotoxic and helper T cells

The two most important and well-described cells of the cellular arm of the immune system are **cytotoxic T cells/lymphocytes** (T_c) and helper T cells/lymphocytes (T_h). In contrast to antibodies, these T cells usually detect the presence of intracellular pathogen, through recognition of chopped-up protein fragments (epitope peptides) derived from the pathogen's proteins, which are presented on the surface of the infected human cell. Cytotoxic T_c cells recognise the foreign antigens and then mature into active killer T cells, and develop the ability to lyse the cells carrying these antigens. T_h helper T cells respond to antigen by producing **cytokines** that have downstream effects on T_c action.

T cells recognise antigen through their **T-cell receptors** (TCRs). As with antibodies, T-cell receptors with multiple different specificities are required to produce competent immune surveillance in the human host. Indeed, the genetic recombination and generation within the foetus, of many thousands of T_c and T_h cell specificities are very similar to the process already described for antibody antigen-binding site diversity. However, there are some structural differences between antibodies and T-cell receptors. First, TCRs are firmly implanted in the T cell membrane producing downstream signalling effects to the T cell, rather than being secreted and performing a humoral function. Second, the T-cell receptor (TCR) is equivalent to a single antigen-binding fragment of an antibody (Fig. 2.5). There are two chains, generally α and β. Each chain has a constant region (C) and a variable region (V). A minority of T cells carry an alternative pair of polypeptide chains but the function of this subset is not completely clear.

T_c and T_h cells are differentiated at a molecular level by cell surface expression of specific signalling molecules. T_c express **CD8** and T_h express CD4. Of note, the CD8 and CD4 molecules are called co-receptors because they are integral to the formation of a strong contact (the immunological synapse) between T cells and the cell presenting the foreign antigen. Their presence enhances the resultant T cell activation by at least 100-fold.

T-cell receptors of T_c and T_h cells recognise short contiguous regions of the pathogen protein (epitopes), which are only exposed and presented when the protein undergoes processing within the human cell. This processing cleaves pathogenic protein into small peptide fragments. The foreign proteins recognised by T cells are presented on the cell surface in association with **major histocompatibility complex** (MHC) proteins. The TCR cannot 'see' the epitope peptide by itself and it is the stoichiometric structure of the peptide lying in the

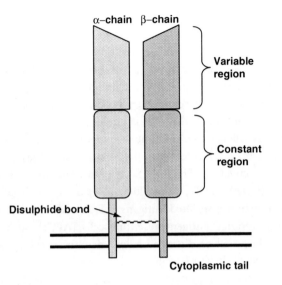

Fig. 2.5 The T-cell receptor. There are two chains, each with a constant and a variable region. These are linked by a disulphide bond.

peptide-binding groove of the MHC molecule that triggers T-cell recognition. In order to understand the T-cell recognition of antigen fully, one needs to be aware of MHC proteins and the processing/presentation pathways.

3.2 Major histocompatibility proteins

Major histocompatibility proteins were so-called because they were first recognised through their potential deleterious effect on the outcome of trans-planted organs. There are two classes of MHC molecule (**class I** and **class II**) differing in their structure and their tissue distribution in the body—MHC class I on most nucleated cells of the body and MHC class II only on specialised presenting cells (e.g. **dendritic cells**) and B cells of the immune system. MHC class I and II also differ in terms of their interactions with subsets of T cells and hence their final effector functions. Class I molecules present peptides from pathogens, commonly viruses, to CD8+ cytotoxic T_c cells and class II molecules present peptide to CD4+ helper T_h cells.

It is important to note that MHC antigens are highly polymorphic and each person can have a fairly unique **HLA** (human leukocyte antigen) type, inherited from his or her parents. So, for example, each individual carries six class I **alleles**, two each of A, B, and C. More importantly, different alleles or haplotypes (e.g. A2, A11) will bind different epitopes from a single antigen. The epitopes bound will depend upon the anchor-position requirements (usually amino acid positions 2 and 9 of a class I epitope) of the particular MHC molecule. Thus, A11 molecules prefer the amino acid valine at position 2 and lysine at position 9 of the epitope peptide. These are the amino acid residues that most closely interact with the peptide-binding groove in the class I molecule, hence the strict regulation of their size and shape (Fig. 2.6).

It is also worthy of note here that even this intricate interaction between the MHC/epitope complex and the TCR is often insufficient for T-cell priming. Additional cross-talk between co-stimulatory molecules on the presenting cell and the CD28 family of molecules on the surface of the T-cells, is required for maximal T-cell activation (Fig. 2.7). Such co-stimulatory molecules include the B7 family (CD80, CD86), intercellular adhesion molecule (ICAM) group, lymphocyte function associated antigens (LFA), and vascular cell adhesion molecules. Professional **antigen-presenting cells** (APCs), such as dendritic cells (DCs), which will be discussed below, demonstrate very high levels of expression of these critical molecules.

3.3 **The generation of T cell epitopes for TCR recognition (processing and presentation)**

We have noted that, in order for proteins to be recognised by a TCR, antigen processing and presentation must occur. Antigen processing is the modification

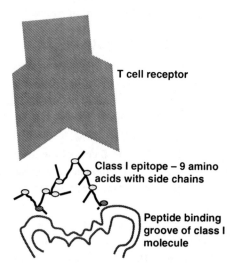

T cell receptor

Class I epitope – 9 amino acids with side chains

Peptide binding groove of class I molecule

Fig. 2.6 Class I epitope lying within the MHC class I binding groove. Amino acid residues 2 and 9 are in closest proximity to the bed of the groove and their exact structure is paramount for effective binding. Residues 4 to 7 of the epitope are more important in terms of the interaction with the T-cell receptor.

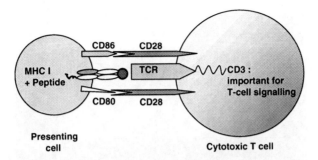

Fig. 2.7 Maximal T-cell activation often requires additional cross-talk between the T cell and the presenting cell. The CD28 molecules on the T cell bind to CD80 (B7.1) and CD86 (B7.2) molecules on the presenting cell to allow this to happen. Specialised presenting cells, such as dendritic cells, are rich in these co-stimulatory molecules.

of native proteins from a pathogen into a form (the epitope) that can be recognised by a TCR. Presentation is the displaying of this epitope on the cell surface in association with MHC molecules.

In general terms, viruses and certain bacteria that replicate in the **cytosol** are processed and presented through the class I presentation pathway (Fig. 2.8). In this pathway, viral proteins are generally synthesised *de novo* when the virus hijacks the cell's protein machinery for its own gain. These proteins are then cleaved by the immunoproteasome. This is a specialised form of the standard multicatalytic protease complex—the proteasome—and it is explicitly induced under the direction of the interferons (particular cytokines) that are produced in excess during infection. The immunoproteasome has specific cleaving activity, which produces peptides that appear to have an enhanced potential for take up into the **endoplasmic reticulum**. These peptides are usually approximately 8 to 11 amino acids long. Once generated, the peptides are then transported by the transporter associated with antigen processing-1 and −2 (TAP1 and TAP2) complex into the endoplasmic reticulum (ER). Again the TAP complex holds some specificity and peptides that are 8 or more amino acids long with hydrophobic or basic amino acids at the carboxy terminus are preferred. In the ER, the peptides are complexed with class I MHC molecules. Finally, they are transported to the cell surface for recognition by CD8+ T_c cells leading to T_c activation. Of note, empty class I molecules are not efficiently transported to the cell surface and therefore if TAP mutations are present, a deficiency of class I molecules at the cell surface is observed.

Alternatively, several classes of pathogen replicate inside macrophage vesicles and are processed through the class II pathway because they are not

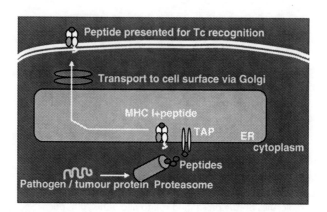

Fig. 2.8 Viruses and certain bacteria replicate in the cytosol and are processed and presented through the class I presentation pathway. It is also believed that tumour proteins are presented in the same fashion.

accessible to the proteasome in the normal fashion. However, after a macrophage is activated, proteases within the vesicles break down the proteins into small fragments, usually 10 to 22 amino acids in length. These then bind to class II molecules and are delivered to the cell surface for recognition by CD4+ T_h cells. It is also understood that secreted pathogen protein products may enter specialised antigen-presenting cells through the endosome and be processed and presented on class II molecules (so-called cross-presentation). These products can also then be recognised by CD4+ T_h cells. The T_h cells become activated and can differentiate into cells producing radically different downstream effects.

3.4 The effector actions of Tc and Th cells

When cytotoxic T cells (T_c) recognise their specific epitope presented in association with class I molecules and the required co-stimulatory molecules, they will become activated and proliferate. Progeny-specific T cells can then kill target cells presenting the specific epitope, by programming them to undergo apoptosis (cellular suicide). The process also appears to have a direct effect stimulating the degradation of viral DNA (preventing **virion** escape and infection of new cells during the cell death).

The major mechanism of inducing apoptosis is by the release of **lytic** granules from the T_c, particularly **perforin** (which polymerises to form transmembrane pores in the attacked cell) and proteases called granzymes (which belong to the serine protease family and which appear to trigger a cascade of other enzyme activities resulting in DNA degradation). Activated T_c also express Fas ligand and this can bind to Fas on target cell membranes leading to the activation of **caspases**, which again induce apoptosis in the target cell. This mechanism may also be critical to the regulation of T_c expansion after removal of the pathogen, in order to prevent auto-immunity.

Cytotoxic T cells (T_c) also release a number of cytokines, including γ-interferon (γ-IFN) and α-interferon (α-IFN), as well as tumour necrosis factor (TGF). These cytokines can directly inhibit viral replication, as well as recruiting and activating macrophages and increasing the expression of class I molecules (a positive feedback on presentation in the infected human cells).

When T_h cells recognise their specific epitope in association with class II molecules, they are prompted to differentiate into either a Th1 or Th2 **phenotype**. This phenotypic divergence determines the spectrum of their secreted cytokines and the downstream effector activity. Th1 cells secrete g-interferon (g-IFN) and **interleukin**-2 (IL2) and promote T_c cytotoxicity against the infected cells, while the Th2 cells secrete interleukin-4 (IL4) and interleukin-10 (IL10) and drive B-cell class switching and a magnified humoral response.

3.5 Other important components in the cellular immune system

Although much effort has been made to tease out the detailed functions of T_c and T_h cells, a number of other cells are crucial to the fine coordination of the immune system. These include NK cells, dendritic cells, and regulatory T cells.

3.5.1 NK cells

NK cells were originally thought to be solely a constituent of the innate immune system. However, recent evidence suggests that they play a critical role in adaptive immunity especially with respect to their interactions with dendritic cells (DCs). NK cells display and act through a restricted variety of receptors but do not undergo the recombination diversity of T_c and T_h receptor generation. One of the receptors that is felt to be particularly important, recognises a non-variant part of class I molecules, i.e. a part seen on all haplotypes. This receptor is inhibitory to the killer activity of the cell and is felt to be critical in determining cells that are non-self. This means that if class I molecules are down-regulated or absent, as is the case with many viral infections and with organ transplants, then this receptor on the NK cell will not be engaged and its natural killer activity will be unleashed. This concept is termed missing-self recognition; it is recognising that the 'self' antigen is absent and acting accordingly.

Another NK receptor, NKG2D, recognises up-regulated self-proteins, such as MHC class I chain-related A chain (MICA), a protein that is only usually up-regulated in the presence of infection. Increased expression of these receptor ligands again induces the NK cells to attack the target cells and also stimulates the NK cells to produce interferons, which activate cytotoxic T cells.

3.5.2 Dendritic cells

Dendritic cells (DCs) are known as professional antigen-presenting cells. They are highly specialised and their function is to ingest and present antigen (Fig. 2.9). They ingest antigen when they are in their immature state in the periphery. They then migrate back to draining lymph nodes, where they mature into highly effective presentation cells with expression of specific co-stimulatory molecules and up-regulation of class I and class II molecules. Mature DCs are the most potent activators of naïve T cells and therefore play an important role in immune rejection. They can prime and activate T_c cells directly but also have an important role in inducing T_h cells to produce the relevant cytokines to skew the response along the cytotoxic pathway rather than the inflammatory route.

3.5.3 Regulatory T cells

Regulatory T cells (T_{regs}) are T cells that express CD4 (like T_h cells) but also express high levels of the CD25 molecule. They can produce transforming growth factor (TGF) and interleukin 10 (IL10)—both are immunosuppressive

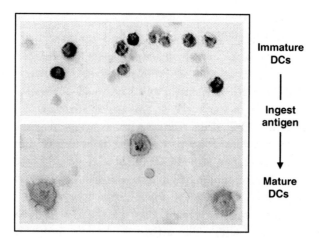

Fig. 2.9 Immature DCs ingest antigen in the periphery, then migrate back to the draining lymph nodes, maturing and processing the antigen. In the lymph node they can present their antigen to the T cells.

cytokines. However, they also seem to interact by cell–cell contact. T_{regs} appear critical in maintaining homeostasis in the equilibrium between immunity (important to fight off pathogens) and **tolerance** (important to prevent tissue damage through auto-immunity), and specifically they appear to have a suppressive role in immune activation.

4 Cancer and the immune system

4.1 Does the immune system have a role in cancer?

Observational human and mouse studies have suggested a possible role for the immune system in rejecting cancer cells. Thus, patients with acquired immune deficiency syndrome suffer a higher rate of lymphoma and other solid cancers. Patients who are heavily immuno-suppressed following transplantation are also at increased risk of lymphoma. Knock-out mouse models have confirmed the importance of the integrated activity of both T_h and T_c cells in mounting an effective anti-tumour response and preventing anergy or tolerance. Furthermore, in some tumours, **tumour-infiltrating T cells (TILs)** have been seen and their presence correlated with improved prognosis. For these reasons particularly, many scientists believe that the cellular component of the immune system plays a greater role than the humoral arm, although this evidence is not conclusive.

Certainly, the possibility of using the immune system to combat established cancer has been attempted for many years. Initially non-specific immunostimulatory agents, such as levamisole and **Bacillus Calmette-Guérin (BCG)**, were utilised. More recently investigators have attempted general immune stimulation with systemic cytokine administration. Others have attempted to increase the frequency of NK cells in the body. Many cancers down-regulate class I molecules and therefore should become more susceptible to NK activity. Most recently, specific vaccination has been attempted.

But why should the immune system recognise cancer? The last fifteen years have demonstrated that there are proteins that are over-expressed, expressed in a mutant form, or exclusively expressed in tumour cells compared to their normal cellular counterparts. With this knowledge, it is tempting to perceive a potential benefit in trying to raise an immune response against these particular proteins, which would allow specific attack of cancer cells leaving normal cells intact.

Opponents of **immunotherapy** theory argue that if the immune system was capable of halting the carcinogenic process, then tumours should not occur; all tumours should be recognised at an early stage and should be extinguished by the ensuing immune response. There are two counter-arguments to this.

Unfortunately, because a large proportion of the specific antigens expressed in tumours are also expressed during foetal life, then many of the specific T-cell precursors for these antigens will have undergone clonal deletion during immune development. That is, the T cells will have been registered as recognising self-antigen and will have been deleted in the thymus. This means these precursors are likely to be at very low level during adult life. In addition, raising an immune response to tumour antigens is very difficult in the non-vaccinated situation because, although the tumour is expressing these proteins (**tumour-associated antigens**), it is also harnessing a number of mechanisms to subvert or evade the immune response. These are detailed below. It is likely that, in order to raise an effective response, the antigens will need to be expressed on professional antigen-presenting cells such as dendritic cells. Immuno-therapists believe that if we can raise the frequency of specific T cells (or anti-body titre) against tumour antigens to a critical threshold level, then there is a possibility that immune suppression may be overcome and tumour cells destroyed.

4.2 Examples of tumour immune escape mechanisms

Many tumours exhibit a total loss or reduction in expression of MHC class I molecules leading to decreased presentation of antigens. This loss is frequently progressive as the stage of the tumour increases. Metastases demonstrate least expression and therefore may be the hardest to treat with immunotherapy. In mismatch repair-defective colorectal cancers, the class I molecule reduction appears in part due to mutations in b_2 microglobulin, the 12-kDa polypeptide that is non-covalently associated with the heavy chain of the MHC molecule and which is essential for the interaction between the MHC complex and the TCR. Further upstream in the processing pathway, mutations in the trans-porter molecules (TAP1/TAP2) have been reported in a number of solid tumours and this would of course adversely affect antigen presentation.

Some tumour-associated antigens, in addition to acting as potential targets for immune attack, can also contribute to immune evasion. For example, mucin-1 (a tumour-associated antigen with documented antibody and T_c-recognition elements) is redistributed on colorectal cancer cells from its normal luminal polarisation to pan-membrane expression, potentially cloaking surface immuno-regulatory molecules and inhibiting T-cell–tumour-cell inter-actions, as well as antibody–tumour-cell interactions. Secretion of Muc-1 from the cancer cells also induces **apoptosis** of surrounding tumour-infiltrating T cells (TILs). Interestingly, also in colorectal cancer, during progression from normal epithelium via adenoma to established carcinoma, there is gradual up-regulation of Fas ligand. Excessive surface-expressed Fas-L binds to its receptor (Fas) on TILs, again inducing apoptotic cell death, providing a further mechanism of immune tolerance. In addition, decreased expression of CD3 zeta chains (important for signalling in the TCR) of both peripheral blood T cells and TILs, leading to signal **transduction** defects, has been reported in patients with solid tumours. Some solid tumours also secrete transforming growth factor β (TGFβ), interleukin 10, leukaemia-inhibitory factor, and prostaglandins, all of which have immuno-suppressive effects.

5 Conclusion

This chapter has given an overview of some of the important components of the immune system in its historical and major function combating infection. The evidence for a role of the immune system in rejecting tumours has been outlined. It is clear that immune responses directed against solid tumours do exist and these can be measured. However, anti-tumour antigen-specific T cells (or B cells in the case of antibodies) are usually at low frequency and proliferation and activation cannot be induced by the tumour itself, because of a variety of inhibitory mechanisms.

Immunotherapeutic strategies aim to convert these latent immune responses into effective anti-tumour rejection. Such strategies will be described in detail in the ensuing chapters, including methods and success of inducing **monoclonal antibodies** against tumours (Chapter 7); how antibodies can be used in **antibody-directed enzyme pro-drug therapy** (**ADEPT**, Chapter 8); the role of exogenous cytokines (Chapter 9); and active and passive vaccination techniques (Chapters 11 and 12).

Further reading

Mapara M, Sykes M (2004) Tolerance and cancer : mechanisms of tumour evasion and strategies for breaking tolerance. *J. Clin. Oncol.* 22: 1136–51.

Midgley RS, Kerr DJ (2003) Immunotherapy for colorectal cancer. *Expert Rev. Anticancer Ther.* 3: 63–78. (Review.)

Midgley R, Kerr D (2000) Immunotherapy for colorectal cancer: a challenge to clinical trial design. *Lancet Oncol.* 1: 159–68. (Review.)

Raulet D (2004) Interplay of NK cells and their receptors with the adaptive immune response. *Nat. Immunol.* 5: 996–1002.

Chapter 3

The clinical development of biologic therapies

David Kerr

1 Introduction

In contrast to what you will read elsewhere in this book, I do not want to say here that cancer is a disease of cells: it is not. For our purposes, cancer is a disease of people. It is the potential to extend and save human lives that drives our interest in cancer and at some point in our research we are bound to attempt to translate interesting developments in our biological understanding into real therapies for people with cancer.

The process of devising and testing a new therapy in patients is called clinical research or clinical development, and the form of test used is called a clinical trial. It is the purpose of a clinical trial to establish what the benefits and risks of a therapy are to patients and how the former can be maximised while the latter are kept to a minimum. Clinical research is not 'soft' science; clinical trials must be rigorously devised and ethically valid; they must be conducted in a controlled, methodical way with careful recording of relevant data, but without placing excessive demands on, frequently vulnerable, patients. In addition we should note that clinical trial evidence is a requirement for new therapies to be licensed for routine therapeutic use. Clinical trials are invariably subject to independent scientific and ethical review, depending on the legislation applying in the countries involved.

2 Ethical considerations in clinical research

It is imperative that clinical research be conducted ethically. The cornerstone of clinical research ethics for more than 40 years has been the World Medical Association Declaration of Helsinki (World Medical Association 1964), which places greatest emphasis on respect for human life and dignity, and stresses the importance of formulating a clear and scientifically sound protocol for any clinical trial. A full review of the ethical conduct of clinical trials is probably outside the scope of this chapter; some topics, however, will be considered here.

2.1 Informed consent process

Voluntary informed consent of patients participating in clinical trials is considered essential under most circumstances, a principle that is increasingly covered by national laws (see, for example, article 2, point j of the EU GCP Directive 2001/20/EC), and one that predates the Declaration of Helsinki (Nuremberg Code 1947). Generally, the collecting of informed consent involves discussing the trial with the patient, and giving a consent form, to be signed, together with written information about the trial—the patient information sheet. It is a process, however, and the dialogue between patient and clinician on all aspects of the trial goes on for the duration of the trial and beyond. Several studies have called into question the quality of informed consent in clinical research in general (reviewed in Edwards *et al.* 1998), and cancer trials in particular (Olver *et al.* 1995; Joffe *et al.* 2001). The quality of informed consent is, unsurprisingly, linked to the quality of the procedures used in informing the patient and in the information provided in the patient information sheet. Joffe *et al.* (2001) noted that patient understanding was enhanced, and so quality of consent improved by:

> careful reading of consent forms and patient information sheets;
> having a nurse present during discussions about the trial;
> giving patients more time to consider their decisions, e.g. by allowing them to
> take consent forms and patient information sheets home overnight for consideration;
> using simplified consent forms that focus on key information rather than every single detail.

The UK Central Office for Research Ethics Committees (COREC 2001) recommends that the information detailed in Table 3.1 should be included in consent forms and patient information sheets. In the end, and despite all the regulatory requirements, the only way to drive up the quality of the informed consent process is to emphasise the key role of open and honest communication between the clinicians involved and the patient.

2.2 Ethics committees

Research ethics committees (RECs), or institutional review boards (IRBs), serve to provide independent review and recommendations to the people running a clinical trial, both at the outset, when their formal approval must be given before the trial can proceed, and throughout the trial period. The

Table 3.1 COREC guidance on consent forms and patient information sheets

1. An understandable study title.

2. An invitation to the patient to participate in the trial.

3. A description of the purpose of the study.

4. An explanation of how the patient has been chosen to participate.

5. An explanation that participation is voluntary.

6. An explanation of what participation in the trial involves.

7. Specific explanations of what the patient will have to do on trial.

8. Details of the drug or procedure being tested.

9. Details of the available alternatives for diagnosis or treatment.

10. An explanation of possible side-effects of any treatment received in the trial.

11. An explanation of the possible disadvantages and risks of taking part.

12. An explanation of the possible benefits of taking part.

13. An explanation of how new information will be handled if it becomes available during the trial.

14. An explanation of how treatment will proceed when the trial stops.

15. An explanation of how complaints and claims for compensation will be handled.

16. An explanation of how the patient's medical records will be used and the extent to which confidentiality will be maintained.

17. An explanation of how the results of the trial will be used.

18. Details of who is organising and funding the research.

19. Details of who and how the trial has been reviewed.

20. Contact details for Further Information.

The Patient Information Sheet should state that the patient will be given a copy of the information sheet and a signed consent form to keep.

legal requirements for ethical review of clinical research may vary from country to country, but this independent ethical review is a key element of the international standard known as good clinical practice (GCP; ICH 1996). The primary concerns of a REC are the ethics of the clinical research itself and patient safety. The defining feature of a REC is that its members must have no connection with the trial other than as a member of the committee. They can, however, be members of the general public, or patients, nurses, doctors, statisticians, pharmacists, and academics, as well as people with particular ethical expertise. The predominantly voluntary work of the REC includes, among other things, reviewing and approving the trial protocol, the suitability of the clinical investigator(s), the facilities to be used, and the consent forms and patient information sheets. Daugherty (1999) suggests that ethics committee members should become an educational resource for matters related to the informed consent process and research ethics in general. In this way, they could focus on educating and mentoring investigator, rather than on the fine print of consent forms.

2.3 Equipoise

A key component of later stage clinical development, is randomisation, the comparison of two or more different therapies, often the standard therapy versus the experimental therapy, by allocating patients to receive them on a random basis (of which, more below). For such a process of random allocation of therapies to be ethical, uncertainty must exist as to which is the most effective therapy. Clearly, if the treating physicians had little doubt as to which was the more effective therapy, they would be acting unethically in allocating patients to the therapy they believed was less effective. This uncertainty is called equipoise, originally defined by Fried (1974). However, research has suggested that personal clinical equipoise is difficult to achieve, with physicians and patients often having important biases towards experimental therapies, and that it should perhaps only exist within a specified medical community as opposed to an individual (reviewed in Edwards *et al.* 1998).

3 'Classical' clinical development for cancer therapies

Generally, clinical trials for all types of disease, not just cancer, can be divided into four consecutive categories, or phases, with each phase acting as a checkpoint, whereby progression to the next phase is dependent on the collection of sufficient evidence to support further testing.

Phase I is the initial stage of testing, usually when a therapy is tested in people for the first time. The primary aim of such a phase I clinical trial is to test safety, to establish toxicities, and to recommend a dose schedule for subsequent use. Sometimes, however, phase I trials are performed when an established therapy is being used for a different disease or is being administered in combination with other agents or via a different route.

Phase II clinical trials test therapies that have been shown to be acceptably safe in phase I trials. Importantly, a phase II trial will usually involve more participants than a phase I trial, so affording a better understanding of the therapy's safety profile. In addition a phase II allows a preliminary assessment of how effective the therapy may be.

Phase III trials involve hundreds to thousands of people, to help to decide how an intervention should be used in standard practice; for example, by comparing a new intervention that has shown promise in a phase II trial, with an existing intervention.

Phase IV trials involve hundreds of thousands of patients. Phase IV trials aim to get a better understanding of a medical intervention after it has been licensed. Information may be gathered on rarer side effects, better dosage and cost effectiveness.

3.1 Phase I clinical trials

Outside of the oncology setting, most phase I clinical trials are conducted in healthy volunteers. However, because of the toxicities generally associated with new **cytotoxic** anticancer agents, phase I studies in oncology are almost always conducted in patients with advanced cancers, though not always the same cancer, for whom no standard therapy is suitable. The purpose of a phase I trial is to test safety and toxicity. Published reviews of phase I trials in cancer report that tumours respond in only 4–6% of patients in these trials and that about 0.5% of patients die as the result of toxicity (see, for example, Sekine *et al.* 2002).

Generally, in phase I oncology studies, small groups of patients are treated with increasing doses according to their chronological entry into the study. This is based on the assumption that activity increases with dose, and the primary aim of most cancer-agent phase I trials is to establish the **maximum tolerated dose** (MTD) (ASCO 1997). The starting dose is usually based on pre-clinical testing, with a standard measure of toxicity in such testing being the percentage of animals (rodents) who die because of treatment. The dose at which 10% of the animals die is known as the LD_{10}, which has in the past often correlated with the maximum-tolerated dose (MTD) in humans, adjusted for body-surface area (Freireich *et al.* 1966). A number of schemes for dose escalation are commonly in use but these normally allow for large increases in the early doses, but much smaller increases once toxicities start to emerge. If the agent being tested is ultimately considered suitable for phase II studies, the dose that may be used in those phase II trials may not be the MTD but the prior dose (recommended dose schedule), which causes moderate but reversible toxicity in most patients (Carter 1977).

The MTD of an agent is defined by its **dose-limiting toxicity** (DLT), the toxicity caused by the agent which, if the dose were increased further, the damage caused would be irreversible or life-threatening. DLTs vary from agent to agent and can be, for example, myelosuppression, cardiotoxicity, dermatologic toxicity, or neurologic toxicity. To ensure patient safety and vouchsafe the quality of phase I trial results, careful monitoring and recording of toxicities are required. The US NCI's *Common Terminology Criteria for Adverse Events* (CTCAE; NCI 2003) provides standard scales for the assessment of a wide variety of toxicities, with the scales running from 1, asymptomatic, to 4, life-threatening or disabling, and 5, death. The CTCAE are commonly used to assess toxicities through all phases of cancer agent clinical development.

Phase I trials may also provide an opportunity to assess the pharmacokinetics of the new agent being studied. Pharmacokinetics is the study of how the body acts on the drug, and the processes involved are frequently short-handed to ADME: the Absorption, Distribution, Metabolism and Excretion of the drug by the body.

A key issue for patients to understand is that a phase I trial can offer no guarantee of benefit to an individual patient. The consent process is therefore complex due to many factors including the vulnerability of the patient and the expectations and interest of the guiding clinician (see Chapter 13, Gene therapy).

3.2 Phase II clinical trials

Once the safety of an experimental cancer agent has been established and a suitable 'therapeutic' dose determined, phase II trials represent the first real attempt to evaluate the agent's anticancer activity. Phase II trials aim to assess the activity, feasibility, and toxicity of a given dose and schedule of the experimental agent. Phase II trials include more patients than phase I trials, typically from 20 to 50 patients. As a consequence of these increased numbers, and the need for extended periods of patient recruitment, phase II trials may be conducted over longer periods than phase I trials. Phase II trials typically take several months to several years to complete.

There are a number of commonly used phase II trial designs (see Thezenas *et al.* 2004), but all are dependent on prospective recruitment of patients, to avoid potential bias caused by retrospective patient selection, and on accurate and consistent measurement of patient responses to the experimental agent.

A standard phase II trial design, that of Fleming (Fleming 1982) assumes that, for any new treatment, there is a response rate below which the treatment will not be considered for further testing and a higher response rate above which it will certainly qualify for further testing. The sample size, the number of patients that must be entered into the trial and evaluated for response, is then calculated on the basis of minimising the probabilities of concluding that response is above the lower response level, when that is false, or below the higher response level, when that is false.

Phase II trials may also be the first phase in which the concepts of a control group and randomised assignment to therapy groups arise. Randomisation assigns patients to different groups in a trial so that valid results can be obtained for comparison of treatments. A control group may be included to allow evaluation of efficacy. There is a trend of increasing use of randomised phase II designs in cancer research but the accrual rate and success rate of the trials remain low. More innovative, flexible designs are needed to address study population enrichment, selection, and validation of the most appropriate target-based endpoints and early stopping rules for futility and so on (Lee and Feng 2005).

Response evaluation is obviously a key component of all clinical trials that aim to assess the activity of anticancer agents, be they phase II trials or later phase trials. The commonly used response evaluation criteria in solid tumours (RECIST; Therasse *et al.* 2000) allow for consistent measurement and recording of responses, so allowing comparisons between studies. RECIST is based on the measurement of specific, so called, target lesions and on the counting of the overall number of tumour lesions. Consequently, shrinkage of target lesions and reduction in the overall number of lesions are indicative of high response. Response itself is classified as complete response (CR), partial response (PR), stable disease (SD), or progressive disease (PD).

3.3 Phase III clinical trials

In the sequence of clinical development of new agents, phase III trials represent the first direct comparison of the new agent with the existing standard care, which may in some cases be no active treatment at all. Phase III trials aim to clarify the efficacy, best doses, and methods of administration of an experimental agent. As phase III trials typically enrol several hundred to thousands of patients, they also provide an opportunity to identify less frequently occurring toxicities and adverse events. Again, because of this requirement for increased numbers of patients, phase III trials may recruit patients over several months or even years. Increasingly, to speed recruitment of the necessary numbers of patients, phase III trials are being run over multiple institutions and even countries. The need for standardised operating procedures and quality control, to ensure that patients treated in different institutions within the trial are treated comparably, is obvious.

In addition to randomisation for the allocation of patients to the two, or more, treatment groups, one of which is usually a control group, phase III trials may also include blinding, i.e. concealing from patients and/or researchers which treatment group a particular patient is in. The purpose of such blinding is to eliminate the possibility of 'wish bias', patients responding better simply because they are aware they are receiving the experimental agent and researchers, similarly, evaluating the responses of the experimental agent more positively simply in the expectation that it is better (Wynder *et al.* 1990).

Entire books have been written on clinical trials in cancer and their statistical design (see, for example: Pu and Crowley 2001; Girling *et al.* 2003) with much of the emphasis resting on the design of phase III randomised controlled trials. In essence, patients are recruited and randomised in sufficient number that an assumed but specific difference in efficacy between the groups would only be found falsely with a significantly low probability, frequently 0.05, i.e. a 1 in 20 probability of returning a false positive result. Many of the key elements of phase III randomised controlled trial design have been incorporated into a specific checklist for the reporting of such trials, the consolidated standards of reporting trials (CONSORT), which form a major part of the CONSORT Statement (Moher *et al.* 2001). The checklist details 22 items (see Table 3.2), mainly dealing with the reporting of methods, results, and discussion, which the CONSORT group consider essential to the external and internal validity of a trial report.

The question then arises as to how efficacy is measured in phase III cancer trials. Rather than simply measure tumour response in the manner detailed by the RECIST criteria, phase III trials have historically focused on patient survival as the key measure of efficacy, the key endpoint. In a trial with two groups, the control group and the trial group, a comparison can be made between the median survival times of the two groups. This measurement of survival produces time-to-event data, where the event in question is the death of the patient; this is usually called overall survival. However, other time-to-event measures may also be used, these include time to disease progression (TTP) or time to local recurrence.

An additional endpoint that is increasingly considered in phase III cancer trials is quality of life (QoL). There are a plethora of definitions for QoL, most of which include the two concepts of 'subjective' (QoL can only be understood from the patient's perspective) and multi-dimensional (the various human dimensions that may be affected by cancer (Cella 1994). Again, a wealth of measures have been developed for assessing QoL—single (one tool or measurement) and multiple tools. Some measures are specific for patients with cancer, whilst other are more general. Measures should be chosen that will make a clear and important difference to patient care, whilst not causing an excessive burden to patients, and sufficiently refined to pick up any differences in the treatment experience in clinical trials. Combining QoL data with survival data now permits statistical approaches to determine quality-adjusted life years. A comprehensive list of QoL measures commonly used in cancer clinical trials is provided by Cella and Tulsky (1990).

Table 3.2 CONSORT Checklist of items to include when reporting a randomised trial

PAPER SECTION and topic	Item	Description	Reported on Page #
Title and Abstract	1	How participants were allocated to interventions (*e.g.* 'random allocation', 'randomised', or 'randomly assigned').	
Introduction Background	2	Scientific background and explanation of rationale.	
Methods Participants	3	Eligibility criteria for participants and the settings and locations where the data were collected.	
Interventions	4	Precise details of the interventions intended for each group and how and when they were actually administered.	
Objectives	5	Specific objectives and hypotheses.	
Outcomes	6	Clearly defined primary and secondary outcome measures and, when applicable, any methods used to enhance the quality of measurements (e.g. multiple observations, training of assessors).	
Sample size	7	How sample size was determined and, when applicable, explanation of any interim analyses and stopping rules.	
Randomisation Sequence generation	8	Method used to generate the random allocation sequence, including details of any restrictions (e.g. blocking, stratification).	
Allocation concealment	9	Method used to implement the random allocation sequence (e.g. numbered containers or central telephone), clarifying whether the sequence was concealed until interventions were assigned.	
Implementation	10	Who generated the allocation sequence, who enrolled participants, and who assigned participants to their groups.	
Blinding (masking)	11	Whether or not participants, those administering the interventions, and those assessing the outcomes were blinded to group assignment. When relevant, how the success of blinding was evaluated.	
Statistical methods	12	Statistical methods used to compare groups for primary outcome(s); methods for additional analyses, such as subgroup analyses and adjusted analyses.	

(continued)

Table 3.2 (*continued*) CONSORT Checklist of items to include when reporting a randomised trial

PAPER SECTION and topic	Item	Description	Reported on Page #
Results Participant flow	13	Flow of participants through each stage (a diagram is strongly recommended). Specifically, for each group report the numbers of participants randomly assigned, receiving intended treatment, completing the study protocol, and analysed for the primary outcome. Describe protocol deviations from study as planned, together with reasons.	
Recruitment	14	Dates defining the periods of recruitment and follow-up.	
Baseline data	15	Baseline demographic and clinical characteristics of each group.	
Numbers analysed	16	Number of participants (denominator) in each group included in each analysis and whether the analysis was by 'intention-to-treat'. State the results in absolute numbers when feasible (e.g. 10/20, not 50%).	
Outcomes and estimation	17	For each primary and secondary outcome, a summary of results for each group, and the estimated effect size and its precision (e.g. 95% confidence interval).	
Ancillary analyses	18	Address multiplicity by reporting any other analyses performed, including subgroup analyses and adjusted analyses, indicating those pre-specified and those exploratory.	
Adverse events	19	All important adverse events or side-effects in each intervention group.	
Discussion Interpretation	20	Interpretation of the results, taking into account study hypotheses, sources of potential bias or imprecision and the dangers associated with multiplicity of analyses and outcomes.	
Generalisability	21	Generalisability (external validity) of the trial findings.	
Overall evidence	22	General interpretation of the results in the context of current evidence.	

4 Challenges presented by cancer biotherapies for clinical development

Cancer biotherapies present a number of challenges to the standard pattern of cancer drug development described above. These challenges relate to the appropriate strategies for selection of patients, study design, and choice of more appropriate endpoints. Since the activities of many new cancer biotherapies are targeted to cancer cells, increasing the dose to toxicity may be ineffective, and determining MTD may be an inappropriate method of establishing an effective dose in phase I trials. Lower doses of some of these agents may be just as effective as higher doses. Similarly, some of the biotherapies, e.g. kinase inhibitors (see Chapter 4), may act through amelioration of growth stimulation rather than by induction of cell death (and may therefore not necessarily shrink the tumour). These agents may be regarded as **cytostatic** rather than cytotoxic, and under these circumstances, response evaluation by measuring reductions in lesion size or numbers of lesions may also be inappropriate.

Korn *et al.* (2001) recommend the choice of trial designs for cytostatic agents, which depends on what is known pre-clinically about the agent (e.g do you have a validated and reproducible biologic endpoint that can be used to guide dose escalation?), what is known about the patient population being studied (e.g. do you have a well-documented historical progression free survival rate at one year for comparison with the experience of the new agent?), and the numbers of agents and patients available for the trial. For example, statistical designs for a dose that maximises the biologic response (optimum biologic dose) would likely require many more patients than are studied in a typical phase I trial. Serum markers of tumour progression were studied in 312 patients treated with a **matrix metalloproteinase** inhibitor (MMPI) (see Chapter 10) to try and establish an appropriate dose for phase II studies (Nemunaitis *et al.* 1998). For **anti-angiogenic** trials, the biologic response criteria should be included along with conventional criteria for assessment of efficacy as the expected advantage of anti-angiogenic therapies is to achieve long-term biologic benefits by inducing a dormant state in residual tumour foci without unacceptable toxic effects (Isner and Asahara 1999). The improvement of clinical study design is crucial as new therapeutic approaches may fail if inappropriate clinical trials are performed (Betensky *et al.* 2002).

5 Conclusion

Current systems of drug development have not much changed in the last two decades but trials probably take longer to complete due to the regulatory necessities outlined above. Patients, rather than the laboratory, still seem to be the most valuable and efficient way of testing new therapies, although the spectrum of types of tumours (e.g. HER-2 positive) for which a specific biotherapy will have an application is becoming narrower, resulting in greater patient selectivity but also the exclusion of others. The efficacy of these new agents, measured by survival, overall, has been modest but new biologic endpoints may be more efficacious. There is a rapidly expanding programme of promising agents being utilised currently, many of which are been discussed in this book; patients expect that they will be made available for their care in a timely manner. So, as well as testing new trial designs with specific patient populations, it is imperative to build new trial networks for streamlining and speeding up the 'bench to bedside' pathway. International collaboration, including the developing world, in accrual of patients for phase III trials, will help achieve this goal.

References

ASCO (1997) Critical role of phase I clinical trials in cancer treatment. *J Clin Oncol*; 15: 853–9.

Betensky RA, Louis DN, Cairncross JG (2002) Influence of unrecognised molecular hetergeneity on randomised clinical trials. *J Clin Oncol*; 20: 2495–9.

Carter SK (1977) Clinical trials in cancer chemotherapy. *Cancer*; 40: 544–57.

Cella DF (1994) Quality of life concepts and definition. *J Pain and Symptom Manage*; 9(3): 186–92.

Cella DF and Tulsky DS (1990) Measuring quality of life today: methodological aspects. *Oncology*; 4(5): 29–38.

Central Office for Research Ethics Committees (2001) *Guidelines for researchers – patient information sheet & consent form* (available online at: www.**corec**.org.uk/applicants/help/ docs/Guidance_on_ Patient_Information_Sheets_and_Consent_Forms.doc; last accessed 20 June 2005).

Daugherty C (1999) Impact of therapeutic research on informed consent and the ethics of clinical trials: a medical oncology perspective. *J Clin Oncol*; 17(5): 1601–17.

Directive 2001/20/EC of the European Parliament and of the Council of 4 April 2001 on the approximation of the laws, regulations and administrative provisions of the Member States relating to the implementation of good clinical practice in the conduct of clinical trials on medicinal products for human use. Official Journal L 121 , 01/05/2001 P. 0034–0044.

Edwards SJL, Lilford RJ, Hewison J (1998) The ethics of randomised controlled trials from the perspectives of patients, the public, and healthcare professionals. *BMJ*; 317: 1209–12.

Fleming TR (1982) One-sample multiple testing procedure for phase II clinical trials. *Biometrics*; 38: 143–51.

Freireich EJ, Gehan EA, Rall DP *et al.* (1966) Quantitative comparison of toxicity of anticancer agents in mouse, rat, hamster, dog, monkey, and man. *Cancer Chemother Rep*; 50: 219–44.

Girling DJ, Parmar MKB, Stenning SP *et al.* (2003) *Cancer clinical trials: principles and practice.* Oxford: Oxford University Press.

International Conference on Harmonisation of Technical Requirements for Registration of Pharmaceuticals for Human Use (1996) *ICH Harmonised Tripartite Guideline for Good Clinical Practice.*

Isner J, Asahara T (1999) Angiogenesis and vaxculogenesis as herapeutic strategies for postnatal neovascularization. *J Clin Invest*; **103**: 1231–6.

Joffe S, Cook EF, Cleary PD *et al.* (2001) Quality of informed consent in cancer clinical trials: a cross-sectional survey. *Lancet*; **358**: 1772–7.

Korn EL, Arbuck SG, Pluda JM *et al.* (2001) Clinical trial designs for cytostatic agents: are new approaches needed? *J Clin Oncol*; **19**(1): 265–72.

Lee JJ, Feng L (2005) Randomized phase ii designs in cancer clinical trials: current status and future directions. *J Clin Oncol*; **23**(19): 4450–7.

Moher D, Schulz KF, Altman DG *et al.* (2001) The CONSORT statement: revised recommendations for improving the quality of reports of parallel group randomized trials. *JAMA*; **285**: 1987–91.

National Cancer Institute (2003) *Common Terminology Criteria for Adverse Events* v3.0 (CTCAE). National Cancer Institute. *http://ctep.cancer.gov/forms/CTCAEv3.pdf* (last accessed 20 June 2005)

Nemunaitis J, Poole C, Primrose J *et al.* (1998) Combined analysis of studies of the matrix metalloproteinase inhibitor maromastat on serum tumor markers in advanced cancer: selection of a biologically active and tolerable dose for longer-term studies. *Clin Cancer Res*; **4**: 1101–9.

The Nuremberg Code 1947 (1996) *BMJ*; **313**: 1448.

Olver IN, Buchanan L, Laidlaw C, Poulton G (1995) The adequacy of consent forms for informing patients entering oncological clinical trials. *Ann Oncol*; **6**: 867–70.

Pu J, Crowley J (2001) *Handbook of statistics in clinical oncology.* New York: Marcel Dekker Ltd.

Sekine I, Yamamoto N, Kunitoh H *et al.* (2002) Relationship between objective responses in phase I trials and potential efficacy of non-specific cytotoxic investigational new drugs. *Ann Oncol*; **13**: 1300–6.

Therasse P, Arbuck SG, Eisenhauer EA *et al.* (2000) New guidelines to evaluate the response to treatment in solid tumors. European Organization for Research and Treatment of Cancer, National Cancer Institute of the United States, National Cancer Institute of Canada. *J Natl Cancer Inst*; **92**: 205–16.

Thezenas S, Duffour J, Cotine S, *et al.* (2004) Five-year change in statistical designs of phase II trials published in leading cancer journals. *Eur J Cancer*; **40**: 1244–9.

World Medical Association (1964) *World Medical Association Declaration of Helsinki. Ethical principles for medical research involving human subjects* (amended in 1975, 1983, 1989, 1996, 2000 and 2004). *http://www.wma.net/e/policy/pdf/17c.pdf* (last accessed 28 May 2005)

Wynder EL, Higgins IT, Harris RE (1990) The wish bias. *J Clin Epidemiol*; **43**: 619–21.

Chapter 4

Kinase inhibitors

Stefan Sleijfer, Kees Nooter, and Jaap Verweij

1 Introduction

Normal cell growth is a strictly regulated process with well-balanced activity between growth-stimulating and growth-inhibiting factors. In tumour cells, mechanisms of growth control are severely altered, shifting the balance towards uncontrolled proliferation. In addition, tumour cells are characterised by resistance against triggers for programmed cell death (**apoptosis**), growth into adjacent structures and the ability to form metastases. This abnormal situation develops through mutations in genes involved in pivotal cellular processes such as proliferation, **differentiation**, migration, adhesion, and apoptosis. Over recent years, an expanding number of products from these mutated genes have been identified. Simultaneously, our knowledge on the mechanisms by which these, as well as normal proteins, transduce signals has considerably increased. Essential for signal **transduction** of many proteins, and thereby for their function, are enzymes called kinases. Selective inhibition of the kinases of mutated proteins accounting for malignant behaviour, while leaving normal cells relatively unaffected, obviously forms an attractive strategy to treat cancer. Recently, several such kinase inhibitors have been developed and have emerged as a novel class of anti-tumour drugs.

This chapter focuses on the role of altered kinase activity in tumour cells and on several aspects of kinase inhibitors used in oncology.

2 Kinases and protein function

The activity of many proteins is controlled by their state of phosphorylation. Phosphorylation is the substitution of phosphate groups for hydroxyl groups on the amino acids serine, tyrosine, or threonine on substrate proteins. Enzymes called kinases and phosphatases, responsible for binding and removing of phosphate groups, respectively, mediate this process. Kinases are named after the amino acids to which they bind phosphate groups. Consequently, there are three groups of kinases: tyrosine, serine, and threonine kinases. Sequencing has revealed that the human **genome** contains more than 500 different **protein kinases** (Manning *et al.* 2002).

Kinases are involved in internal and external cellular communication. For external communication with the environment, the cell membrane is covered with receptors of which many exert their effects through kinases. These receptors consist of an extracellular **ligand**-binding domain, a transmembrane region, and an intracellular region containing a kinase domain. After attachment of a ligand, a protein that is able to bind specifically to a corresponding receptor, the kinase associated with the receptor is activated followed by recruitment and binding of an adenosine triphosphate (**ATP**) molecule. By transferring a phosphate group from ATP to a substrate protein, kinases mediate phosphorylation of the receptor itself (autophosphorylation) and receptor-associated proteins. This results in activation of numerous downstream signalling pathways and finally activation of **transcription** factors (Fig. 4.1). These transcription factors bind to **promoter** regions in the chromosomal DNA, thereby affecting the transcription of genes critical for the function of the receptor that was initially activated by ligand binding. The number of receptors that use kinases for signal transduction is large and includes the members of the epithelial growth factor receptor (EGFR), vascular endothelial growth factor receptor (VEGFR), and platelet-derived growth factor receptor (PDGFR) families (Blume-Jensen and Hunter 2001; Madhusudan & Ganesan 2004).

Many non-receptor proteins involved in internal cellular communication depend on kinase activity for their function as well. They comprise a kinase domain linked to a region that regulates its activity but, in contrast to receptors, they lack an extracellular ligand-binding and a transmembrane region. Following modulation of the regulatory domain, for example by phosphorylation, kinase activity is enhanced (Irby and Yeatman 2000). Numerous non-receptor proteins with kinase activity have been described (Table 4.1). All these proteins are involved in important cellular functions (Blume-Jensen and Hunter 2001; Madhusudan & Ganesan 2004).

3 Kinase-dependent proteins and cancer

Similar to normal proteins, products from mutated genes frequently depend on kinase activity. The first tumour type in which the importance of increased kinase activity from a mutated protein was recognised was chronic myeloid leukaemia (CML). CML is characterised by the presence of the so-called **Philadelphia chromosome** in approximately 95% of the cases. Through exchange of genetic material, this Philadelphia chromosome comprises a shortened chromosome 22 and a part of chromosome 9. At the fusion region of

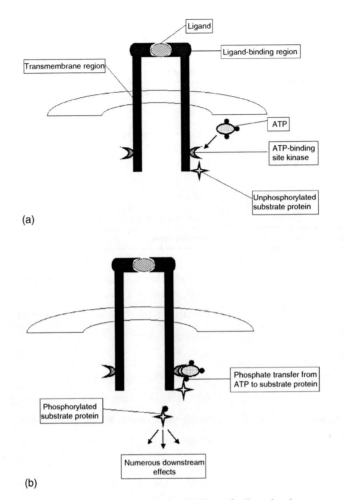

(a)

(b)

Fig. 4.1 Kinase-containing receptor. (a) After binding of a ligand to its receptor, the kinase domain is activated followed by recruitment of an ATP molecule.
(b) Subsequently, the kinase mediates the transfer of a phosphate from the ATP molecule to a substrate protein. The phosphorylated substrate protein induces multiple downstream effects, ultimately resulting in altered transcription of genes essential for the function of the receptor that was initially activated by ligand binding.

these two chromosomes, a new gene arises consisting of parts of the genes BCR from chromosome 22 and ABL from chromosome 9. In normal cells, the tyrosine kinase-dependent ABL is involved in proliferation and is tightly controlled. The tyrosine kinase activity from the fusion gene BCR–ABL, however, is deregulated and continuously enhanced. The importance of this fusion gene in the pathogenesis of CML is supported by the observation that introduction of BCR–ABL into haematologic cell lines induces uncontrolled cell

Table 4.1 Examples of kinase-dependent proteins implicated in human malignancies

Non-receptor proteins	Tumour type
BCR-ABL	CML, ALL, AML
JAK-family	leukaemias
SRC-family	leukaemias, melanoma, colon, breast
SYK-family	breast
PKC-family	many tumours
BRAF	melanoma
Akt	many malignancies
Receptors	**Tumour type**
EGFR-family	
EGFR	head and neck, lung, gliomas, breast, colon, prostate, cervix, kidney, endometrium, and others
HER2	breast, lung, colon, stomach, ovary, and others
HER3	breast
HER4	breast
PDGFR-family	gliomas, leukaemias, ovary
KIT	GIST, seminoma, lung, melanoma, leukaemias
VEGFR-family	tumour angiogenesis (many malignancies)
FGFR-family	leukaemias, lymphomas, prostate, breast
IGFR	cervix, sarcomas
HGFR	hepatocellular carcinoma, rhabdomyosarcoma, thyroid, kidney

growth and resistance to apoptotic triggers (Savage and Antman 2002). In addition, inhibition of the BCR–ABL kinase activity in these cell lines yields anti-proliferative activity. Besides ABL kinase activity, overexpression of other non-receptor proteins using kinases also plays a role in human cancers (Table 4.1). For example, elevated levels and kinase activity of proteins such as SRC, PKC, and others, have been demonstrated in several tumour types, while these levels were not increased in surrounding normal tissue (Irby and Yeatman 2000). For most of these proteins, it is not fully elucidated yet how their expression and increased kinase activity leads to cellular transformation.

Receptors using kinases have also been implicated in the development of malignant cells. Of these, the EGFR-family is probably the most extensively studied. This family consists of four members, EGFR (HER1), HER2 (Neu), HER3, and HER4. Deregulated signalling in particular of EGFR and HER2 is commonly seen in human cancers. Overexpression of EGFR has been demonstrated in several human tumour types including non-small cell lung, head and neck, ovarian, breast, cervical, colorectal, bladder, gastric, and oesophageal carcinoma. In pre-clinical models, overexpression of both EGFR and HER2 confers resistance against chemotherapy and radiotherapy. Accordingly, increased expression of EGFR is associated with a poor prognosis (Nicholson *et al.* 2001) and also HER2 overexpression renders a poor prognosis in breast, lung, ovarian, bone, and prostate cancer (Ranson 2004). Next to members of the EGFR family, other kinase-containing receptor families for which a role in cancer has been demonstrated include among others PDGFR, VEGFR, Fibroblast Growth Factor Receptor, and the Insulin Receptor family (Blume-Jensen and Hunter 2001; Madhusudan & Ganesan 2004) (Table 4.1).

Several mechanisms have been reported to enhance kinase activity in tumour cells. Tumour cells can overexpress ligands that induce enhanced receptor kinase activity in the tumour cell itself or neighbouring cells in an **autocrine** and paracrine manner, respectively. For example, overexpression of transforming growth factor-a (TGF-a), one of the ligands for EGFR, has been demonstrated in head and neck cancer. Also increased circulating levels of VEGF, the ligand of VEGFR, are frequently seen in many tumour types.

Genetic alterations by mutations, amplifications, or **translocations** may also lead to constitutive expression of a kinase. Through mutations in kinase-regulating domains, so-called gain-of-function mutations yield constitutive kinase activation without the normally required binding of a ligand. Such gain-of-function mutations have been found in the genes encoding the c-KIT receptor and EGFR in gastrointestinal stromal tumours (GIST) (Hirota *et al.* 1998) and non-small cell lung cancers, respectively (Lynch *et al.* 2004). The BCR–ABL gene found in CML is an example of kinase activation through translocation. In addition, this gene is also prone to amplification.

In conclusion, increased kinase activity of many proteins is thought to play a pivotal role in the pathogenesis of several human cancers. Obviously, inhibition of the function of these proteins by targeting kinase activity is an attractive approach to treat these cancers.

4 Inhibition of kinase activity

There are currently three clinical approaches to inhibit kinase activity. One way is by targeting the ligand of a receptor by use of **monoclonal antibodies**. A successful example of this strategy is bevacizumab, an antibody directed against VEGF, the ligand of VEGFR (Hurwitz *et al.* 2004). Kinase activity can also be abrogated by monoclonal antibodies targeting the ligand-binding region of a receptor. Examples with proven clinical activity are cetuximab (Cunningham *et al.* 2004) and trastuzumab (Slamon *et al.* 2001), which bind the EGFR and the HER2 receptor, respectively. The use of monoclonal antibodies is further discussed in another chapter (see Chapter 7).

A strategy to block receptor, as well as non-receptor, kinases is the application of agents that directly target the kinase domain. In recent years, an enormous number of small compounds have been identified that bind in the vicinity of the ATP-binding region of the kinase. Attachment of ATP to the kinase is thereby competitively prevented, as a consequence of which phosphorylation and protein functions are inhibited (Fig. 4.2). Since the ATP-binding regions of the various kinases differ slightly, it is possible to develop specific inhibitors for the individual kinases. This enables us, at least in theory, to develop therapies that will affect tumour cells by specifically targeting those kinases that play an important role in tumour growth.

5 Clinical studies with kinase inhibitors

Following many years of pre-clinical investigation, kinase inhibitors have entered the clinic only recently. When studying kinase inhibitors, it must be kept in mind that there are some important differences compared with studies testing conventional agents such as chemotherapy. One of these is the duration of therapy. Since kinase inhibition is reversible for most of the currently available drugs, kinase inhibitors should be administered (semi-)continuously. This contrasts treatment

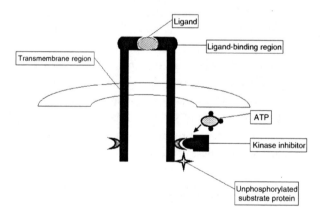

Fig. 4.2 Through binding to the ATP-binding domain of a kinase, a kinase inhibitor prevents binding of ATP to a kinase thereby inhibiting phosphorylation and consequently the function of the targeted kinase.

with conventional **cytotoxic** agents that induce an irreversible effect and can already exert anti-tumour activity when administered for a limited period of time. Therefore, important requisites for kinase inhibitors are that they can be given safely for prolonged periods of time and are convenient for the patients.

In addition, there are strong indications that higher doses of conventional chemotherapy yield better anti-tumour efficacy. Consequently, assessment of anti-tumour activity occurs at the highest doses that can be tolerated. The maximum tolerated dose of a cytotoxic drug is established in early clinical trials and is based on the occurrence of dose-limiting toxicities. For kinase-inhibitors, the inhibition of the target may happen at doses much lower than the highest tolerable dose. Doses above the level that adequately inhibits the targeted kinases will mainly add toxicity without yielding improved anti-tumour efficacy. Establishment of the optimal dose in cancer patients will preferably be done by looking at the specific molecular targets in tumour biopsies. Since taking biopsies are cumbersome procedures for patients with solid tumours, this has not been achieved for most kinase inhibitors tested up to now. An alternative could be the use of surrogate tissues. These tissues may harbour molecules that are structurally or functionally almost identical as the ones that are aimed to be targeted in the tumour. An illustrative example is the use of skin biopsies in the case of EGFR kinase inhibition. The efficacy of systemically applied EGFR kinase inhibitors can be followed in the skin by assessing the inhibition of substrate phosphorylation by normal EGFR using immunohistochemistry (Albanell *et al.* 2002). It is obvious, however, that this surrogate-tissue approach has its difficulties, by finding easily accessible tissues with right surrogate target molecules. Moreover, effects of kinase inhibitors against such normal proteins will not always accurately reflect effects on their mutated counterparts.

Furthermore, in view of the working mechanisms of kinase-inhibitors, it is questionable whether efficacy can be adequately established on basis of response rates achieved, an end point frequently used in the assessment of conventional chemotherapy. Kinase inhibitors are thought to exert their anti-tumour activity mainly through amelioration of growth stimulation and less through induction of cell death. Therefore, these agents should be regarded as **cytostatic** rather than cytotoxic. In these circumstances, the most accurate parameter to establish efficacy is probably time to progression.

6 Efficacy of kinase inhibitors

Numerous inhibitors directed towards kinases of (mutated) proteins are assessed in various stages of clinical studies. Currently, more than 100 clinical studies are underway. At present, two kinase inhibitors, imatinib and gefitinib, have been approved for clinical use. Since for these two the reported experience is largest, they are discussed in greater detail, serving as examples.

6.1 Imatinib

The first kinase inhibitor that was clinically applied is imatinib (STI-571, Glivec[R], Gleevec[TM]). Imatinib was initially developed as an inhibitor of the PDGFR, but appeared to target the tyrosine kinases of ABL and the receptor c-KIT as well. Kinases of other proteins such as EGFR were not affected (Buchdunger et al. 2000).

A logical first choice for exploring the activity of imatinib was CML. As previously discussed, the vast majority of CML cases is characterised by a specific chromosomal translocation yielding increased ABL kinase activity. In the first phase I trial in chronic phase CML, patients not responding to, or not tolerating, standard treatment, a rapid response was observed in those receiving at least 300 mg imatinib daily (Druker et al. 2001a). Phosphorylation of substrate proteins of BCR–ABL was clearly impaired at these doses, indicating adequate inhibition of BCR–ABL kinase. Subsequent phase II studies have confirmed these encouraging results and a recent phase III study showed superiority for imatinib over the combination of interferon and cytarabine in terms of response, time to progression, and toxicity (O'Brien et al. 2003). Imatinib also possesses anti-tumour activity in patients with other BCR–ABL harbouring leukaemias. These include acute lymphoblastic leukaemia and CML in more advanced stages than the chronic phase, the so-called accelerated phase and blast phase. Although imatinib had substantial activity, anti-tumour efficacy in these subsets is less than in chronic phase CML, while relapses occur earlier (Druker et al. 2001; Sawyers et al. 2002; Talpaz et al. 2002).

Prompted by the favourable outcomes in CML, another tumour type in which imatinib has been studied is gastrointestinal stromal tumour (GIST). GIST is a mesenchymal tumour primarily arising in the gastrointestinal tract and is characterised by overexpression of the c-KIT receptor. It has been shown that in about 90% of the patients, this receptor harbours a mutation causing constitutive kinase activation. In those few cases without c-KIT mutations, activating mutations in PDGFRa, another tyrosine kinase-dependent receptor, or no mutations at all can be detected (Heinrich et al. 2003). Joensuu et al. were the first to apply imatinib for GIST (Joensuu et al. 2001). In a heavily pretreated patient with metastatic GIST, daily administration of imatinib resulted in a rapid response and improvement of symptoms. Several subsequent trials have established the efficacy of imatinib in patients with unresectable GIST (Demetri et al. 2002; Van Oosterom et al. 2001; Verweij et al. 2004).

Over 80% of the patients obtain a rapid clinical improvement with 5%, 45–50%, and 25–30% achieving complete response, partial response, and stable disease, respectively (Demetri *et al.* 2002; Verweij *et al.* 2004). In general, responses are durable frequently with a median progression free survival of approximately two years (Verweij *et al.* 2004). Since other systemic treatment options have previously failed to yield benefit with regard to survival, imatinib has become first-line treatment for patients with unresectable GIST. Studies exploring the efficacy of imatinib, either following complete resection of GIST to prevent recurrences or as pre-operative treatment to facilitate removement of large GISTs, are ongoing.

Another disease that can be treated successfully with imatinib is dermatofibrosarcoma protuberans, a tumour type harbouring a constitutively activated PDGFR kinase (Rubin *et al.* 2002). The reported number of patients treated with imatinib, however, is limited, as metastatic disease is rare.

Besides these tumour entities, several other disease conditions have overexpression of kinases potentially susceptible for imatinib. C-KIT overexpression is found in melanoma, seminoma, mastocytosis, and small-cell lung cancer, while PDGFR overexpression has been found in high-grade gliomas, melanoma, and certain sarcomas. Although the kinases of these proteins in theory can be inhibited by imatinib, overexpression does not automatically imply that such tumours will respond to imatinib. For example, hardly any anti-tumour activity was demonstrated in patients with extensive stage small-cell lung cancer (Johnson *et al.* 2003) or sarcomas other than GIST (Verweij *et al.* 2003). Several mechanisms probably underlie the failures of imatinib in these disease conditions. Importantly, most models suggest that imatinib mainly affects a mutated tyrosine kinase domain, while the above mentioned diseases without exception overexpress wild-type c-KIT (Burger *et al.* 2003). Another important prerequisite for anti-tumour activity is that tumours must highly rely on single increased kinase activity for malignant behaviour. In most tumours, numerous pathways are deregulated due to multiple mutations. In such cases, inhibition of only one pathway will frequently not suffice for inducing clinically relevant anti-tumour effects. Accordingly, treatment efficacy of imatinib in patients with BCR–ABL positive CML in advanced stages, which are featured by the accumulation of multiple genetic abnormalities, is less than in CML in chronic phase (Druker *et al.* 2001; Sawyers *et al.* 2002).

6.2 Gefitinib

Gefitinib (ZD1839, Iressa[R]) is a potent EGFR tyrosine kinase inhibitor that has lower activity against related proteins such as HER2 (Woodburn 1999). The first tumour type in which the tolerability and efficacy of gefitinib was assessed, was in advanced non-small-cell lung cancer (NSCLC). EGFR is highly expressed in about 40–80% of the patients with NSCLC and has been shown to be a poor prognostic feature (Lynch *et al.* 2004). In two randomised trials, pretreated patients with advanced NSCLC were allocated to receive oral doses of 250 mg or 500 mg gefitinib (Fukuoka *et al.* 2003; Kris *et al.* 2003). About 10% and 30–35% of the patients experienced partial response, and stable disease, respectively, while improvement of symptoms was observed in approximately 40%. Both doses were equivalent in terms of efficacy, while greater toxicity was encountered in the high-dose group.

Gefitinib has also been studied in other tumour types associated with EGFR overexpression. Efficacy in a phase II study in unselected patients with recurrent glioblastoma was considered promising, leading to initiation of randomised phase III studies (Rich *et al.* 2004). In patients with metastatic squamous cell carcinoma of the head and neck, a response rate of 5–10% was achieved while up to a third of the patients experienced stable disease (Cohen *et al.* 2003). By contrast, gefitininb was inactive in advanced renal cell carcinoma (Drucker *et al.* 2003).

6.3 Toxicities of imatinib and gefitinib

Both imatinib and gefitinib can be orally administered and are well-tolerated. The most frequent imatinib-induced toxicities are oedema, skin rash, fatigue, nausea, pleuritic pain, and diarrhoea. The most common haematologic adverse event is anaemia (Demetri *et al.* 2002; Van Oosterom *et al.* 2001; Verweij *et al.* 2004). The toxicity profile of gefitinib consists predominantly of skin reactions, elevated liver enzymes, and diarrhoea (Fukuoka *et al.* 2003; Kris *et al.* 2003).

7 Predictive factors for response to kinase inhibitors

Knowledge about factors determining sensitivity to kinase inhibitors is of utmost importance, since this may enable identification of patients who are likely to benefit from treatment. Thereby, over- or under-treatment can be avoided. Overexpression of the targeted protein alone does clearly not suffice to select patients, since there is a lack of correlation between the level of expression of the targeted protein and the observed efficacy (Ranson 2004). At present, several factors have been identified that may more adequately serve this purpose.

One of the most important determinants of sensitivity to kinase inhibitors is the mutation site in the kinase-containing protein. In GIST, it has been revealed that tumours with activating mutations in exon 11 of the c-KIT gene, which encodes the juxtamembrane domain, are most sensitive. Response rate and overall survival in patients with mutations in another site, exon 9, are significantly less, while patients lacking c-KIT mutations have the worst treatment outcome (Heinrich *et al.* 2003). Also for NSCLC patients treated with gefitinib targeting the EGFR kinase, mutational status has been demonstrated to affect efficacy. Of the nine patients who had a response on gefitinib, eight had specific activating mutations in EGFR gene, while none of seven non-responding patients had such mutations. Additionally, in a group of untreated patients, approximately 10% of the NSCLC patients appeared to have activating EGFR mutations, a percentage that resembles the 10% obtaining a response on gefitinib in clinical studies. In line with these observations is the finding that cell lines with such activating EGFR mutations are highly sensitive to gefitinib (Lynch *et al.* 2004).

Surrogate markers for gain-of-function mutations are probably formed by parameters reflecting the activity of the targeted kinase. Patients with NSCLC had better outcome on gefitinib treatment when one of the substrates of EGFR was phosphorylated indicating the presence of an activated EGFR (Cappuzzo *et al.* 2004).

Collectively, the available data strongly suggest that predominantly the site of mutation in the targeted kinase-containing protein affects treatment outcome. This and other not yet unravelled factors may enable to restrict treatment to only those who are at chance to respond.

8 Mechanisms conferring resistance against kinase inhibitors

Acquired resistance against kinase inhibitors while on treatment is a common phenomenon with the currently available agents. Unfortunately, the vast majority of CML and GIST patients eventually relapse after initially obtaining a durable response. Defining the underlying mechanisms may allow the development of strategies to overcome this resistance. Presently, several mechanisms have been elucidated (Table 4.2).

In tumour samples from imatinib-treated patients with progressive CML or GIST, it appeared that a high rate of tumour cells bears mutations in the ATP-binding site of the targeted kinase, whereas these mutations could not be found prior to treatment initiation. Due to conformational changes of the ATP-binding site, such mutations impair the binding of the inhibitor whereas binding of ATP and, consequently, kinase activity remains intact (Fletcher *et al.* 2003; Shah and Sawyers 2003; Von Bubhoff *et al.* 2002).

Another mechanism of drug resistance is chromosomal amplification of the locus on which the mutated gene resides. This results in a higher number of

Table 4.2 Resistance mechanisms against kinase inhibitors

Mutations in ATP-binding site	reduced drug binding
Amplification of targeted protein	excess of targeted protein
Activation of alternative pathways	independence from the targeted protein
Increased expression of drug efflux pumps	reduced intracellular drug concentration
Elevated levels of a_1-acid glycoprotein	reduced circulating drug levels
Decreased systemic drug levels by yet unknown mechanisms	reduced drug exposure

targets than actually can be inhibited by the drug (Fletcher *et al.* 2003; Le Coutre *et al.* 2000). Also, activation of alternative pathways next to the initially activated one may confer resistance. This will render tumour cells no longer dependent on the initial activated kinase, as a consequence of which inhibitors targeting this kinase become ineffective (Fletcher *et al.* 2003).

Overexpression of drug-efflux pumps, such as P-glycoprotein (Mahon *et al.* 2000) and BCRP (Burger *et al.* 2004), causes resistance in pre-clinical models. Imatinib has been reported as a substrate for these pumps resulting in reduction of intracellular drug levels and consequently efficacy (Mahon *et al.* 2000). The clinical relevance of drug efflux pump overexpression however, remains to be established. In addition, pharmacologic factors may impair efficacy of imatinib. For example, high levels of the blood protein a_1-acid glycoprotein have been shown to bind imatinib and to reduce availability of the drug (Gambacorti-Passerini *et al.* 2002). Finally, despite sustained drug doses, imatinib blood levels decrease over time through yet unravelled mechanisms (Judson *et al.* 2004).

In conclusion, several underlying mechanisms affecting sensitivity to the currently available kinase inhibitors have been revealed, but it is unlikely that all have been elucidated. Hopefully, better insight in these resistance mechanisms will lead to approaches potentiating the efficacy of kinase inhibitors.

9 Kinase-inhibitor-containing multi-drug therapy

Overexpression of kinase-dependent proteins confers resistance against anti-tumour treatments such as chemotherapy, hormonal treatment, **immunotherapy**, and radiotherapy in pre-clinical models. Accordingly, overexpression of some kinase-dependent proteins has been shown to negatively affect response to treatment in humans. In pre-clinical models, modulation of these factors by kinase inhibitors is able to overcome resistance and to potentiate the anti-tumour efficacy of other strategies. In line with these data are observations that the application of chemotherapy combined with monoclonal antibodies directed against VEGF, and HER2 renders greater anti-tumour efficacy than chemotherapy alone (Hurwitz *et al.* 2004; Slamon *et al.* 2001).

In two randomised trials in patients with advanced NSCLC, the combination of gefitinib and chemotherapy was compared with chemotherapy alone. In both studies, efficacy of both treatments was equivalent (Giaconne *et al.* 2004; Herbst *et al.* 2004). The lack of a positive outcome of the combinations in these studies is probably due to the fact that only approximately 10% of this unselected group of patients harbours EGFR mutations susceptible for inhibition by gefitinib (Lynch *et al.* 2004). Furthermore, possible negative interactions between the applied drugs were inappropriately assessed prior to initiating these large phase III studies. Nevertheless, combinations of kinase inhibitors and chemotherapy remain an interesting strategy, especially either using more potent multi-targeting inhibitors or in selected tumours types known to be susceptible for the particular drug. To prove the latter, studies have been initiated exploring the efficacy of imatinib combined with cytarabine in CML patients in chronic phase (Gardembas *et al.* 2003).

10 Conclusions and future directions

The insight that many tumours are characterised by deregulated kinase-dependent protein signalling and the ability to inhibit kinase activity by small compounds have provided medical oncologists with a novel class of anti-tumour agents. In particular for unresectable GIST, for which no effective treatment was available, and CML, for which imatinib has superior efficacy compared with standard therapy, the introduction of kinase inhibitors is a major breakthrough. It must be noted, however, that CML and GIST have several features that are essential to the successes obtained with kinase inhibitors. Increased BCR–ABL and c-KIT tyrosine kinase activity in CML and GIST, respectively, have been shown convincingly to be essential in the pathogenesis of both diseases. In contrast, most other malignancies have multiple deregulated pathways accounting for malignant behaviour and do not solely rely on the kinase activity of one mutated product. In such cases, inhibition of a single pathway will not yield anti-tumour efficacy. Therefore, more potent inhibitors that simultaneously target several kinases implicated in human cancers have been developed.

Next to dependence on a particular kinase-activated pathway, another important determinant for the success of a kinase inhibitor is the precise cause of the kinase activation. It has been revealed that the site of mutation greatly affects sensitivity to kinase inhibitors. This may allow identification of patients who are likely to respond to a particular kinase inhibitor and to individualise treatment. An example of such approach may be SU11248, a multi-targeted tyrosine kinase inhibitor. GIST patients with exon 9 mutations in the c-KIT gene have a relatively low chance to benefit from imatinib whereas preliminary results suggest that SU011248 has greater efficacy (Demetri *et al.* 2004). So, in the near future, it can be anticipated that not only the clinicopathological presentation, but also the underlying genetic abnormalities will determine treatment.

Acquired resistance during treatment with single-agent imatinib is a frequently encountered phenomenon in GIST and CML patients. Increased insight into the underlying mechanisms offers possibilities to overcome this. When resistance occurs through amplification of the targeted kinase or through decreased drug levels, increasing the dose can be anticipated to induce secondary responses. Accordingly, such an approach yields clinical benefit for approximately 30% of the GIST patients progressive using standard doses of imatinib (Zalcberg *et al.* 2004). In case of either mutations in c-KIT conferring imatinib resistance or activation of other kinase-dependent pathways, more potent drugs, which simultaneously target multiple kinases, may yield anti-tumour activity (Demetri *et al.* 2004). Randomised studies assessing such drugs are underway in GIST patients with imatinib-refractory disease.

As single-agent treatment with kinase inhibitors will probably not cure patients and increased activity of kinase-containing factors frequently contributes to resistance against other anti-tumour agents, there is a clear rationale to explore kinase inhibitors in multi-drug combination treatment. The first studies in patients with NSCLC did not yield a benefit for such combinations over chemotherapy alone. However, it may be possible that these combinations will be fruitful either in more selected patients likely to respond to kinase inhibition or using more potent kinase inhibitors.

Currently, an overwhelming number of trials assessing new potent kinase inhibitors both as single agents and as part of multi-drug regimens is ongoing in many different tumour types in various clinical stages. Hopefully, these studies will provide better understanding in the mechanisms of action of these drugs which will enable the individualisation of treatment in the future.

Nevertheless, despite the fact that much remains to be revealed and that kinase inhibitors have only recently been introduced into clinical practice, the advent of these drugs has already proved to be a valuable addition to the armamentarium against cancer. It can be envisioned that the application of kinase inhibitors will considerably expand in the coming years.

References

Albanell J, Rojo F, Averbuch S et al. (2002). Pharmacodynamic studies of the epidermal growth factor receptor inhibitor ZD1839 in skin from cancer patients: histopathological and molecular consequences of receptor inhibition. *J Clin Oncol*, 20, 110–24.

Blume-Jensen P, Hunter T (2001) Oncogenic kinase signalling. *Nature*, 411, 355–65.

Buchdunger E, Cioffi CL, Law N et al. (2000). Abl protein-tyrosine kinase inhibitor STI571 inhibits in vitro signal transduction mediated by c-Kit and platelet-derived growth factor receptors. *J Pharmacol Exp Ther*, 295, 139–45.

Burger H, Den Bakker MA, Stoter G, Verweij J, Nooter K (2003) Lack of c-kit exon 11 activating mutations in c-KIT/CD117-positive SCLC tumour specimens. *Eur J Cancer*, 39, 793–9.

Burger H, van Tol H, Boersma AWM et al. (2004). Imatinib mesylate (STI571) is a substrate for the breast cancer resistance protein (BCRP)/ABCG2 drug pump. *Blood*, 104, 2940–42.

Cappuzzo F, Magrini E, Luca G et al. (2004). Akt phosphorylation and gefitinib efficacy in patients with advanced non-small-cell lung cancer. *J Natl Cancer Inst*, 96, 1133–41.

Cohen EEW, Rosen F, Stadler WM et al. (2003). Phase II trial of ZD1839 in recurrent or metastatic squamous cell carinoma of head and neck. *J Clin Oncol*, 21, 1980–7.

Cunningham D, Humblet Y, Sienna S et al. (2004). Cetuximab monotherapy and cetuximab plus irinotecan for irinotecan-refractory colorectal cancer. *New Engl J Med*, 351, 337–45.

Demetri GD, von Mehren M, Blanke CD et al. (2002). Efficacy and safety of imatinib mesylate in advanced gastrointestinal stromal tumors. *New Engl J Med*, 347, 472–80.

Demetri GD, Desai J, Fletcher JA et al. (2004). SU11248, a multi-targeted tyrosine kinase inhibitor, can overcome imatinib (IM) resistance caused by diverse genomic mechanisms in patients (pts) with metastatic gastrointestinal stromal tumor (GIST). *Proc ASCO*, 22, 3001.

Druker BJ, Talpaz M, Resta DJ et al. (2001a). Efficacy and safety of a specific inhibitor of the BCR–ABL tyrosine kinase in chronic myeloid leukemia. *New Engl J Med*, 344, 1031–7.

Druker BJ, Sawyers CL, Kantarjian H et al. (2001b). Activity of a specific inhibitor of the BCR–ABL tyrosine kinase in the blast crisis of chronic myeloid leukemia and acute lymphoblastic leukemia with the Philadelphia chromosome. *New Engl J Med*, 344, 1038–42.

Drucker B, Bacik J, Ginsberg M et al. (2003). Phase II trial of ZD1839 (Iressa[TM]) in patinets with advanced renal cell carcinoma. *Invest New Drugs*, 21, 341–5.

Fukuoka M, Yano S, Giaccone G et al. (2003). Multi-institutional randomized phase II trial of gefitinib for previously treated patients with advanced non-small-cell lung cancer. *J Clin Oncol*, 21, 2237–46.

Fletcher JA, Corless CL, Dimitrijevic et al. (2003). Mechanisms of resistance to imatinib mesylate (IM) in advanced gastrointestinal stromal tumor (GIST). *Proc ASCO*, 22, 815.

Gambacorti-Passerini C, Zucchetti M, D'Incalci M (2002). Binding of imatinib by alpha (1)-acid glycoprotein. *Blood*, 367–8.

Gambacorti-Passerini C, Zucchetti M, Russo D et al. (2003). Alpha1 acid glycoprotein binds to imatinib (STI571) and substantially alters its pharmacokinetics in chronic myeloid leukemia patients. *Clin Cancer Res*, 9, 625–32.

Gardembas M, Rousselot P, Tulliez M et al. (2003). Results of a prospective phase 2 study combining imatinib mesylate and cytarabine for the treatment of Philadelphia-positive patients with chronic myelogenous leukemia in chronic phase. *Blood*, 102, 4298–305.

Giaconne G, Herbst RS, Manegold C et al. (2004). Gefitinib in combination with gemcitabine and cisplatin in advanced non-small-cell lung cancer: a phase III trial—INTACT 1. *J Clin Oncol*, 22, 777–84.

Heinrich MC, Corless CL, Demetri GD *et al.* (2003). Kinase mutations and imatinib response in patients with metastatic gastrointestinal stromal tumor. *J Clin Oncol*, 21, 4342–9.

Herbst RS, Giaconne G, Schiller JH *et al.* (2004). Gefitinib in combination with paclitaxel and carboplatin in advanced non-small-cell lung cancer: a phase III trial—INTACT 2. *J Clin Oncol*, 22, 785–94.

Hirota S, Isozaki K, Moriyama Y *et al.* (1998). Gain-of-function mutations of c-kit in human gastrointestinal stromal tumors. *Science*, 279, 577–80.

Hurwitz H, Fehrenbacher L, Novotny W *et al.* (2004). Bevacizumab plus irinotecan, fluorouracil, and leucovorin for metastatic colorectal cancer. *New Engl J Med*, 350, 2335–42.

Irby RB, Yeatman TJ (2000). Role of Src expression and activation in human cancer. *Oncogene*, 19, 5636–42.

Joensuu H, Roberts PJ, Sarlomo-Rikala M *et al.* (2001). Effect of the tyrosine kinase inhibitor STI571 in a patient with a metastatic gastrointestinal stromal tumor. *New Engl J Med*, 344, 1052–7.

Johnson BE, Fischer T, Fischer B *et al.* (2003). Phase II study of imatinib in patients with small cell lung cancer. *Clin Cancer Res*, 9, 5880–7.

Judson IR, Ma P, Peng B *et al.* (2005). Imatinib pharmacokinetics in patients with gastrointestinal stromal tumour: a retrospective population pharmacokinetic study over time. *Cancer Chemother Pharmacol*, 55, 117–28.

Kris MG, Natale RB, Herbst RS *et al.* (2003). Efficacy of gefitinib, an inhibitor of the epidermal growth factor receptor tyrosine kinase, in symptomatic patients with non-small-cell lung cancer: a randomised trial. *JAMA*, 290, 2149–58.

Le Coutre P, Tassi E, Varella-Garcia M *et al.* (2000). Induction of resistance to the Abelson inhibitor STI571 in human leukemic cells through gene amplification. *Blood*, 95, 1758–66.

Lynch TJ, Bell DW, Sordella R *et al.* (2004). Activating mutations in the epidermal growth factor receptor underlying responsiveness of non-small-cell lung cancer to gefitinib. *New Engl J Med*, 350, 2129–39.

Madhusudan S, Ganesan TS (2004). Tyrosine kinase inhibitors in cancer therapy. *Clin Biochem*, 37, 618–35.

Mahon FX, Deininger MW, Schultheis B *et al.* (2000). Selection and characterisation of BCR–ABL positive cell lines with differential sensitivity to the tyrosine kinase inhibitor STI571: diverse mechanisms of resistance. *Blood*, 96, 1070–9.

Manning G, Whyte DB, Martinez R, Hunter T, Sudarsanam S (2002). The protein kinase complement of the human genome. *Science*, 298, 1912–34.

Nicholson RI, Gee JM, Harper ME (2001). EGFR and cancer prognosis. *Eur J Cancer*, 37 (Suppl 4), S9–S15.

O'Brien SG, Guilhot F, Larson RA *et al.* (2003). Imatinib compared with interferon and low-dose cytarabine in newly diagnosed chronic-phase chronic myeloid leukemia. *New Engl J Med*, 348, 994–1004.

Ranson M. (2004). Epidermal growth factor receptor tyrosine kinase inhibitors. *Br J Cancer*, 90, 2250–5.

Rich JN, Reardon DA, Peery T *et al.* (2004). Phase II trial of gefitinib in recurrent glioblastoma. *J Clin Oncol*, 22, 133–42.

Rubin BP, Schuetze SM, Eary JF *et al.* (2002). Molecular targeting of platelet-derived growth factor B by imatinib mesylate in a patients with metastatic dermatofibrosarcoma protuberans. *J Clin Oncol*, 20, 3586–91.

Savage DG, Antman KH (2002). Imatinib mesylate-A new oral targeted therapy. *New Engl J Med*, **346**, 683–93.

Sawyers CL, Hochhaus A, Feldman E *et al.* (2002). Imatinib induces hematologic and cytogenetic responses in patients with chronic myelogenous leukemia in myeloid blast crisis: results of a phase II study. *Blood*, **99**, 3530–9.

Shah NP, Sawyers CL (2003). Mechanisms of resistance to STI571 in Philadelphia chromosome-associated leukaemias. *Oncogene*, **22**, 7389–95.

Slamon DJ, Leyland-Jones B, Shak S *et al.* (2001). Use of chemotherapy plus a monoclonal antibody against HER2 in metastatic breast cancer that overexpress HER2. *New Engl J Med*, **344**, 783–92.

Talpaz M, Silver RT, Druker BJ *et al.* (2002). Imatinib induces durable hematologic and cytogenetic responses in patients with accelerated phase chronic myeloid leukemia: results of a phase 2 study. *Blood*, **99**, 1928–37.

Van Oosterom AT, Judson I, Verweij J *et al.* (2001). Safety and efficacy of imatinib (STI571) in metastatic gastrointestinal stromal tumours: a phase I study. *The Lancet*, **358**, 1421–3.

Verweij J, Casali PG, Zalcberg J *et al.* (2004). Progression-free survival in gastrointestinal stromal tumours with high-dose imatinib: randomised trial. *The Lancet*, **364**, 1127–34.

Verweij J, Van Oosterom A, Baly J-Y *et al.* (2003). Imatinib mesylate (STI-571, Glivec®, Gleevecs™) is an active agent for gastrointestinal stromal tumours, but does not yield responses in other soft-tissue sarcomas that are unselected for a molecular target: Results from an EORTC Soft Tissue and Bone Sarcoma Group phase II study. *Eur J Cancer*, **39**, 2006–11.

Von Bubnoff N, Schneller F, Peschel C, Duyster J (2002). BCR–ABL gene mutations in relation to clinical resistance of Philadelphia-chromosome-positive leukaemia to STI571: a prospective study. *The Lancet*, **359**, 487–91.

Woodburn JR (1999) The epidermal growth factor receptor and its inhibition of cancer therapy. *Pharmacol Ther*, **82**, 241–50.

Zalcberg JR, Verweij J, Casali P *et al.* (2004) Outcome of patients with advanced gastrointestinal stromal tumors (GIST) crossing over to a daily imatinib dose of 800 mg after progression on 400 mg: an international intergroup study of the EORTC, ISG, and AGITG. *Proc ASCO*, **23**, 2004.

Chapter 5

The RAS pathway—a target for anticancer therapy
Monica M. Mita and Eric K. Rowinsky

1 Introduction

Cellular signalling is critical for embryonic development, tissue **differentiation**, and cellular response to the environment. The complex signalling network is initiated in large part by extracellular **ligands**, including growth factors and other various stimuli, which interact with membrane receptors and then activate a cascade of intracellular molecules known as secondary messengers that ultimately are responsible for the cellular response. De-regulated cellular signalling is a common feature of cancer cells, which leads to uncontrolled proliferation and increased survival. Identification of the molecular abnormalities in cancer cells, particularly key proteins that play a role in abnormal cell proliferation, have led to the development of anticancer strategies that disrupt the synthesis or function of these proteins. As a large body of data about the cellular signalling network is accumulating, the complexities related to these strategies are being recognised and it is becoming increasingly clear that the redundancies in cellular signalling are very important in cancer cells, making approaches to therapy that involve any single pathway more challenging.

The *ras* **proto-oncogene** is an attractive target for anticancer therapy, as aberrant Ras function occurs in as many as 30% of human cancers (Barbacid 1987; Bos 1989). Ras plays a critical role as an intermediate protein in the signal **transduction** pathway that mediates signals from the cell membrane via receptor tyrosine kinases (RTK) to downstream cascades of **protein kinases** that control growth and proliferation (Bogusky and McCormick 1993). Several drugs that disrupt Ras function are currently being evaluated in clinical studies. Among these, farnesyltransferase inhibitors (FTIs) have been the most thoroughly studied class of anticancer drugs that were designed to target Ras.

However, the FTIs may operate by inhibiting the farnesylation of many critical proteins. This chapter will review the upstream and downstream elements of Ras, as well as the preliminary results and implications of therapeutic strategies targeting Ras.

2 The *ras* gene and Ras protein: structure and normal function

Ras mediates proliferative signals from upstream RTK, such as the erbB family of receptors and insulin growth factor receptor (IGFR), to downstream cascades of protein kinases. So far, Ras appears to be strategically positioned as an upstream mediator in these essential signal transduction pathways (Fig. 5.1) (Barbacid 1987; Bogusky and McCormick 1993) and therefore represents an important and strategic target for therapeutic development against cancer.

2.1 Structure

The *ras* proto-oncogenes identified to date include three closely related members of the same family, H-*ras*, K-*ras*, and N-*ras*, which was first isolated from a neuroblastoma cell line. The H-, N-, and K-*ras* genes are located on the short arms of **chromosomes** 1, 11, and 12, respectively (Bogusky and McCormick 1993; Leonard 1997; Lowy and Willumsen 1993). The *ras* superfamily of **oncogenes** encodes four small 21-kDa proteins, called p21^{ras} or Ras (H-ras, N-ras, and K-ras 4A and K-ras 4B). These guanosine triphosphatases (GTPases) are members of a yet larger family, which includes proteins involved in protein synthesis and signal transduction, and are typically located on the inner surface of the plasma membrane in mammalian cells. The four Ras proteins contain 188 to 189 amino acids and show high sequence similarity (Leonard 1997; Lowy and Willumsen 1993). Their structure is highly conserved across mammalian species, indicating that Ras proteins serve specific, essential cellular functions. All Ras proteins have a specific amino acid sequence motif at their carboxy-terminal domain, known as the CAAX box, comprising a cysteine residue (C), two aliphatic amino acids (AA), usually valine, leucine or isoleucine, and a methionine or serine (X) (Gibbs *et al.* 1994). This motif plays an important role in determining the subcellular localisation of Ras. Ras proteins are synthesised as biologically inactive precursors, located in the **cytosol** and must undergo a series of modifications to be converted into the lipophilic molecules capable of attaching to the cell membrane and being activated. The post-translational modifications involve four steps: farnesylation, **proteolysis**, carboxymethylation, and palmitoylation (Fig. 5.2). Farnesylation is the first and most critical step, and involves

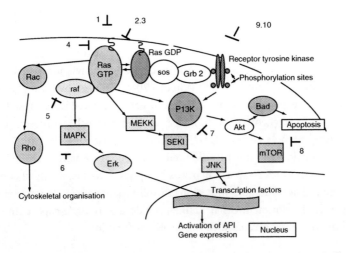

Fig. 5.1 RAS signalling pathway and possible therapeutic targets. 1, Ras association with cell membrane; 2, restoring GTPase; 3, gene therapy; 4, farnesyltransferase inhibitors (FTIs); 5, Raf inhibitors; 6, MAPK inhibitors; 7, PI3K inhibitors; 8, mTOR inhibitors; 9, anti-receptor antibodies; 10, receptor tyrosine kinase inhibitor. Abbreviations: PI3K, phosphoinositide 3 kinase; Akt, protein kinase B (PKB); MAPK, mitogen activated protein kinase; MEKK, mitogen activated protein kinase kinase; JNK, Jun amino-terminal kinase; mTOR, mammalian target of Rapamycin; GDP, guanosine diphosphate; GTP, guanosine triphosphate; SOS, son of sevenless; BAD, pro-apoptotic protein of the bcl-2 family.

addition of a hydrophobic farnesyl isoprenoid (15-carbon) group to the cysteine residue in the CAAX box (Prior and Hancock 2001). This rate-limiting process is catalysed by the enzyme farnesyltransferase (FTase). Other proteins involved in signal transduction, control of cell proliferation, and

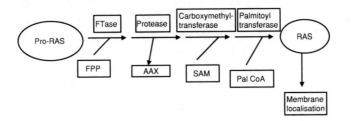

Fig. 5.2 The steps for Ras post-translational modification. Ras post-translational modifications include the addition of a farnesyl transferase, then the removal of AAX group by CAAX protease, and finally the methylation of the C-terminal by methyl-transferase. Palmytoylation is a fourth step that occurs in some Ras proteins before membrane localisation. Abbreviations: FPP, farnesyl pyrophospahate; SAM, S-adenosyl methionine.

nuclear structural integrity such as Rho, Rac, nuclear laminins, Akt2, CENP-E, and -F, and retinal proteins, are also farnesylated (Sinensky *et al.* 1994), implying that inhibition of FTase will interfere with multiple molecules important to the cell's economy. Another type of prenylation reaction, ger-anylgeranylation, involves the addition of a 20-carbon geranylgeranyl group to the forming Ras protein and is catalysed by geranylgeranyl transferase I and II (GGT I and II) (Leonard 1997). Ras and several other proteins can be alternatively prenylated by GGT-I, creating a functional K-Ras protein that is able to contribute to uncontrolled cell proliferation (Zhang *et al.* 1997). The efficiency of this process, particularly as it applies to K-Ras, the most common Ras protein that undergoes mutations in solid malignancies, is important for therapeutic development, as it could provide a sort of 'escape pathway' if inhibitors of FTase were used to inhibit K-ras function.

2.2 Activation and downstream effectors

Ras proteins are not functionally redundant despite strong similarities, as suggested by the fact that deletion of the K-*ras* gene, but not H-*ras* or N-*ras* genes, is embryonically lethal, reflecting differences in tissue expression or signalling potential (Reuther and Der 2000). Each Ras protein functions as a biochemical switch cycling between inactive guanosine diphosphate (GDP) bound and active guanosine triphosphate (GTP) bound states. The activation of membrane-anchored Ras occurs either by cell stimulation by extracellular growth factors such as erbB or IGF, or by intracellular signalling proteins such as oestrogen receptor-a, both of which lead to transient conversion of Ras proteins to the GTP-bound active form (Ras-GTP) (Migliaccio *et al.* 1996). The sequence of activation includes phosphorylation of the growth factor bound RTK, followed by the binding of adaptor proteins such as the growth factor receptor binding protein (Grb-2) to the phosphorylated receptor. The multiprotein complex formed allows the binding of yet another protein, the beautifully-named guanine dissociation stimulator son of sevenless (SOS) with Ras, which results in the key switch of Ras from its GDP-bound to its GTP-bound state. In its GTP-bound state, Ras then activates several down-stream effectors including Raf-1 and **mitogen**-activated proteins (MAP) kinase kinase (MEK), p21$^{wafl/cip1}$, Rac and Rho—small GTP-binding proteins (called G proteins), phosphatidylinositol 3 kinase (PI3K)/Akt, and also nu-clear transcription factors such as Fos (Marshall 1996; Vojtek and Der 1998). The pathway involving the serine-threonine kinase Raf-1 has been thoroughly elucidated. Activated Raf phosphorylates MEK1 and MEK2, which in turn phosphorylate the MAP kinases extracellular signal-regulated kinase 1 (ERK1) and 2 (ERK2). Translocation of ERK1 and ERK2 to the **nucleus** allows the phosphorylation of several nuclear **transcription** factors, leading to the activation of other kinases and transcription factors such as c-fos, and other target genes associated with proliferation. There is therefore a cascade of events, subsequent to switching the Ras pathway on, which amplifies the original signal and increases the cell's commitment to proliferate. The signalling pathway mediated by Rho and Rac ultimately regulates the organisation of the actin cytoskeleton, gene expression, cell cycle progression, and cell proliferation (Qiu *et al.* 1995). Another downstream effector of Ras, the PI3K/Akt pathway, plays an important role in cell cycle progression, increase in cell motility, invasiveness, and prevention of **apoptosis**, all key events that contribute further to oncogenic Ras' capacity to transform cells (Rodriguez Viciana *et al.* 1997).

2.3 Farnesyltransferases and other enzymes involved in prenylation

Prenylation is the most important step of the post-translational modification of Ras protein. Farnesylation alone is sufficient to anchor Ras sufficiently firmly to the membrane and to confer transforming potential. FTases catalyse the transfer of a 15-carbon farnesyl isoprenoid from farnesyl diphosphate (FDP) to Ras after recognising the CAAX motif at the C-terminus of Ras (Omer *et al.* 1997). As previously discussed, two other structurally related protein prenyltransferases, geranylgeranyltransferase I and II (GGTase), have similar roles of catalysing the attachment of one or two 20-carbon geranylgeranyl groups to the C-terminal end of several critical proteins including K-Ras (Andres *et al.* 1993). The results of several studies indicated that prenylation of Ras by GGTase-I can result in a functional Ras protein and that no specific isoprenoid group is essential for Ras function. The potential of cross-prenylation of Ras by GGTases implies that the function of Ras and other similar proteins following FTase inhibition could be alternatively 'rescued' by GGTases, and could therefore explain the lack of relevant clinical activity in malignancies with K-*ras* mutations following treatment with inhibitors of FTase (Armstrong *et al.* 1995; Gibbs and Oliff 1997; James *et al.* 1995).

Several other mammalian proteins besides Ras have a CAAX motif and are substrates for FTase or GGTase, or both. It is still not completely known why some proteins have a preference for being farnesylated or geranylgeranylated. Protein farnesylation is considered essential for many physiological processes, including muscle function and vision (Qiu *et al.* 1995). Thus, disrupting prenylation may have an inhibitory role in many other processes causing a range of unwanted side-effects and should be taken into consideration in developing therapeutics targeting FTase and/or GGTase.

3 Ras dysregulation in human malignancies

Ras proteins—also called G-proteins—are activated following binding to GTP, which results in interactions with downstream effectors and the activation of signalling cascades. The hydrolysis of GTP to GDP, which is mediated by the intrinsic GTPase activity of the Ras protein, inactivates Ras-dependent signalling. In normal cells, wild-type Ras rapidly reverts to its inactive, GDP-bound form. Although wild-type Ras has low intrinsic GTPase activity, the hydrolysis of bound GTP to GDP and conversion to the inactive form of Ras is enhanced by the GTPase activator protein (Gap). Maintaining Ras in an activated GTP-bound state requires the continuous stimulation by extracellular growth factors (say during a period of intense cellular growth), intracellular signalling proteins, or the sort of mutations seen in cancer cells that lead to constitutive activation of Ras (i.e. mutant Ras genes in tumours are 'permanently switched on') (Barbacid 1987; Lowy and Willumsen 1993). The common effect of these processes is to activate downstream pathways, leading to markedly enhanced proliferation and survival (Rowinsky et al. 1999). Biochemical studies have suggested that the principal functional effect conferred by mutant Ras is a marked decrease in its ability to interact with Gap proteins. Consequently, Ras remains in an active GTP-bound state and continues to activate downstream effectors in the absence of growth factor stimulation (Rowinsky et al. 1999).

Although *ras* mutations with activating potential are mainly associated with myeloid malignancies and carcinomas of the colon, pancreas, lung, and thyroid, the mutations have also been described in many other tumour types and occur in approximately 30% of human malignancies (Barbacid 1987). Of the three *ras* genes, K-*ras* mutations are the most common in human tumours and H-*ras* the least common and the type of mutation seems to relate to the specific type of malignancy (Table 5.1) (Alemany 1996; Coffety et al. 1998). Although there are subtle differences in the signalling pathway that they activate, and in their subcellular distribution, the three Ras proteins all promote proliferation and cell-cycle progression. Several lines of evidence indicate that *ras* mutations are early events in carcinogenesis compared with other oncogenic processes (Reddy et al. 1982). This is supported by the fact that non-malignant human colon polyps bear *ras* mutations and their oncogenic transformation depends on other events such as p53 mutations (Vogelstein et al. 1988). Ras mutations may remain silent for long periods of time until other proliferative events or genetic aberrations occur and trigger neoplastic transformation, since *ras* genes transform cells only when they are in the proliferative state (Kloog et al. 1999). Overexpression of normal Ras is a much less common cause of malignant transformation than

Table 5.1 Ras mutations in human cancers

Cancer type	Type of mutated Ras	Frequency of mutation (%)
Pancreatic carcinoma	K-ras	90
Colorectal carcinoma	K-ras	40–50
Thyroid carcinoma		50–80
Follicular	H, K, N-ras	50
Non-differentiated	H, K, N-ras	60
Non-small cell lung cancer	K-ras	30–50
Head and neck carcinoma	H, K, N-ras	25
Bile duct carcinomas	N-ras	>50
Seminoma	K, N-ras	40
Hepatocellular carcinoma	N-ras	30
Acute myelogenous leukemia	N-ras	30
Myelodysplastic syndrome	N, K-ras	30
Renal clear cell carcinoma	H-ras	10
Endometrial carcinoma	K-ras	20–40
Ovary carcinoma	K-ras	25
Glioma	WT, overexpression	< 5
Breast carcinoma	H, K -ras	< 5

Compiled from: Khosravi-Far and Der 1994; Clark and Der 1995; Rowinsky *et al.* 1999; Ghobrial and Adjei 2002

mutations. In addition, tumours with no *ras* mutations may depend indirectly on activation of normal Ras pathway for signal transduction, due to the overexpression of RTKs or increased secretion of growth factors. For example, epithelial growth factor (EGF) receptors are commonly overexpressed in glioblastomas, breast carcinoma, non-small lung carcinoma (NSCLC), and melanomas, and may also induce Ras activation (End 1999). In breast cancers, a strong positive relationship between ErbB2 and Ras expression have been documented, with overexpression of both proteins resulting in an aggressive, poor-prognosis **phenotype** (Slamon *et al.* 1989).

Although many components of the Ras signalling networks have been identified and their function understood, the precise roles of these elements in carcinogenesis and their relevance as targets for anticancer therapeutics require further clarification.

4 Targeting the Ras pathway: therapeutic implications

Hypothetically, the Ras signalling pathway can be disrupted at several different levels (Crul *et al.* 1993; Ghobrial and Adjei 2002) including the inhibition of Ras protein expression by gene therapy, **antisense oligonucleotides** (ASONs) or intracellular antibodies, inhibition of Ras association with the cell membrane, inhibition of Ras trafficking and stimulation of Ras inactivation, and inhibition of downstream effectors of Ras. Among these strategies aiming to inhibit Ras, antisense compounds and FTIs are discussed below.

4.1 Antisense compounds

Although inhibition of FTase has been the principal focus of pre-clinical research and numerous clinical studies aiming to block the activation of Ras, ASONs designed to inhibit Ras function have also been evaluated. ASONs hybridise to complementary sequences on the target messenger **RNA** (mRNA), which is followed by RNase H-mediated degradation of the mRNA. A principal advantage of this approach is the specificity of the ASON in blocking the expression of the cancer-specific mutated forms of Ras. Most research efforts have focused on short ASONs to target H-*ras* and K-*ras* RNA. The therapeutic use of these compounds was initially limited, since earlier ASONs were rapidly degraded by intracellular nucleases. More recently, chemical modifications of the oligonucleotide backbone have been performed to overcome this problem. Another concern about the use of ASONs is their unique toxicity profile, which includes hypersensitivity reactions and constitutional toxicities. ISIS 2503 (Isis Pharmaceuticals, Carlsbad, CA), which is currently under clinical development, is a 20-**nucleotide** phosphorothioate oligonucleotide that binds to H-Ras and leads to its degradation by RNase H. In pre-clinical studies, ISIS 2503 discriminated between the mRNA of H-Ras and that of K-Ras and N-Ras. The compound showed a good overall tolerability profile in phase I trials on a 14-day intravenous continuous infusion (CIVI) schedule, which has been recommended for disease-oriented clinical studies. Toxicities have included fever, fatigue, and nausea. However, no objective responses have been observed despite evidence of biologic activity as manifested by reduced H-*ras* mRNA expression in the peripheral blood mononuclear cells (PBMC) even at the lowest dose level (Dorr *et al.* 1999). The 24-h weekly infusion schedule for ISIS 2503 was also determined to be well-tolerated; however, hypersensitivity manifestations, including fever, chills, and urticaria, were relatively common. No objective responses were noted (Gordon *et al.* 1999). Several phase II studies using the 14-day CIVI schedule were completed in patients with metastatic colorectal carcinoma (CRC), advanced NSCLC, and untreated advanced pancreatic carcinoma. The schedule was tolerated at 6 mg/kg/day, but there were no objective responses (Dang *et al.* 2001; Perez *et al.* 2001; Saleh *et al.* 2000). Additionally, studies of ISIS 2503 in combination with gemcitabine, docetaxel, or paclitaxel have been performed in patients with metastatic carcinomas of the pancreas, lung (non-small cell), and breast, respectively (Burch *et al.* 2003; Goldsmith *et al.* 2003; Saleh *et al.* 2003). Encouraging preliminary activity was reported for breast carcinoma patients with the combination ISIS 2503 and weekly paclitaxel, with eight (47%) of the 17 evaluable patients achieving partial responses (PR) (Saleh *et al.* 2003). Similarly, anti-tumour activity was seen in patients with pancreatic carcinoma, with seven (14.6%) out of 48 evaluable patients achieving major responses, and 28 patients (57.5%) surviving more than 6 months (Goldsmith *et al.* 2003). Nevertheless, the contribution of the ASON to the activity observed in these studies cannot be determined.

4.2 Farnesyltransferase inhibitors

FTIs have been developed under the premise that farnesylation is an essential step in the maturation of functional Ras, and that inhibition of farnesylation would abolish the proliferative activity of Ras. Investigators began to evaluate FTIs as a potential strategy for targeting Ras more than a decade ago. One developmental strategy has been the rational design of FTIs, based on the crystalline structure of their target, FTase. To date, three types of small-molecule inhibitors of FTase have been designed including: farnesyl diphosphonate analogues that compete with the FDP (e.g. hydroxyfarnesyl phosphonic acid), peptidomimetics (or CAAX mimetics) that compete with the CAAX portion of Ras for FTase, and bisubstrate analogues that possess features of both FDP analogues and peptidomimetics. The second strategy has been directed towards the identification of non-peptidomimetic, small molecules inhibitors. Several non-peptidometic FTIs are currently being evaluated in clinical trials including R115,777 (tipifarnib, Zarnestra™, Johnson & Johnson, New Brunswick, NJ), SCH66336 (lonafarnib, Sarasar™, Schering-Plough, Kenilworth, NJ), and BMS 214662 (Bristol-Myers Squibb, New York, NY), all of which will be reviewed in this chapter. Another compound, L-778,123 (Merck & Co, Whitehouse Station, NJ) was developed as a dual FTase and GGTase inhibitor but its clinical development was discontinued because it failed to demonstrate inhibition of both enzymes in the clinic and because of cardiac conduction abnormalities, principally prolongation of QTc interval. Other FTIs or dual FTase and GGTase inhibitors are in late pre-clinical development (Ashar *et al.* 2000; deSolms *et al.* 2003).

4.2.1. Pre-clinical studies (*in vitro* and *in vivo*)

Most developmental efforts have been focused on agents with preferential activity against FTase than either GGTase-I or II. As a large number of physiological proteins are known to be substrates for GGTase-I, this strategy was undertaken to avoid undesirable toxicity due to GGTase inhibition. The FTIs do not only inhibit the farnesylation of Ras, but also block the farnesylation of many other protein substrates of FTase. Several studies have suggested that inhibiting the farnesylation of other critical proteins, such as RhoB, the centromeric proteins CENP-E and CENP-F, and/or signalling elements of the PI3K/Akt pathway, may contribute to the anti-tumour activity of the FTIs (Sebti and Hamilton 2000). Although most FTIs developed to date inhibit FTase activity *in vitro* with IC_{50} values in the subnanomolar to low micromolar range (Cox and Der 1997), much higher concentrations (usually at high micromolar concentrations) are required to block the farnesylation of most of these substrates (Garcia *et al.* 1993).

The FTIs have principally demonstrated anti-tumour activity, including complete tumour regressions in human tumour **xenografts**, against malignancies with H-*ras* mutations (Kohl *et al.* 1995). Activity has been less impressive in tumours that are dependent on mutant K-*ras* (Sepp-Lorenzino *et al.* 1995). One possible explanation for these findings is that K-ras is alternatively prenylated by GGTase-I when farnesylation is blocked, which implies that combinations of GGTase and FTase inhibitors may be more effective against tumours harbouring mutant K-*ras*. However, such combinations may also produce much more toxicity than the FTIs as single agents (Whyte *et al.* 1997). FTIs block the farnesylation of Ras in a dose-dependent manner in cancer cells growing in tissue culture, although most initial studies were performed in tumour cells with mutated H-*ras* (Garcia *et al.* 1993). It has also been established that FTIs can inhibit the growth of human cancers with either activated or mutated forms of Ras (End *et al.* 2001), including tumour with K-*ras* mutations (Kelland *et al.* 2001). One explanation for these findings may be that, in addition to Ras, the FTIs are inhibiting the farnesylation of other proteins that are essential for growth (James *et al.* 1993).

Other studies demonstrated that the FTIs inhibit survival, **angiogenesis**, and cell-cycle traverse. For example, the FTIs have been shown to augment the expression of the apoptosis-promoting proteins Bax and Bcl-Xs, thereby resulting in apoptosis by suppressing the Akt pathway (Chun *et al.* 2003). The potential importance of angiogenesis inhibition for the anti-tumour effects of FTIs has also been demonstrated *in vivo* (Smets *et al.* 1998).

Pre-clinical studies have demonstrated synergistic anti-tumour activity between the FTI and inhibitors of tubulin depolymerisation such as the taxanes and epothilones (Moasser *et al.* 1998). The findings that lonafarnib prevents farnesylation of centromere-binding proteins raises the possibility that FTIs may inhibit microtubule formation, which may lead to enhanced sensitivity to the microtubule stabilising action of the taxanes. Furthermore, at least additive interactions have been noted between FTIs and other **cytotoxic** agents such as cisplatin, cyclophosphamide, doxorubicin and 5-fluorouracil (Adjei *et al.* 2001; Bishop *et al.* 2003). Combination pre-clinical studies revealed that lonafarnib displays synergy with paclitaxel and gemcitabine in NSCLC (Adeji *et al.* 2001b; Loprevite *et al.* 2004). Additionally lonafarnib was found to have multi-drug protein 1 and 2 inhibitory effects (Wang and Johnson 2003). Therefore, these data concur to support the use of FTIs in combination with chemotherapy in future clinical trails.

Interestingly, the FTIs appear to be devoid of growth inhibitory activity against non-malignant cells *in vitro* and they demonstrated a high degree of safety in animal toxicology studies (Manne *et al.* 1995). Histological examination of tissues from animals treated with FTIs for protracted periods did not reveal any significant abnormalities either in rapidly dividing tissues or in tissues in which farnesylated proteins appear to play critical physiologic roles such as the retina and skeletal muscles (Kohl *et al.* 1994). The major clinical implication of this finding is the potential for high therapeutic indices of the FTIs in patients with malignant diseases, allowing treatment at potentially biologically active dosages, as well as the combination of high doses of FTIs with cytotoxic and/or other anticancer agents.

4.2.2 Clinical studies: phase I

The development of a new targeted therapy, such as the FTIs, represents a challenge, especially in the phase I stage when an optimal dosage for disease-directed studies must be determined. Toxic effects may not be evident at doses that inhibit Ras farnesylation or may not be quantifiable or even related to FTase inhibition. Thus, **pharmacokinetic** (PK) and **pharmacodynamic** (PD) studies have been used to identify relationships between plasma concentrations associated with maximal inhibition of Ras farnesylation and anti-tumour activity (Adeji *et al.* 2000a). Furthermore, determining the optimal schedule of administration of FTIs is also challenging. Although some experimental evidence suggests that continuous drug exposure may be optimal for maximal efficacy, the use of protracted dosing schedules raises concerns about drug resistance and toxicity. Rigorous monitoring of pertinent physiological processes that require farnesylation, such as vision and muscular function, is therefore required in initial clinical studies. Phase I studies of FTIs administered alone and in combination are presented in Tables 5.2 and 5.3, respectively.

Table 5.2 Phase I studies with farnesyltransferase inhibitors administered as single agent

FTI	Tumor type	Recommended dose and schedule	Dose-limiting toxicity	Anti-tumor activity	Reference
Tipifarnib	Solid tumors	500 mg twice daily for 5 days every 14 days	Neuropathy, fatigue	1/27 SD (CRC)	Zujewski et al. 2000
	Solid tumors	300 mg twice daily, uninterrupted	Neutropenia, thrombocytopenia, neurosensory, neuromotor	1/18 PR (NSCLC) 4/18 SD (CRC, pancreas)	Crul et al. 2002
	Solid tumors	300 mg twice daily, days 1–7 and 15–21 every 28 days (dose escalation ongoing)	Neutropenia	6/17 SD	Lara et al. 2003
	Poor-risk leukaemias	900 mg twice daily for 21 days every 28 days	Central neurotoxicity (ataxia, confusion)	2/34 CR, 8 /34 PR	Karp et al. 2001
	Acute leukaemia (paediatric)	200 mg twice daily for 21 days every 28 days	Hyperbilirubinaemia, rash, AST elevation, neutropenia	2/20 SD	Wideman et al. 2003

(continued)

Table 5.2 (continued) Phase I studies with farnesyltransferase inhibitors administered as single agent

FTI	Tumor type	Recommended dose and schedule	Dose-limiting toxicity	Anti-tumor activity	Reference
Lonafarnib	Solid tumors	400 mg twice daily for 7 days every 21 days	Nausea, vomiting, diarrhea, fatigue	1/ 20 PR (NSCLC); 8/20 SD	Adjei *et al.* 2000
	Solid tumors	200 mg twice daily, uninterrupted	Neutropenia, neurocortical toxicity, fatigue	2/24 SD (peritoneal, thyroid)	Eskens *et al.* 2001
	Solid tumors	300 mg once daily, uninterrupted	Nausea, vomiting, diarrhoea, fatigue, renal failure	-	Awada *et al.* 2002
BMS214662	Solid tumors	One-hour IV infusion every 21 days (MTD not reached)	Nausea, vomiting, diarrhoea, AST elevation	1/38 MR (NSCLC); SD (breast, CRC)	Ryan *et al.* 2004
	Solid tumors	50 mg twice daily for 14 days every 21 days	Nausea, diarrhoea, vomiting	1/23 SD	Camacho *et al.* 2001
	Solid tumors	278 mg/m² weekly IV	Vomiting, hypotension	1/30 MR (breast)	Voi *et al.* 2001
	Solid tumors	300 mg/m² as 24 h CIVI weekly for 3 weeks every 28 days	Transaminase elevation, neuropathy	-	Zhu *et al.* 2002

Abbreviations: FTI, farnesyltransferase inhibitor; DLT, dose limiting toxicity; MTD, maximum tolerated dose; SD, stable disease; MR, minor response; PR, partial response; NSCLC, non-small cell lung cancer; SCLC, small cell lung cancer; MBC, metastatic breast cancer; CRC, colorectal carcinoma; IV, intravenous; h, hour; CIVI, continuous intravenous infusion

Table 5.3 Phase I combination studies with farnesyltransferase inhibitors

FTI	Combination drug	Recommended dose and schedule	Dose-limiting toxicity	Anti-tumor activity	Reference
Tipifarnib	Docetaxel	Tipifarnib 200–300 mg twice daily for 7–14 days every 21 days (MTD not reached) Docetaxel 75 mg/m² every 21 days	Neutropenia, fatigue	1/32 CR (MBC); 7/32 PR; 6/32 SD	Piccart et al. 2001
	Paclitaxel	Tipifarnib 200 mg twice daily for 21 days every 28 days Paclitaxel 60 mg/m² weekly for 3 weeks every 28 days	Neutropenia	4/35 PR (MBC, SCC); 3/35 MR	Patnaik et al. 2004
	Capecitabine	Tipifarnib 300 mg twice daily for 14 days every 21 days Capecitabine 2250 mg/m²/day for 14 days every 21 days	Diarrhea, hand/foot syndrome, neutropenia	3/27 PR (CRC, MBC, H&N); 9/27 SD	Adjei et al. 2001
	5FU/LV	Tipifarnib 200–500 mg twice daily for 21 days every 28 days 5FU/LV (de Gramont schedule)	Neutropenia, fatigue	–	Haluska et al. 2002
	Gemcitabine and Cisplatin	Tipifarnib 300 mg twice daily for 14 days every 21 days Gemcitabine 1,000 mg/m² weekly for 2 weeks every 21 days Cisplatin 75 mg/m² every 21 days	Neutropenia, thrombocytopenia, gastrointestinal toxicity	1/15 CR (NSCLC); 4/15 PR (NSCLC);	Adjei et al. 2003
	Irinotecan	Tipifarnib 300 mg twice daily for 14 days every 21 days Irinotecan 350 mg/m² every 21 days	Neutropenia, thrombocytopenia, nausea, vomiting	3/35 PR 14/35 SD	Spareeboom et al. 2004

(continued)

Table 5.3 (*continued*) Phase I combination studies with farnesyltransferase inhibitors

FTI	Combination drug	Recommended dose and schedule	Dose-limiting toxicity	Anti-tumor activity	Reference
	Topotecan	Tipifarnib 200 mg twice daily for 21 days every 28 days Topotecan 1 mg/m^2/day for 5 days every 28 days	Neutropenia, thrombocytopenia	-	Liebes *et al.* 2001
	Trastuzumab	Tipifarnib 400 mg twice daily for 21 days every 28 days Trastuzumab 2 mg/kg weekly (4 mg/kg first week)	Febrile neutropenia, thrombocytopenia	1PR; 4 SD	De Bono *et al.* 2002
	Tamoxifen	Tipifarnib 200 mg twice daily, uninterrupted Tamoxifen 20 mg daily	Gastrointestinal symptoms	3/11 PR; 1/11 SD	Lebowitz *et al.* 2004
Lonafarnib	Gemcitabine	Lonafarnib 100–150 mg twice daily, uninterrupted Gemcitabine 1,000 mg/m^2 weekly for 3 weeks every 28 days	Nausea, vomiting, diarrhoea, myelosuppression	2/25 PR (pancreas); 2/25 MR (pancreas, mesothelioma); 11/25 SD	Hurwitz *et al.* 2000
	Paclitaxel	Lonafarnib 100 mg twice daily, uninterrupted Paclitaxel 175 mg/m^2 every 21 days	Febrile neutropenia, dehydration, hyperbilirubinaemia	8/21 PR (NSCLC, salivary gland); 7/21 SD	Khuri *et al.* 2001
	Gemcitabine and Cisplatin	Lonafarnib 75 mg twice daily, uninterrupted Gemcitabine 1000 mg/m^2 weekly for 3 weeks every 28 days Cisplatin 100 mg/m^2 every 28 days	Myelosuppression, gastrointestinal symptoms	-	Pierson *et al.* 2002

(*continued*)

Table 5.3 (continued) Phase I combination studies with farnesyltransferase inhibitors

FTI	Combination drug	Recommended dose and schedule	Dose-limiting toxicity	Anti-tumor activity	Reference
	Paclitaxel and Carboplatin	Lonafarnib 75–100 mg twice daily for 21 days Paclitaxel 125 mg/m^2 every 21 days Carboplatin AUC 5 every 21 days	Neutropenia, diarrhoea	-	Sprague et al. 2002
BMS 214662	Cisplatin	BMS 214662 200 mg/m^2 IV every 21 days Cisplatin 75 mg/m^2 every 21 days	Transaminase elevation	15/29 SD	Mackay et al. 2004
	Paclitaxel	BMS 214662 120 mg/m^2 IV weekly Paclitaxel 80 mg/m^2 weekly	Febrile neutropenia	2/6 PR (laryngeal, prostate);	Bailley et al. 2002
	Paclitaxel and Carboplatin	BMS 214662 160 mg/m^2 IV every 21 days Paclitaxel 225 mg/m^2 every 21 days Carboplatin AUC 6 every 21 days	Neutropenia, nausea, vomiting	2/32 PR (ovarian, esophageal); 10/32 SD	Dy et al. 2004

Abbreviations: FTIs, farnesyltransferase inhibitors; MTD, maximum tolerated dose; SD, stable disease; MR, minor response; PR, partial response; NSCLC, non-small cell lung cancer; SCLC, small cell lung cancer; MBC, metastatic breast cancer; CRC, colorectal carcinoma; H&N, head and neck carcinoma; SCC, squamous cell carcinoma; AUC, area under the curve; IV, intravenously; G-CSF, granulocyte colony stimulator factor

Table 5.4 Phase II studies with farnesyltransferase inhibitors

(a) Lung cancer

FTI	Dose	Number of Patients	Antitumor Activity	References
Tipifarnib	300 mg twice daily for 21 days every 28 days	44 NSCLC	7 SD	Adjei et al. 2003
Tipifarnib	400 mg twice daily for 14 days every 21 days	22 SCLC	No objective responses	Heymach et al. 2004
Lonafarnib with Paclitaxel	400 mg twice daily for 7 days every 21 days	33 NSCLC (taxane refractory)	5 PR; 4 MR; 10 SD	Kim et al. 2002
L,778, 123	560 mg/m^2/day CIVI for 14 days every 21 days	23 NSCLC (1st line)	No objective responses	Evans et al. 2002

(b) Breast cancer

FTI	Dose	Number of Patients	Antitumor Activity	References
Tipifarnib	400–300 mg twice daily, uninterrupted (CD) 300 mg twice daily for 21 days every 28 days (ID)	41 patients MBC 35 patients MBC	4 PR; 6 SD 5 PR; 3 SD	Kelland et al. 2001
Tipifarnib with Doxorubicin and Cyclophosphamide (AC regimen)	Tipifarnib 200 mg twice daily on days 1–7 every 14 days AC every 14 days with G-CSF support	patients with MBC	8 objective responses	Sparano et al. 2004

Abbreviations: FTI, farnesyltransferase inhibitor; DLT, dose limiting toxicity; MTD, maximum tolerated dose; SD, stable disease; MR, minor response; PR, partial response; NSCLC, non-small cell lung cancer; SCLC, small cell lung cancer; MBC, metastatic breast cancer; CD, continuous dosing; ID, intermittent dosing; CIVI, continuous intravenous infusion.

The principal FTI that is undergoing clinical development is the orally available quinolone analogue tipifarnib (Zarnestra™, Johnson & Johnson, New Brunswick, NJ) (Fig. 5.3), which was initially developed as an antifungal agent. Two phase I studies established that the recommended doses of tipifarnib for phase II trials in patients with solid malignancies are 500 mg orally twice daily for five consecutive days every other week, and 300 mg orally twice daily on an uninterrupted continuous dosing schedule (Crul *et al.* 2002; Skrzat *et al.* 1998; Zujewski *et al.* 2000). Dose-limiting toxicities for the five-day schedule were neuropathy and fatigue. The most frequent side-effects included nausea, vomiting, headache, fatigue, hypotension, and myelosuppression. For the continuous dosing schedule, the dose-limiting toxicities were myelosuppression and neurotoxicity. The pharmacokinetic behaviour was characterised by dose-proportionality, limited drug accumulation, and the achievement of steady state within 2 to 3 days. One patient with metastatic colon cancer who was treated with tipifarnib 500 mg orally twice daily on the 5-day schedule had a reduction in carcinoembrionic antigen and stable disease (SD) lasting 5 months. In the phase I study of tipifarnib administered continuously, one patient with platinum-refractory NSCLC had a partial response (PR) lasting 5 months and four patients with carcinomas of the pancreas, colon, and cervix, had stable disease (SD) lasting at least 3 months. In another phase I study of tipifarnib administered twice daily weeks 1 and 3 every 4 weeks, the principal toxicities included myelosuppression and fatigue, and two patients experienced minor response and SD, respectively (Lara *et al.* 2003).

A phase I trial in patients with poor-risk acute leukaemias evaluated tipifarnib administered twice daily for up to 21 days. Dose-limiting central neurotoxicity, consisting of ataxia, confusion, and dysarthria, occurred at

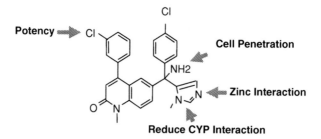

Fig. 5.3 Tipifarnib. Nonpeptide CAAX peptidomimetic, oral quinolone analogue of imidazoles (antifungals). Inhibits farnesylation of Ras, lamin B and other proteins. Primarily growth inhibitory: low-sub nM range. Least effective against K-*ras*–mutated tumours.

the 1200 mg twice-daily dose level. Nausea, myelosuppression, and renal dysfunction were also observed. Pharmacokinetic studies revealed dose-proportionality and weekly bone marrow aspirates demonstrated that the drug accumulated in the bone marrow in a dose-dependent fashion. Clinical responses occurred in 10 (29%) of 34 evaluable patients, including two complete responses (CRs). Eight of the ten responders were patients with acute myelogenous leukaemia (AML), and none harboured *ras* mutations (Karp *et al.* 2001).

A phase I of tipifarnib administered orally twice daily on a 3-week-on/1-week-off schedule for 8 weeks has been also completed in patients with myelodysplastic syndrome (MDS) (Kurzrock *et al.* 2003). Twenty-one patients, including four patients with *ras* mutations, were treated. Objective responses were observed in 6 (30%) of 20 evaluable patients. The **maximum tolerated dose** (**MTD**) was established at 400 mg twice daily. Consistent dose-limiting fatigue and confusion occurred at the 450 mg twice-daily dose level. Pharmacodynamic studies indicated that the tipifarnib inhibited the prenylation of chaperone protein HDJ-2 and suppressed FTase activation at clinically-relevant dosages. The authors concluded that tipifarnib markedly inhibits FTases and has anti-tumour activity in MDS at tolerable doses.

Tipifarnib was also evaluated in a paediatric phase I trial involving 20 children with refractory leukaemia (Widemann *et al.* 2003). Dose-limiting toxicities included hyperbilirubinaemia, transaminitis, rash, and neutropenia. The best responses consisted of two patients with SD out of 12 evaluable patients in spite of consistent drug-induced decrements in FTase activity in leukemic blasts.

The feasibility of administering tipifarnib in combination with a number of cytotoxic agents, including topotecan, capecitabine, and 5-FU/leucovorin, has also been evaluated (Adjei *et al.* 2001a; Haluska *et al.* 2002; Holden *et al.* 2001; Patnaik *et al.* 2003). Combination regimens, consisting of tipifarnib and docetaxel (Piccart-Gebhart *et al.* 2001) or paclitaxel (Patnaik *et al.* 2004), have demonstrated acceptable safety profiles, and objective responses, principally in patients with metastatic breast carcinoma that failed to respond to taxanes, were noted. In addition, a well-tolerated combination regimen, consisting of gemcitabine, cisplatin, and tipifarnib, demonstrated clinical activity in patients with NSCLC in a phase I study, with 5 (33%) of 15 patients experiencing objective responses. At the MTD, the principal toxicity was myelosuppresion (Adjei *et al.* 2003a). Two phase I studies with tipifarnib in combination with irinotecan have also been published (Cohen *et al.* 2004; Spareboom *et al.* 2004). In one study, clinically relevant doses of irinotecan, 350 mg/m^2 IV every 3 weeks, and tipifarnib 300 mg orally twice daily for 14 days every 3 weeks, were determined to be safe, with neutropenia and thrombocytopenia being the principal dose-limiting effects. In a phase I study of tipifarnib and trastuzumab, the combination was well-tolerated and a patient with metastatic colorectal cancer experienced a PR, and four additional patients had prolonged SD as their best response (deBono *et al.* 2002). Protracted grade 4 neutropenia, fever, and thrombocytopenia precluded further dose escalation of tipifarnib above 400 mg twice daily in combination with clinically relevant doses of trastuzumab. Based on pre-clinical studies in MCF-7 xenografts suggesting that combinations of tipifarnib and either tamoxifen or oestrogen deprivation were significantly more active than each individual therapy (Johnston *et al.* 2002), a phase I trial combining tipifarnib (200 and 300 mg orally twice daily for 21 days every 28 days) and tamoxifen (20 mg daily) was designed for patients with metastatic breast cancer whose tumours expressed oestrogen and/or progesterone receptors (Lebowitz *et al.* 2004). Toxicities included diarrhoea, nausea, vomiting, constipation, fatigue, rash, neutropenia, thrombocytopenia, and anaemia. All patients treated with tipifarnib 300 mg twice-daily required dose reduction due to toxicity, although no significant change in the pharmacokinetic profile of tipifarnib was observed. Four (36%) of 11 evaluable patients had clinical benefit, including three PRs and one SD. Pharmacodynamic analysis showed that FTase inhibition in PBMCs was enhanced by the combination regimen compared with tipifarnib alone. The combination was considered well tolerated and a phase II trial is in progress.

Lonafarnib (SCH66336, Sarozar^{TM}; Schering-Plough, Kenilworth, NJ) (Fig. 5.4) is an oral, nonpeptidyl, nonsulfhydryl tricyclic FTI that has been shown to inhibit the farnesylation of H- and N-ras in nanomolar concentrations (Sternberg *et al.* 1998). Phase I studies have explored the feasibility of administering lonafarnib twice daily for 7 days every 3 weeks, as well as uninterrupted, continuous dosing (Adjei *et al.* 2000b; Eskens *et al.* 2001). On the interrupted dosing schedule, dose-limiting toxicities, which included nausea, vomiting, diarrhoea, and fatigue, were, noted at the 400 mg orally twice daily dose level. A patient with NSCLC experienced a PR. The uninterrupted dosing schedule was well-tolerated at lonafarnib doses up to 200 mg orally twice daily, which was recommended for phase II studies. At 300 mg orally twice daily, an unacceptably high incidence of dose-limiting toxicities, consisting of neutropenia, neurocortical toxicity, and fatigue, were noted. The pharmacokinetics were dose-proportional, with steady state achieved within 7 days. SD lasting longer than 9 months was noted in patients with pseudomyxoma peritonei and thyroid carcinoma. In a phase I study of lonafarnib administered once daily on an uninterrupted schedule, in which 12 patients were enrolled, principal toxicities included nausea, vomiting, diarrhoea, fatigue, and renal

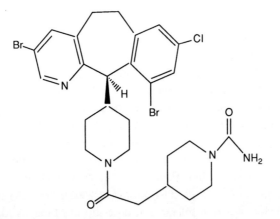

Fig. 5.4 Lonafarnib. Oral non-peptide, tricyclic competitive inhibitor of FT. Purified FTI (IC_{50}): H-Ras (1.9 nmol/l) and K-Ras (IC_{50}, 5.2 nmol/l). Potent enhancer of the cellular uptake and cytotoxicity of Pgp substrates. Abbreviations: FT, farnesyltransferase; FTI, farnesyltransferase inhibitor; IC_{50}, 50% inhibitory concentration.

dysfunction. The dose recommended for phase II studies in patients with solid malignancies was determined to be 300 mg daily (Awada *et al.* 2002). The pharmacokinetics were characterised by plasma half-life values ranging from 5 to 9 h and a large volume of distribution at steady state, suggesting extensive tissue distribution. No objective responses were observed.

Based on the encouraging pre-clinical data, the feasibility of administering lonafarnib and paclitaxel was evaluated. Myelosuppression, gastrointestinal toxicity, and cumulative neurotoxicity were the principal toxicities (Khuri *et al.* 2001). The MTD level was established at 100 mg orally twice daily of lonafarnib and 175 mg/m^2 every three weeks of paclitaxel. Anti-tumour activity was demonstrated in patients with advanced breast cancer and NSCLC, including patients who received prior therapy with taxanes. Additionally, the combination of lonafarnib with paclitaxel and carboplatin was demonstrated to be tolerable at clinically relevant doses (Sprague *et al.* 2002). The combination of lonafarnib, cisplatin, and gemcitabine was also evaluated in patients with advanced solid malignancies. The dose of lonafarnib was escalated up to 75 mg twice daily in combination with gemcitabine 1000 mg/m^2 weekly for 3 weeks every 4 weeks and cisplatin 100 mg/m^2 every 4 weeks, which exceeded the MTD (Pierson *et al.* 2002). Diarrhoea, nausea, vomiting, and neutropenia were the principal toxicities. No objective responses were observed in the first 14 patients.

BMS-214662 (Bristol-Myers Squibb, New York, NY), a benzodiazepine derivative is a highly selective inhibitor of FTase with potent pro-apoptotic properties. An oral formulation was not demonstrated to be feasible because of gastrointestinal intolerance and therefore the agent was evaluated as a parenteral formulation (Camacho et al. 2001; Hunt et al. 2000). BMS-214662 has been evaluated as a 1-h IV infusion administered every 3 weeks and daily for 5 days every 3 weeks (McDermott et al. 2004; Sonnichsen et al. 2000). The single 1-h infusion schedule was modified to a 24-h IV infusion schedule, which appeared to be much better tolerated at doses up to $300 \, \text{mg/m}^2$. Diarrhoea, nausea, vomiting, and abdominal cramping were the principal toxicities. Although no major responses were documented, minor responses and prolonged SD were observed in patients with non-small cell lung, colorectal, and breast carcinomas (Ryan et al. 2004; Zhu et al. 2002). The daily-for-5-day IV infusion schedule was well-tolerated at doses up to $81 \, \text{mg/m}^2/\text{day}$, but only transient inhibition of tissue FTase was noted (McDermott et al. 2004). In another phase I study, BMS-214662 was evaluated in patients with refractory or relapsed acute leukaemias and high-risk MDS. The MTD was $118 \, \text{mg/m}^2$ weekly. Of the six MDS patients, three had more than 50% reduction in bone marrow blasts (Cortes et al. 2001). The combination of BMS-214662 and cisplatin was also demonstrated to be well-tolerated in patients with advanced solid malignancies, and there was no evidence of adverse drug–drug interactions at the recommended dose level, consisting of $200 \, \text{mg/m}^2$ of BMS 214662 as a 1-h IV infusion and $75 \, \text{mg/m}^2$ of cisplatin. Fifteen of the 29 patients enrolled in the study had SD as their best response, but no major responses were observed (Mackay et al. 2004). The combination of BMS 214662 with paclitaxel and carboplatin was also demonstrated to be well-tolerated (Dy et al. 2004). Dose-limiting toxicities included neutropenia, nausea, and vomiting. Two patients with ovarian and oesophageal carcinomas experienced PRs and seven patients with NSCLC experienced SD as their best response.

The membrane-permeable agent L-778,123 (Merck, Nutley, NJ), a dual inhibitor of both FTase and GGTase, was evaluated as a 7-day CIVI administered every 3 weeks in patients with advanced solid malignancies. The agent appeared to be well-tolerated at doses up to $560 \, \text{mg/m}^2/\text{day}$. At $1120 \, \text{mg/m}^2/\text{day}$, however, an unacceptably high incidence of dose-limiting toxicities, consisting of thrombocytopenia, QTc interval prolongation, and profound fatigue, were observed. The pharmacokinetic behaviour was linear and the $560 \, \text{mg/m}^2/\text{day}$ dose resulted in biologically-relevant concentrations and consistent inhibition of HDJ2 chaperon protein prenylation in PBMCs (Britten et al. 2001). Another phase I study evaluated the feasibility of administering L-778,123 as a CIVI for either 2 or 4 weeks followed by 1-week drug-free period (Rubin et al. 2000). The dose-limiting toxicities included QTc interval prolongation and neutropenia. No objective responses were observed. The recommended phase II dose of the 2 week CIVI schedule was $560\,\mathrm{mg/m^2}$, whereas it was not determined for the 4-week schedule. Pharmacodynamic studies from these two phase I studies indicated that GGTase-I inhibition did occur; however, no inhibition of K-Ras prenylation was detected in patients PBMCs (Lobell *et al.* 2002). These findings suggested that although L-788,123 inhibited FTase, sufficient GGTase inhibitory activity could not be achieved *in vivo*, and therefore it could not adequately inhibit K-ras prenylation *in vivo*. However, pre-clinical animal studies with GGTIs that were more potent than L-788,123 demonstrated that the agents were quite toxic (Lobell *et al.* 2002). The development of L-788,123 was discontinued due to a high incidence of QTc prolongation and lack of significant activity in phase II evaluations.

4.2.3 Clinical studies: phases II and III

Lung cancer In a phase II study of tipifarnib 300 mg orally twice daily for 21 days every 28 days in 44 previously untreated patients with stages IIIB and IV NSCLC, there were no objective responses; however, seven patients had SD lasting longer than 6 months as their best response (Adjei *et al.* 2003). The principal toxicity was neutropenia. Other toxicities included anaemia, anorexia, and peripheral neuropathy. Although no objective responses were documented, significant FTase inhibition, as manifested by accumulation of pre-laminin A in buccal mucosa cells and accumulation of unfarnesylated HDJ-2 in PBMCs, was noted in 83% of patients. Similarly, no objective responses were noted in a phase II study of L-778,223 in 23 patients with previously untreated NSCLC (Evans *et al.* 2002). In a phase I/II study of lonafarnib and paclitaxel in 33 patients with metastatic taxane-refractory NSCLC, there were five PRs and four minor responses, and 10 patients had SD as their best response (Kim *et al.* 2002). Toxicity, consisting of neutropenia, diarrhoea, and fatigue, was minimal. In addition, preliminary clinical activity has been noted in pts with NSCLC in phase I feasibility trials of combinations of FTIs with taxanes, gemcitabine, and cisplatin, providing a rationale for subsequent phase II studies (Adjei *et al.* 2001a; Dy *et al.* 2004; Khuri *et al.* 2001; Kim *et al.* 2002; Piccart-Gebhart *et al.* 2001). Tipifarnib 400 mg twice daily for 14 days every 3 weeks has also been evaluated in 22 patients with relapsed small cell lung cancer (SCLC). Toxicities included neutropenia, thrombocytopenia, acute renal failure, fatigue, anorexia, and nausea. No objective responses were observed (Heymach *et al.* 2004).

The role of the FTIs in the chemoprevention of NSCLC and other solid tumours in high-risk patients is also being evaluated. In one such study, the role of the FTIs in preventing the progression of pre-malignant lesions in former or current smokers with histories of smoking-related cancer is being studied (Khuri 2003).

Breast carcinoma Although *ras* is rarely mutated in breast carcinoma (<2%), aberrant activation of the Ras pathway is common because of enhanced upstream growth factor receptor activity, such as erbB1 and erbB2 (Clark and Der 1995). In pre-clinical studies, tipifarnib demonstrated potent growth inhibition of hormone-sensitive, wild-type Ras MCF-7 breast cancer xenografts, and induced apoptosis and expression of the cell-cycle inhibitor p21 (Kelland *et al.* 2001). In view of these results, 76 patients with metastatic breast carcinoma were enrolled in a phase II study of tipifarnib (Johnston *et al.* 2003). The first 41 patients were treated with tipifarnib at 400 or 300 mg twice daily on an uninterrupted schedule. Another group of 35 patients received tipifarnib 300 mg twice daily for 21 days every 28 days. Since patients treated with tipifarnib on the uninterrupted schedule experienced an unacceptably high incidence of haematological and neurological toxicities, the intermittent schedule was the principal focus of subsequent efforts. In the first cohort, four (10%) patients experienced PRs and six (15%) patients had SD as their best response. On the intermittent schedule, five (14%) patients had PRs and three (9%) patients had SD as their best response. Interestingly, erbB2 gene amplification was documented in six of the nine patients who experienced PRs. The activity of tipifarnib in breast cancer, in which wild-type Ras may be driven by upstream growth factor over-expression, suggested that Ras mutations were not essential for the activity of the FTIs. Evaluations of tipifarnib combined with other relevant agents in patients with advanced breast carcinoma are in progress.

Given the fact that the majority of patients with erbB2 expressing breast cancer do not respond to trastuzumab as a single agent (Vogel *et al.* 2002), the possibility of augmenting trastuzumab sensitivity by inhibiting FTase was evaluated. Early clinical data suggest that dual erbB2 blockade with trastuzumab and FTIs may result in additive activity, and that the combination can be safely administered at clinically relevant doses of both agents (de Bono *et al.* 2002). The combination of tipifarnib with doxorubicin and cyclophosphamide administered on a dose-dense schedule has also been evaluated in patients with metastatic breast cancer (Sparano *et al.* 2004). The recommended phase II dose of tipifarnib is 200 mg orally twice daily for seven days when combined with doxorubicin 60 mg/m^2 and cyclophosphamide 600 mg/m^2 administered on day 1 every 2 weeks with filgastrim. The dose-limiting toxicities included severe neutropenia with fever and thrombocytopenia. Objective responses occurred in eight of nine evaluable patients. The regimen is being further explored in patients with locally advanced breast cancer. Other evaluations are exploring the feasibility of administering the FTIs in combination with relevant cytotoxic or hormonal therapies in patients with advanced breast cancer. Tipifarnib is explored in combination with capecitabine for patients with taxane-resistant metastatic breast cancer, as well as in combination with tamoxifen and with fulvestrant as first- and second-line therapy in patients with metastatic breast cancer expressing oestrogen and/or progesterone receptors. Lonafarnib is also being evaluated for the treatment of advanced breast cancer in a placebo-controlled, randomised phase II study in combination with anastrozole.

Colon carcinoma In a phase II study of lonafarnib 200 mg orally twice daily on an uninterrupted, continuous schedule, there were no responses among 21 patients with metastatic CRC who were previously treated with fluoropyrimidines. Three patients experienced SD as their best response (Sharma *et al.* 2002). The principal side-effects were fatigue, nausea, and diarrhoea. Although the investigators did not recommend further evaluations of lonafarnib in this patient population, a phase III, randomised, double-blind, placebo-controlled study was performed in 368 patients with metastatic CRC who had received at least two prior chemotherapy regimens. Patients were randomised in a 2:1 fashion to treatment with either tipifarnib 300 mg orally twice daily for 21 days every 28 days or placebo (Rao *et al.* 2004). The results were disappointing, as the median overall survival of patients receiving tipifarnib was 5.7 months versus 6.1 months for those receiving placebo. Only one (0.4%) of the 235 patients treated with tipifarnib achieved a PR, and 57 patients (24%) had SD as their best response, compared with 17 patients (12.8%) who had SD as their best response in the placebo arm. Disappointing anti-tumour activity was also noted in a phase II trial performed by Southwest Oncology Group (SWOG) using an identical schedule of tipifarnib in previously untreated patients with metastatic CRC. Of 51 evaluable patients, one confirmed and two unconfirmed PRs were noted and the median time to treatment failure was 1.7 months (Whitehead *et al.* 2003). As previously discussed, one possible explanation for these disappointing results is the predominance of K-*ras* mutations in this malignancy and the potential of GGT-1 to prenylate K-ras.

Pancreatic carcinoma The role of tipifarnib as first-line treatment in patients with advanced pancreatic adenocarcinoma has been evaluated. In one phase II trial, 20 patients were treated with 300 mg of tipifarnib twice daily for 21 days every 28 days. Several patients experienced grade 3–4 neutropenia, transaminitis, and rash. No objective responses were observed and the median time to progression and median survival were 4.9 and 19.9 weeks, respectively (Cohen *et al.* 2003). In another phase II study performed by the SWOG, which evaluated tipifarnib on the same schedule in 56 patients with previously untreated advanced pancreatic carcinoma, no objective responses were noted (Macdonald *et al.* 2002). Furthermore, the drug was poorly tolerated, as 43% of the patients experienced grade 3–4 toxicities including fatigue, malaise, emesis, and anaemia. However, the combination of tipifarnib and gemcitabine was well tolerated at doses of 200 mg twice daily continuously and 1000 mg/m^2 day 1, 8 and 15 every 4 weeks, respectively (Patnaik *et al.* 2003). Myelosuppression was the principal toxicity. PRs were observed in patients with advanced pancreatic and nasopharyngeal carcinomas. These results led to a phase III trial, in which 688 previously untreated patients with advanced pancreatic cancer were randomised to treatment with either tipifarnib plus gemcitabine or gemcitabine plus placebo (Van Cutsem *et al.* 2004). No differences in time to progression and survival endpoints were observed. The median survival and progression-free survival for the experimental arm were 193 days and 112 days versus 182 days and 109 days for the control arm, respectively. The objective response rates were 6% and 8%, and the 1-year survival was 27% and 24%, respectively.

The activity of lonafarnib was also evaluated in a multicentre phase II randomised study, in which 63 previously untreated patients with advanced pancreatic cancer were treated with either lonafarnib 200 mg twice daily or gemcitabine 1000 mg/m^2 weekly for 7 weeks every 8 weeks (Lersch *et al.* 2001). The median survival was 3.3 and 4.4 months for patients treated with lonafarnib and gemcitabine, respectively. In the lonafarnib arm, two patients had PRs and six patients had SD as their best response, whereas there was 1 PR and 11 SD in the gemcitabine arm.

Haematologic malignancies

Acute leukaemia Based on the encouraging activity noted in a phase I study in patients with acute leukaemia (Karp *et al.* 2001), 252 patients with relapsed and refractory AML were enrolled into a phase II multicentre study to further characterise the activity of tipifarnib in this indication. The rate of CRs was the primary endpoint of the study (Harrousseau *et al.* 2003). Tipifarnib was administered at 600 mg twice daily for 21 days every 4 weeks. In a preliminary report, 19 (14%) of 138 evaluable patients had demonstrated reductions in bone marrow blasts to less than 5%, and 25 (18%) additional patients had >50% reduction in bone marrow blasts. Upon an independent review, CR was achieved in ten (6%) of 169 patients with evidence of sustained response for at least 28 days in three (1.8%) patients. The most common toxicities were hypokalaemia, skin rash and hyperbilirubinaemia. These results confirmed that single-agent tipifarnib is well-tolerated and induces CR in heavily pretreated patients with relapsed and refractory AML. Evaluation of the same regimen in newly diagnosed elderly patients is ongoing.

Interestingly, a dose-ranging pharmacodynamic study performed in 34 patients with refractory haematological malignancies has demonstrated that inhibition of farnesylation in bone marrow cells relates to clinical activity. Furthermore, the inhibition of farnesylation in PBMCs also appears to correlate with the inhibition of farnesylation in the bone marrow. In contrast, the inhibition of farnesylation in post-treatment bone marrow was noted at all dose levels tested with no relationship between dose and inhibition of farnesylation (Zimmerman *et al.* 2003). Whether the blood concentration of FTIs is informative for the FTase inhibition in peripheral tissues, and specifically in tumour cells, and which plasma concentration threshold is necessary to achieve biological effectiveness, are important questions. Tipifarnib is currently being evaluated in a randomised phase III study in patients with AML in remission (ECOG 2902 trial), as well as in a randomised phase II trial in patients with AML and MDS in complete remission (JHOC-JO252 trial).

Myelodysplastic syndrome *Ras* mutations occur in up to 20% of patients with MDS. In a phase II study of tipifarnib 600 mg twice daily for 3 weeks every 4 to 6 weeks involving 104 patients with poor-risk AML or MDS, the major response rate was 33% and CRs occurred in 19 (21%) of the 92 evaluable patients (Lancet *et al.* 2003). Inhibition of HDJ-2 protein farnesylation was documented in 17 (74%) of 23 evaluable leukaemic marrow samples, with clinical responses occurring in nearly 50% of these cases. Interestingly, in the six cases in which no inhibition of HDJ-2 occurred, only one patient achieved clinical response, suggesting that failure to inhibit HDJ-2 farnesylation may relate to clinical outcome. Another phase II multicentre study of tipifarnib 600 mg twice daily for 4 weeks every 6 weeks was performed in patients with MDS. Twenty-seven patients were evaluable. Multiple toxicities, including myelosuppresion, fatigue, neurotoxicity, and rash, necessitating dose reductions or discontinuation of treatment in 15 of 27 patients during the first 12 weeks of treatment, were noted. Therefore, the dose of tipifarnib was reduced to 300 mg twice daily. Two patients experienced CR and one patient experienced a PR (Kurzrock *et al.* 2004).

Lonafarnib also showed clinical benefit in patients with haematological malignancies in phase I study (List *et al.* 2002), and was subsequently evaluated in a phase II trial. Three out of 15 patients enrolled had haematological improvement (Cortes *et al.* 2002). Feldman *et al.* reported preliminary results from a phase I/II study of lonafarnib in 32 patients with MDS and 35 chronic myelo-monocytic leukaemia (CMML) patients (Feldman *et al.* 2003). Lona-farnib was administered at doses of 200–300 mg twice daily. Of 42 evaluable patients, two patients had CRs, and haematological improvement was observed in 11 other patients. Toxicities observed were diarrhoea, fatigue, anorexia, and nausea. In another study of lonafarnib involving 12 evaluable patients with MDS and AML treated at a dose of 200 mg twice daily two PRs were observed (Ravoet *et al.* 2002). A phase III trial is planned in patients with advanced MDS.

Multiple myeloma Based on the observation that patients with multiple myeloma bearing *Ras* mutations are less likely to respond to treatment with cytotoxic agents and have shorter survival, a phase II study of tipifarnib 300 mg twice daily was performed in 43 patients with relapsed multiple myeloma (Alsina *et al.* 2004). Overall, tipifarnib was well-tolerated, with most patients experiencing mild fatigue, gastrointestinal toxicity, and myelosuppression. Although no major objective responses occurred, 23 (64%) of 36 evaluable patients had SD (<50% decrease in the M-protein levels) as their best response. The median time to progression for the patients who achieved SD was 4 months (range, 2–26 months). Inhibition of farnesylation of HDJ-2 in unfractionated mononuclear cells and myeloma cells and suppression of FTase in bone marrow and PBMCs were demonstrated but did not correlate with disease stabilisation.

5 Conclusion and perspectives

The high incidence of *ras* mutations in solid malignancies has served as the rationale for the development of specific Ras-targeting ASONs and the FTIs. Although both types of agents have failed to demonstrate relevant anti-tumour activity in clinical studies involving malignancies with high incidences of *ras* mutations, such as pancreatic and colorectal carcinoma, there are many plausible reasons for these failures, which do not entirely relate to the relevance of Ras as a target. With regard to the ASONs, the platform, itself, has not been validated in the treatment of systemic diseases. There are still concerns pertaining to PKs, distribution, and intracellular penetration. On the other hand, the failure of the FTIs to demonstrate relevant anti-tumour activity in malignancies with high incidences of K-*ras* mutations most likely relate to the fact that alternate prenylating enzymes, particularly GGT-I, can prenylate

K-Ras in the face of profound inhibition of FTase. Nevertheless, the FTIs have demonstrated intriguing activity in patients with breast cancer, acute leukaemias, and MDS, most likely due to the dependence of these malignancies on protein farnesylation, which is inhibited by the FTIs. It will be important to identify which farnesylated proteins are being critically affected to develop optimal patient selection strategies as well as superior therapeutics. However, the real challenge is to develop better strategies to inhibit Ras through novel platforms such as siRNA or chemical optimisation.

References

Adjei AA, Davis JN, Erlichman C, Svingen PA, Kaufmann SH (2000a). Comparison of potential markers of farnesyltransferase inhibition. *Clin Ca Res*, **6**, 2318–25.

Adjei AA, Erlichman C, Davis JN *et al*. (2000b) A phase I trial of the farnesyl transferase inhibitor SCH66336: evidence for biological and clinical activity. *Cancer Res*, **60**, 1871–77.

Adjei AA, Bruzek LM, Erlichman C *et al*. (2001a) Combination studies with the farnesyltransferase inhibitor R115777 and chemotherapy agents. *Eur J Cancer*, **37** (Suppl 6), abst 792.

Adjei AA, Davis JN, Bruzek LM, Erlichman C, Kaufmann SH (2001b) Synergy of the protein farnesyltransferase inhibitor SCH66336 and Cisplatin in human cancer cell lines. *Clin Cancer Res*, **7**(5), 1438–1445.

Adjei AA, Croghan GA, Erlichman C *et al*. (2003a) A phase I trial of the farnesyltransferase inhibitor R115777 in combination with gemcitabine and cisplatin in patients with advanced cancer. *Clin Cancer Res*, **9**, 2520–6.

Adjei AA, Mauer L, Bruzek L *et al*. (2003b) Phase II study of the farnesyl transferase inhibitor R115,777 in patients with advanced non-small-cell-lung cancer. *J Clin Oncol*, **21**, 1760–1766.

Alemany R (1996) Growth inhibitory effect of anti-K–Ras adenovirus on lung cancer cells. *Cancer Gene Ther*, **3**, 296–301.

Alsina M, Fonseca R, Wilson EF *et al*. (2004) Farnesyltransferase inhibitor tipifarnib is well tolerated, induce stabilization of disease and inhibits farnesylation and oncogenic/tumour survival pathways in patients with advanced multiple myeloma. *Blood*, **103**, 3271–7.

Andres DA, Goldstein JL, Ho YK, Brown MS (1993) Mutational analysis of a-subunit of protein farnesyltransferase. Evidence for a catalytic role. *J Biol Chem*, **268**, 1383–90.

Armstrong SA, Hannah VC, Goldstein JL, Brown MS (1995) CAAX geranylgeranyl transferases transfers farnesyl as efficiently as geranylgeranyl to RhoB. *J Biol Chem*, **270**, 7864–68.

Ashar HR, Armstrong L, James LJ *et al*. (2000) Biological effects and mechanism of action of farnesyltransferase inhibitors. *Chem Res Toxicol*, **13**, 949–52.

Awada A, Eskens FA, Piccart M *et al*. (2002) Phase I and pharmacological study of the oral farnesyltransferase inhibitor SCH 66336 given once daily to patients with advanced solid tumors. *Eur J Cancer*, **38**, 2272–8.

Barbacid M (1987) Ras genes. *Ann Rev Biochem*, **56**, 779–827.

Bishop WR, Kirschmeier P, Baum C (2003) Farnesyltransferase inhibitors : Mechanism of action, translational studies and clinical evaluation. *Cancer Biol Ther*, 2(4 Suppl 1), S96–S104.

Bogusky MS, McCormick F (1993) Function and regulation of Ras and its relatives. *Nature*, **366**, 643–54.

Bos JL (1989) Ras oncogenes in human cancer: a review. *Cancer Res*, **49**, 4682–89.

Britten C, Rowinsky EK, Soignet S *et al.* (2001) A phase I and pharmacokinetic study of the farnesyl protein transferase inhibitor L-778,123 in patients with solid malignancies. *Clin Ca Res*, **7**, 3894–903.

Burch PA, Alberts SR, Schroeder MT *et al.* (2003) Gemcitabine and ISIS 2503 for patients with pancreatic adenocarcinoma (ACA): A North Central Cancer Treatment Group (NCCTG) phase II study. *Proc Am Soc Clin Oncol*, **22**, abst 1038.

Camacho LH, Soignet SL, Pezzulli S *et al.* (2001) Dose escalation study of oral farnesyltransferase inhibitor BMS214662 in patients with solid tumors. *Proc Am Soc Clin Oncol*, **20**, abst 311.

Chun KN, Lee HY, Hassan K, Khuri F, Hong WK, Lotan R (2003) Implication of protein kinase B/Akt and Bcl-2/Bcl-XL suppression by the farnesyl transferase inhibitor SCH66336 in apoptosis induced in squamos carcinoma cells. *Cancer Res*, **63**, 4796–800.

Clark GJ and Der CJ. (1995) Aberrant function of the Ras signal transduction pathway in human breast cancer. *Breast Cancer Res Treat* **35**(1), 133–44.

Coffety MC, Strong JE, Forsyth PA, Lee PW (1998) Reovirus therapy of tumors with activated Ras pathway. *Science*, **282**,1332–4.

Cohen S, Ho L, Ranganathan S *et al.* (2003) Phase II and pharmacokinetic trial of the farnesyltransferase inhibitor R115,777 as initial therapy in patients with metastatic pancreatic adenocarcinoma. *J Clin Oncol*, **21**, 1301–6.

Cohen SJ, Gallo J, Lewis NL *et al.* (2004) Phase I and pharmacokinetic study of the farnesyltransferase inhibitor R115777 in combination with irinotecan in patients with advanced cancer. *Cancer Chemother Pharmacol*, **53**, 513–8.

Cortes J, Kurzroch R, O'Brien *et al.* (2001) Phase I study of a farnesyltransferase inhibitor (FTI) BMS-214662, in patients with refractory or relapsed acute leukaemias. *Blood*, **98**, 594a.

Cortes J, Holyoake TL, Silver RT *et al.* (2002) Continuous oral lonafarnib (Sarazar™) for the treatment of patients with advanced hematologic malignancies: a phase II study. *Blood*, **100**, 793a, abst 3132.

Cox AD, Der CJ (1997) Farnesyltransferase inhibitors and cancer treatment: targeting simply Ras? *Biochim Biophys Acta*, **1333**(1), F51–71.

Crul M, De Clerk GJ, Beijnen JH, Schellens JH (2001) Ras biochemistry and farnesyl transferase inhibitors: a literature survey. *Anticancer drugs*, **12**, 163–84.

Crul M, de Klerk GJ, Swart M *et al.* (2002) Phase I clinical and pharmacological study of chronic oral administration of the farnesyl protein transferase inhibitor R115777 in advanced cancer. *J Clin Oncol*, **20**, 2726–35.

Dang T, Johnson DH, Kelly K, Rizvi N, Holmlung J, Dorr A (2001) Multicenter phase II trial of an antisense inhibitor of H-raps (ISIS-2503) in advanced non-small cell lung cancer (NSCLC). *Proc Am Soc Clin Oncol*, **20**, abst 1325.

de Bono JS, Schwartz G, Hammond L *et al.* (2002) Concomitant HER2 and farnesyltransferase blockade by R115,777 and trastuzumab in patients with advanced cancer. *Br J Cancer*, **86**(Suppl 1), S110(252).

DeSolms SJ, Ciccarone TM, MacTough SC *et al.* (2003) Dual protein farnesyltransferase-geranylgeranyltransferase I inhibitors as potential cancer chemotherapeutic agents. *J Med Chem*, **46**, 2973–84.

Dorr A, Bruce J, Monia B, *et al.* (1999) Phase I and pharmacokinetic trial of ISIS 2503, a 20-Mer antisense against H-ras by 14-day continuous infusion in patients in patients with advanced cancer. *Proc Am Soc Clin Oncol*, **18**, 603.

Dy GK, Bruzek LM, Croghan GA et al. (2004) A phase I trial of the novel farnesyl protein transferase inhibitor, BMS 214662 in combination with paclitaxel and carboplatin in patients with advanced cancer. Proc Am Soc Clin Oncol, 23, abst 3066.

End DW (1999) Farnesyl protein transferase inhibitors and other therapies targeting the Ras signal transduction pathway. Investig New Drugs, 17(3), 241–58.

End DW, Smets G, Todd A et al. (2001) Characterization of the antitumor effects of the selective farnesyl protein transferase inhibitor R115777 in vivo and in vitro. Cancer Res, 61, 131–7.

Eskens F, Awada A, Cutler DL et al. (2001) Phase I and pharmacokinetic study of the oral farnesyltransferase inhibitor SCH66336 given twice daily to patients with advanced solid tumors. J Clin Oncol, 19, 1167–75.

Evans T, Fidias P, Skarin A et al. (2002). A phase II study of efficacy and tolerability of the farnesyl-protein transferase inhibitor L-788,123 as first line therapy in patients with advanced non-small cell lung cancer. Proc Am Soc Clin Oncol, 21, abst 1861.

Feldman EJ, Cortes J, Holyoake TL et al. (2003) Continuous oral lonafarnib (Sarasar) for the treatment of patients with myelodysplastic syndrome. Blood, 102(11), 421a.

Garcia AM, Rowell C, Ackermann K, Kavalzyc JJ, Lewis MD. (1993) Peptidomimetic inhibitors of Ras farnesylation and function in whole cells. J Biol Chem, 268, 18415–8.

Gibbs JB and Oliff A. (1997) The potential of farnesyltransferase inhibitors as cancer chemotherapeutics. Annu Rev Pharmacol Toxicol, 37, 143–66.

Gibbs JB, Oliff A, Kohl NE (1994). Farnesyltransferases inhibitors: Ras research yields a potential cancer therapeutic. Cell, 77, 175–8.

Ghobrial Im, Adjei AA (2002) Inhibitors of Ras oncogene as therapeutic targets. Hematol Oncol Clin North Am, 16, 1065–88.

Goldsmith G, Larocca RV, Glisson S et al. (2003) Phase 2 of ISIS 2503, an antisense inhibitor of H-ras, in combination with docetaxel for patients with previously treated advanced non-small cell lung cancer. Proc Am Soc Clin Oncol, 22, abst 941.

Gordon MS, Snadler AB, Holmlund JT, et al. (1999) A phase I trial of ISIS 2503, an antisense inhibitor of H-raps administered by a 24-hours infusion in patients with advanced cancers. Proc Am Soc Clin Oncol, 18, 604.

Harousseau J-L, Reiffers J, Lowenberg B et al. (2003) Zarnestra (R115777) in patients with relapsed and refractory acute myelogenous leukaemia-(AML): Results of a multicenter phase 2 study. Blood, 102(11), abst 614.

Haluska P, Dy GK, Adjei AA (2002) Farnesyltransferase inhibitors as anticancer agents. Eur J Oncol, 38, 1685–1700.

Heymach JV, Johnson DH, Khuri FR et al. (2004) Phase II study of the farnesyltransferase inhibitor R115,777 in patients with sensitive relapse small cell lung cancer (SCLC). Ann Oncol, 15, 1187–93.

Holden SN, Eckhardt SG, Fisher S et al. (2001) A phase I pharmacokinetic and biological study of the farnesyl transferase inhibitor (FTI) R115,777 and Capecitabine in patients with advanced solid malignancies. Proc Am Soc Clin Oncol, 20, abst 316.

Hunt JT, Ding CZ, Batorsky R et al. (2000) Discovery of [R]-7-cyano-2, 3,4,5-tetrahydr-1-(1H-imidazol-4-ylmethyl)-3—(phenylmethyl)-4-(2-tienylsulfonyl)-1H-1, 4-benzodiazepine (BMS-214662), a farnesyltransferase inhibitor with potent pre-clinical activity. J Med Chem, 43, 3587–95.

Hurwitz H, Amado R, Prager D et al. (2000) Phase I pharmacokinetic trial of the farnesyltransferase inhibitor SCH66336 plus gemcitabine in advanced cancers. Proc Am Soc Clin Oncol, abst 717.

James GL, Goldstein JL, Brown MS *et al.* (1993) Benzodiazepine peptidomimetics: potent inhibitors of Ras farnesylation in animal cells. *Science*, **260**, 1937–42.

James GL, Goldstein JL, Brown MS (1995) Polylysine and CVIM sequences of K-Ras dictate specificity of prenylation and confer resistance to benzodiazepine peptidomimetics in vitro. *J Biol Chem*, **270**, 6621–6.

Johnston SR, Ellis P, Houston S *et al.* (2002) A phase II study of the farnesyltransferase inhibitor R115, 777 in patients with advanced breast cancer. *Proc Am Soc Clin Oncol*, **19**, abst 318

Johnston S, Hickish T, Ellis P *et al.* (2003) Phase II study of the efficacy and tolerability of two dosing regimens of the farnesyltransferase inhibitor, R115,777 in advanced breast cancer. *J Clin Oncol*, **21**, 2492–99.

Karp J, Lancet JE, Kaufmann SH *et al.* (2001) Clinical and biological activity of the farnesyltransferase inhibitor R115777 in adults with refractory and relapsed acute leukaemias: a phase I clinical-laboratory correlative trial. *Blood*, **97**, 3361–69.

Kelland LR, Smith V, Valenti M, *et al* (2001) Pre-clinical antitumor activity and pharmacodynamic studies with the farnesyl protein transferase inhibitor R115,777 in human breast cancer. *Clin Cancer Res*, **7**, 3544–50.

Khuri FR (2003) Primary and secondary prevention of non-small cell lung cancer SPORE trials of Lung Cancer Prevention. *Clin Lung Cancer*, **5**(Suppl 1), S36–S40.

Khuri F, Glisson B, Meyers M *et al.* (2001) A phase I study of farnesyltransferase inhibitor SCH66336 with paclitaxel in solid tumors: Dose-finding, pharmacokinetics, efficacy/safety. *Proc 11th NCI-EORTC-AACR symposium on new drugs in cancer research*. A403.

Kim ES, Kies MS, Fossella FV *et al.* (2002) A phase I/II study of the farnesyltransferase inhibitor (FTI) SCH66336 (lonafarnib) with paclitaxel in taxane-refractory/resistant patients with non-small cell lung cancer (NSCLC); final report. *Proc Am Assoc Cancer Res*, **43**, 550, abst 2735.

Kloog Y, Cox A, Sinensky M (1999) Concepts in Ras-directed therapy. *Exp Opin Invest Drugs*, **8**, 2121–40.

Kohl NE, Wilson FR, Mosser SD *et al.* (1994) Protein farnesyltransferase inhibitors block the growth of ras-dependent tumors in nude mice. *Proc Natl Acad Sci USA*, **91**, 9141–45.

Kohl NE, Omer CA, Conner MW *et al.* (1995) Inhibition of farnesyltransferase induces regression of mammary and salivary carcinomas in ras transgenic mice. *Nat Med*, **1**(8): 792–7.

Kurzrock R, Kantarjian HM, Corets JE *et al.* (2003) Farnesyltransferase inhibitor R115777 in myelodysplasic syndrome clinical and biologic activities in the phase 1 setting. *Blood*, **102**, 4527–34.

Kurzrock R, Albitar M, Cortes JE *et al.* (2004) Phase II study of R115,777, a farnesyltransferase inhibitor, in myelodysplasic syndrome. *J Clin Oncol*, **22**, 1287–92.

Lancet JE, Gojo I, Gotlib J *et al.* (2003) Zarnestra (R115,777) in previously untreated poor-risk AML and MDS: interim results of a phase II trial. *Blood*, **102**(11), abst 613.

Lara P, Frankel P, Gumerlock H *et al.* (2003) Intermittent dosing of the farnesyltransferase inhibitor R115777 in advanced malignant solid tumors: a phase I California Cancer Consortium Trial. *Proc Am Soc Clin Oncol*, **22**, abst 878.

Lebowitz PF, Eng-Wong J, Ballis B *et al.* (2004) A phase I trial of tipifarnib, a farnesyltransferase inhibitor and tamoxifen in hormone receptor positive metastatic breast cancer. *Proc Am Soc Clin Oncol*, **23**, abst 644.

Leonard DM (1997) Ras farnesyltransferase: a new therapeutic target. *J Med Chem*, **40**, 2971–90.

Lersch C, van Cutsem E, Amado R et al. (2001) Randomized phase II study of SCH66336 and Gemcitabine in the treatment of metastatic adenocarcinoma of the pancreas. *Proc Am Soc Clin Oncol*, 20, abst 608.

Liebes L, Hochster H, Speyer J et al. (2001) Enhanced myelosuppression of Topotecan when combined with the farnesytranferase inhibitor, R115777: a phase I and pharmacodynamic study. *Proc Am Soc Clin Oncol*, abst 321.

List AF, DeAngelo D, O'Brien S et al. (2002) Phase I study of continuous oral administration of lonafarnib (Sarazar™) in patients with advanced hematologic malignancies. *Blood*, 100, 789a, abst 3120.

Lobell RB, Liu D, Buser CA et al. (2002) Pre-clinical and clinical pharmacodynamic assessment of L-778,123, a dual inhibitor of farnesyl-protein transferase and geranylgeranyl-protein transferase type I. *Mol Cancer Ther*, 1, 747–58.

Loprevite M, Favoni RE, De Cupis A et al. (2004) In vitro study of farnesyltransferase inhibitor SCH66336, in combination with chemotherapy and radiation, in non-small cell lung cancer cell lines. *Oncol Rep*, 11, 407–14.

Lowy DR, Willumsen BM (1993) Function and regulation of Ras. *Ann Rev Bioche*, 62, 851–91.

Macdonald JS, Chansky K, Whitehead R, Wade J, Jeffrey G, Abbruzzese JL (2002) A phase II study of farnesyltransferase inhibitor R115,777 in pancreatic cancer. A Southwest Oncology Group (SWOG) study. *Proc Am Soc Clin Oncol*, 21, abst 548.

Mackay HJ, Hoekstra R, Eskens F et al. (2004) A phase I pharmacokinetic and pharmacodynamic study of the farnesyltransferase inhibitor BMS-214662 in combination with cisplatinum in patients with advanced solid tumors, *Clin Cancer Res*, 10, 2636–44.

Manne Y, Yan N, Carboni JM et al. (1995) Bisubstrate inhibitors of farnesyltransferase: a novel class of specific inhibitors of ras transformed cells. *Oncogene*, 10, 1763–79.

Marshall CJ (1996) Ras effectors. *Curr Opin Cell Biol*, 8, 197–204.

McDermott RS, Meroplo NJ, Weiner LM et al. (2004) Phase I clinical and pharmacokinetic study of the farnesyltransferase inhibitor BMS214662 administered intravenously for five consecutive days in patients with advanced malignancies. *Proc Am Soc Clin Oncol*, 23, abst 2033.

Migliaccio A, Di Domenico M, Castoria G et al. (1996) Tyrosine kinase/p21ras/MAP-kinase pathway activation by estradiol receptor complex in MCF-7 cells. *EMBO J*, 15, 1292–1300.

Moasser M, Sepp-Lorenzino L, Kohl NE et al. (1998) Farnesyl transferase inhibitors cause enhanced mitotic sensitivity to taxol and epothilones. *Proc Natl Acad Sci USA*, 95, 1369–74.

Omer CA, Anthony NJ, Buser-Doepner CA et al. (1997) Farnesylprotein transferases inhibitors as agents to inhibit tumor growth. *Biofactors*, 6, 359–66.

Patnaik A, Eckhardt S, Izbicka E et al. (2003) A phase I, pharmacokinetic, and biological study of the farnesyltransferase inhibitor tipifarnib in combination with gemcitabine in patients with advanced malignancies. *Clin Cancer Res*, 9(13), 4761–71.

Patnaik A, Mita AC, Izbicka E et al. (2004) A phase I, pharmacokinetic (PK) and pharmacodynamic (PD) study of the farnesyltransferase inhibitor (FTI) R115777 in combination with weekly paclitaxel in patients (pts) with advanced solid tumors. *Proc Am Soc Clin Oncol*, abst 3136.

Perez R, Smith JW, Alberts SR et al. (2001) Phase II trial of ISIS 2503, an antisense inhibitor of H-ras, in patients with advanced pancreatic carcinoma. *Proc Am Soc Clin Oncol*, 20, abst 628.

Piccart-Gebhart MJ, Brandle F, de Valeriola D *et al.* (2001) A phase I, clinical and pharmacokinetic (PK) trial of the farnesyltransferase inhibitor (FTI) R115,777 and docetaxel: A promising combination in patients with solid tumors. *Proc Am Soc Clin Oncol*, **20**, abst 318.

Pierson AS, Holden SN, Basche M *et al.* (2002) A phase I pharmacokinetic (PK) and biological study of the farnesyltransferase inhibitor (FTI) sarasar (lonafarnib, SCH66336), cisplatin (C), and gemcitabine (G) in patients (pts) with advanced solid tumors. *Proc Am Soc Clin Oncol*, **21**, abst 365.

Prior I, Hancock JF (2001) Compartmentalization of Ras proteins. *J Cell Sci*, **114**, 1603–8.

Qiu RG, Chen J, McCornick F, Symons M (1995) A role for Rho in ras transformation. *Proc Natl Acad Sci USA*, **92**, 11781–5.

Rao S, Cunningham D, de Gramont A *et al.* (2004) Phase II double-blind placebo-controlled study of farnesyltransferase inhibitor R115777 in patients with refractory advanced colorectal cancer. *J Clin Oncol*, **19**, 3950–7.

Ravoet C, Mineur P, Robin V *et al.* (2002) Phase I-II study of a farnesyltransfrase inhibitor (FTI), SCH66336, in patients with myelodysplastic syndrome (MDS) or secondary acute myeloid leukaemia (sAML). *Blood*, **100**, 694a.

Reddy EP, Reynolds RK, Santos E, Barbacid M (1982) A point mutation is responsible for the acquisition of transforming properties by T24 human bladder carcinoma oncogene. *Nature*, **300**, 149–52.

Reuther G, Der C (2000) The ras branch of small GTPases: ras family members don't fall far from the tree. *Curr Opin Cell Biol*, **12**, 157–65.

Rodriguez Viciana P, Warne PH, Khwaja A *et al.* (1997) Phosphatidylinositol-3-OH kinase as a direct target of Raps. *Cell*, **89**, 457–67.

Rowinsky EK, Windle JJ, Von Hoff DD (1999) Ras protein farnesyltransferase: A strategic target for anticancer drug development. *J Clin Oncol*, **17**, 3631–52.

Rubin E, Abbruzzese J, Morisson B *et al.* (2000) Phase I trial of the farnesyl protein transferase (FPTase) inhibitor L-778123 on a 14 or 28-day dosing schedule. *Proc Am Soc Clin Oncol*, **19**, abstr 689.

Ryan DP, Eder JP Jr, Puchlaski T *et al.* (2004) Phase I clinical trial of the farnesyltransferase inhibitor BMS-214662 given as a 1-hour intravenous infusion in patients with advanced solid tumors. *Clin Cancer Res*, **10**, 2222–30.

Saleh MN, Posey J, Pleasant L *et al.* (2000) A phase II trial of ISIS 2503, an antisense inhibitor of H-ras as first line therapy for advanced colorectal carcinoma. *Proc Am Soc Clin Oncol*, **19**, abst 1258.

Saleh MN, Irvin D, Burton G *et al.* (2003) Phase 2 trial of ISIS 2503, an antisense inhibitor of H-ras, in combination with weekly paclitaxel in the treatment of patients with metastatic breast cancer. *Proc Am Soc Clin Oncol*, **22**, abst 829.

Sebti SM, Hamilton AD. (2000) Farnesyltransferase and geranylgeranytransferase I inhibitors as novel agents for cancer and cardiovascular diseases. In *Farnesyltransferase inhibitors in cancer therapy* (ed. Sebti M, Hamilton, AD), pp. 197–220. Totowa, NJ, Humana Press.

Sepp-Lorenzino L, Ma Z, Rands E (1995) A peptidomimetic inhibitor of farnesyl: protein transferase blocks the anchorage-dependent and independent growth of human tumor cell lines. *Cancer Res*, **55**, 5302–9.

Sharma S, Kemeny N, Kelsen DP *et al.* (2002) A phase II trial of farnesyl protein transferase inhibitor SCH66336 given by twice-daily oral administration, in patients with metastatic colorectal cancer refractory to 5-fluorouracil and irinotecan. *Ann Oncol*, **13**, 1067–71.

Sinensky M, Fantle K, Trujilo MA, McLain T, Kupfer A, Dalton M (1994) The processing pathway of prelamin A. *J Cell Sci*, **107**, 61–7.

Skrzat S, Angibaud P, Venet M *et al.* (1998) R115777, a novel imidazole farnesyl protein transferase inhibitor (FTI) with potent oral anti-tumor activity. *Proc Am Assoc Cancer Res*, **39**, 2169A.

Slamon D, Godolphin W, Jones A *et al.* (1989) Studies of the HER2/neu proto-oncogene in human breast and ovarian cancer. *Science*, **244**, 707–12.

Smets G, Xhonneux B, Cornelissen F *et al.* (1998) R115777, a selective farnesyl protein transferase inhibitor (FTI), induces anti-angiogenic, apoptotic and anti-proliferative activity in CAPAN-2 and LoVo tumor xenografts. *Proc Am Assoc Cancer Res*, **39**, abst 2170.

Smith V, Rowlands MG, Barrie E, Workman P, Kelland LR (2002) Establishment and characterization of acquired resistance to the farnesyltransferase inhibitor R115777 in a human colon cancer cell line. *Clin Cancer Res*, **8**, 2002–9.

Sonnichsen D, Damle B, Manning J *et al.* (2000) Pharmacokinetics (PK) and Pharmacodynamics (PD) of the Farnesyltransferase (FT) inhibitor BMS-214662 in patients with advanced solid tumors. *Proc Am Soc Clin Oncol*, **19**, abst 691.

Sparano JA, Hopkins U, Moulder S *et al.* (2004) A phase I trial of the farnesyltransferase inhibitor plus doxorubicin-cyclophosphamide in patients with metastatic breast cancer. *Proc Am Soc Clin Oncol*, **23**, abst 676.

Spareboom A, Kehrer DF, Mathijssen RH *et al.* (2004) Phase I and pharmacokinetic study of irinotecan in combination with R115777, a farnesyltransferase inhibitor. *Br J Cancer*, **90**, 1508–15.

Sprague E, Vokes EE, Garland LL *et al.* (2002) Phase I study of continuous lonafarnib plus paclitaxel and carboplatin in refractory or advanced solid tumors. *Proc Am Soc Clin Oncol*, **21**, abst 1920.

Sternberg PW, Alberola-Ila J (1998) Conspiracy theory: RAS and RAF do not act alone. *Cell* **95**(4), 447–50.

Van Cutsem E, van de VeldeH, Karasek P *et al.* (2004) Phase III trial of gemcitabine plus tipifarnib compared with gemcitabine plus placebo in advanced pancreatic cancer. *J Clin Oncol*, **22**, 1430–8.

Vogelstein B, Fearon ER, Hamilton SR *et al.* (1988) Genetic alterations during colorectal tumor development. *N Engl J Med*, **319**, 525–32.

Vogel CL, Cobleigh MA, Tripathy D *et al.* (2002) Efficacy and safety of trastuzumab as a single agent in first-line treatment of HER2-overexpressing metastatic breast cancer. *J Clin Oncol*, **2**, 719–26.

Voi M, Tabernero J, Cooper MR *et al.* (2001) A phase I study of the farnesyltransferase (FT) inhibitor BMS-214662 administered as a weekly 1-hour infusion in patients with advanced solid tumors: clinical findings. *Proc Am Soc Clin Oncol*, abst 312.

Vojtek AB, Der CJ (1998) Increasing complexity of the Ras signaling pathway, *J Biol Chem*, **273**, 19925–28.

Wang EJ, Johnson WW (2003) The farnesyl protein transferase inhibitor lonafarnib (SCH66226) an inhibitor of multi-drug resistance proteins 1 and 2. *Chemotherapy*, **49**, 303–8.

Widemann BC, Fox E, Goodspeed W *et al.* (2003) Phase I trial of the farnesyltransferase inhibitor (FTI) R115,777 in children with refractory leukaemias. *Proc Am Soc Clin Oncol*, **22**, abst 3250.

Whitehead Pr, McCoy S, Mac Donald J *et al.* (2003) Phase I trial of R115, 777 (NSC#70818) in patients with advanced colorectal carcinoma: A Southwest Oncology Group study. *Proc Am Soc Clin Oncol*, **22**, abst 1092.

Whyte DB, Kirschmeier P, Hockenberry TN *et al.* (1997) K- and N-*ras* are geranylgeranylated in cells treated with farnesylprotein transferase inhibitors. J Biol Chem, **272**, 14459–64.

Zimmerman TM, Harlin H, Odenike T *et al.* (2003) Dose-ranging pharmacodynamic study of R115,777 in patients with refractory hematologic malignancies. *Proc Am Soc Clin Oncol*, **22**, abst 853.

Zhang FL, Kirschmeier P, Carr D *et al.* (1997) Characterization of Ha-Ras, N-Ras, Ki-Ras4A and Ki-Ras4B as *in vitro* substrates for farnesylprotein transferase and geranylgeranylprotein transferase and geranylgeranylprotein transferase type I. *J Biol Chem*, **272**, 10–232–39.

Zhu AX, Supko JG, Ryan DP *et al.* (2002) A phase I clinical, pharmacokinetic and pharmacodynamic study of the farnesyltransferase inhibitor BMS214662 given as a 24 hours continuous intravenous infusion once weekly X 3 in patients with advanced solid malignancies. *Proc Am Soc Clin Oncol*, **21**, abst 366.

Zujewski J, Horak ID, Bol R *et al.* (2000) Phase I and pharmacokinetic study of farnesyl protein transferase inhibitor R115777 in advanced cancer. *J Clin Oncol*, **18**, 927–41.

Chapter 6

The development of cell cycle active agents for cancer therapy

Manish A. Shah, Archie Tse, and Gary K. Schwartz

1 Introduction

With advancements in our understanding of the basic mechanisms of oncogenesis and the induction of **apoptosis**, we have gained a greater appreciation
of the critical role cell cycle regulation plays in malignant transformation and
in the development of resistance to chemotherapy. Perturbations in the cell
cycle are commonly described in carcinogenesis. Furthermore, with our improved understanding of the effects of chemotherapy on normal and cancerous cells, it is increasingly apparent that the cell cycle also plays a critical role in
the development of resistance to chemotherapy. These observations have led
to the development of a new class of anticancer therapeutics in clinical
development today: specifically, those drugs that target the motors of the
cell cycle, the **cyclin-dependent kinases (CDKs)**.

The development of **CDK inhibitors (CDKIs)** has underdone a gradual
evolution. This class of drugs was first primarily applied in the treatment of
malignancy as single agents, in efforts to target the errors of cell cycle regulation
that are already prevalent in malignant cells to achieve tumour-specific cytotoxicity. Presently, these agents are increasingly used in combination with traditional
cytotoxic drugs to overcome cell cycle mediated drug resistance and to improve
cytotoxic efficacy. Along with this shift in development has come an improved
understanding of the role the cell cycle plays in drug resistance.

In this chapter, we describe the cell cycle and its relation to programmed cell
death. We discuss the rationale for cell cycle modulation in drug development, as
well as the emerging concept of cell cycle mediated drug resistance. Specifically,
we describe the cell cycle and the various mechanisms by which novel CDK
inhibitors impact on this cycle. We briefly describe the pre-clinical and clinical

development of these agents, with a particular emphasis on the concept of cell cycle mediated drug resistance and how novel CDK inhibitors are used to overcome this resistance to improve anti-tumour efficacy. We also highlight the importance of sequence of administration of combination chemotherapy as a mechanism to overcome cell cycle mediated resistance.

2 The cell cycle and its regulation

2.1 Cell-cycle machinery

The cell cycle is a critical regulator of the processes of cell proliferation and growth (as mentioned in Chapter 1), as well as of cell division following DNA damage. It governs the transition from quiescence (G_0) to cell proliferation, and through its checkpoints, ensures the fidelity of the genetic transcript. It is the mechanism by which cells reproduce, and is typically divided into four phases. The periods associated with DNA synthesis (S phase) and mitosis (M phase) are separated by gaps of varying length called G_1 and G_2 (Fig. 6.1). Progression of a cell through the cell cycle is promoted by a number of cyclin-dependent kinases (CDKs), which, when complexed with specific regulatory proteins called cyclins, drive the cell forward through the cell cycle. There exist corresponding cell cycle inhibitory proteins (cyclin-dependent kinase inhibitors, CDKIs) that serve as negative regulators of the cell cycle and stop the cell from proceeding to the next phase of the cell cycle (see Fig. 6.1). The INK4 (for inhibitor of CDK4) class of CDKIs, notably $p16^{Ink4a}$, $p15^{Ink4b}$, $p18^{Ink4c}$, and $p19^{Ink4d}$, bind and inhibit cyclin D associated kinases (CDK2, 4, and 6). The KIP (kinase inhibitor protein) group of CDK inhibitors, $p21^{waf1}$, $p27^{kip1}$, and $p57^{kip2}$, negatively regulate cyclin E/CDK2 and cyclin A/CDK2 complexes (Sherr and Roberts 1999).

The pattern of cyclin expression varies with a cell's progression through the cell cycle, and this specific cyclin-expression pattern defines the relative position of the cell within the cell cycle (Grana and Reddy 1995; Johnson and Walker 1999). At least nine structurally related CDKs (CDK1–CDK9) have been identified, though not all have clearly defined cell cycle regulatory roles. A considerable number of cyclins have been identified to date (cyclin A–cyclin T). CDK/cyclin complexes themselves become activated by phosphorylation at specific sites on the CDK by CDK7/cyclin H, also referred to as CDK-activating kinase (CAK) (Kaldis *et al.* 1998). Cyclin D isoforms (cyclin D1-D3) interact with CDK2,4, and 6 and drive a cell's progression through G_1. The association of cyclin E with CDK2 is active at the G_1/S transition and directs entry into S phase. S-phase progression is directed by the cyclin A/CDK2 complex, and the complex of cyclin A with CDK1 (also known as cdc2) is important in G_2. CDK1/cyclin B is necessary for mitosis to occur.

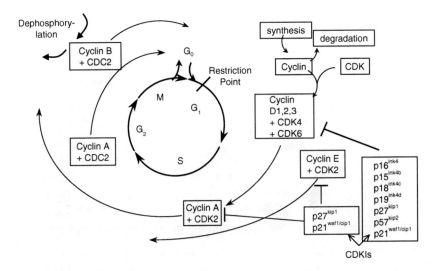

Fig. 6.1 Control of the cell cycle. The cell cycle is divided into four distinct phases (G_1, S, G_2, and M). G_0 represents exit from the cell cycle in which the cell performs its routine functions, including the important function of cell growth. The progression of a cell through the cell cycle is promoted by CDKs, which are positively and negatively regulated by cyclins and CDKIs, respectively. The Restriction Point governs the transition point beyond which a cells progression through the cell cycle is independent of external stimuli.

2.2 Cell cycle regulation: from G_0 to M

Normal cells need to decide when to divide (i.e. enter the cell cycle) and when to stay in G_0. Although often termed a quiescent phase, G_0 is in fact quite an active phase in which, cellular functions and cellular growth occur. It is necessarily tightly regulated because the alternative, i.e. uncontrolled cell division without cell growth, would lead to smaller cells with each division. The entry into the cell cycle (G_1) is historically governed by the Restriction Point—a transition point beyond which cell progression through the cell cycle is independent of external stimuli such as exposure to nutrients or **mitogen** activation (Pardee 1974). This point of determination is thought to divide the early and late G_1 phase of the cell cycle. Mitogenic signalling of a variety of growth signals is mediated by the RAS/RAF/MAPK pathway, whose endpoint is the stimulation of D-type cyclin production. The retinoblastoma **tumour suppressor gene** product (Rb) governs the G_1/S transition (see Fig. 6.2). In its active state, Rb is hypophosphorylated and forms an inhibitory complex with a group of **transcription** factors known as E2F-DP (E2F-1, -2, and -3), thus controlling the G_1/S transition. The activity of Rb is modulated by

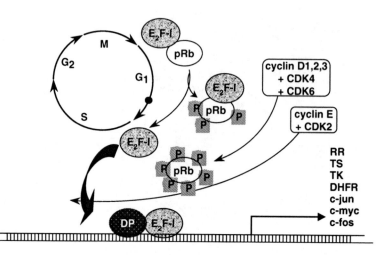

Fig. 6.2 The G_1/S transition and Rb regulation. Retinoblastoma gene product (Rb) governs entry into S phase. In its active state, Rb is hypophosphorylated and forms a complex with a group of transcription factors known as E2F (E2F-1, E2F-2, and E2F-3). CDK4 and CDK6 partially phosphorylate Rb, resulting in partial activation of this transcription factor. Cyclin E is then transcribed and binds to CDK2 to completely hyperphosphorylate Rb, leading to it's complete inactivation and complete release of the E2F transcription factors. This results in the transcription of a wide range of targets involved in chemotherapy sensitivity including ribonucleotide reductase (RR), thymidylate synthase (TS), thymidine kinase (TK), dihydrofolate reductase (DHFR), c-jun, c-myc, and c-fos.

the sequential phosphorylation by CDK4/6-cyclin D and CDK2/cyclin E (reviewed in Malumbres and Barbacid 2001). When Rb is partially phosphorylated by CDK4/6-cyclin D kinases, Rb remains bound to E2F-DP, but this transcription factor is still able to transcribe some genes such as cyclin E. Cyclin E then binds to CDK2 and this active complex then completely hyperphosphorylates Rb, thus releasing the E2F-DP complex and fully activating the E2F transcription factors, resulting in transcriptional activation of numerous S-phase proteins, such as thymidylate synthase (TS) and dihydrofolate reductase (DHFR). In addition to Rb, CDK2 phophorylates other substrates involved in DNA replication (Sherr 2000).

Early in S phase, cyclins D and E are targeted by **ubiquitination** for **proteosome** degradation (Elledge and Harper 1998). The production of cyclin A and its complexing with CDK2 enables S-phase progression, with the production of other enzymes and proteins involved in DNA synthesis, including histones and proliferating cell nuclear antigen (PCNA) (reviewed by Ford and Pardee 1998). During late S and throughout G_2, cells prepare for mitosis by increasing levels of cyclins A and B. As the level of cyclin B rises, it forms a complex with cdc2 (CDK 1) in the cytoplasm, where it remains until mitosis, at which point it shuttles into the **nucleus**. Recently, an S-phase check point has been described, also termed the replication checkpoint (Xu *et al.* 2001; Zhou and Elledge 2000). This checkpoint monitors progression through S phase and slows the rate of on-going DNA synthesis. The S-phase checkpoint is thought to involve activations of ATM and ATR kinases with subsequent activation of Chk1 and Chk2 (Falck *et al.* 2001; Xu *et al.* 2001; Zhou 2002; Zhou and Elledge 2000). These pathways ultimately control the ability of a cell to enter mitosis, which is dependent on the completion of S phase. Entry into mitosis is determined by the activity of the cyclin B/cdc2 complex, which is tightly regulated by its phosphorylation status, both by an activating phosphorylation at Thr161 by CAK and inhibitory phosphorylations at Thr14 and Thr15. At completion of S phase, wee1 kinase is degraded by **proteolysis** in a cdc34-dependent fashion, and the phosphatase, cdc25c, is activated by a regulatory phosphorylation, which leads to cyclin B/cdc2 activation. This complex then rapidly is relocated into the nucleus and mitosis begins (Ford and Pardee 1998, 1999). Upon DNA damage, however, ATM and ATR are activated leading to a checkpoint kinase 1 (Chk1) and Chk2 phosphorylation, and an inhibitory phosphorylation of Cdc-25c, which prevents the activation of cyclin B/cdc 2 and halts further S-phase progression and the entry into mitosis (Xu *et al.* 2001; Zhou *et al.* 2002).

Progression through mitosis is dependent on the anaphase-promoting complex (APC)/cyclosome and the degradation of cyclin B (Ford and Pardee 1999). During mitosis, the assembly of a bipolar spindle by the centrosome is vital to the preservation of genetic fidelity between daughter cells, and is monitored by a checkpoint that senses microtubule defects (Anderson 2000) or aberrant kinetochore attachment (Nicklas 1997; Rudner and Murray 1996). Centrosome abnormalities are often observed in malignancy, responsible for **chromosome** mis-segregation and resultant genomic instability (Salisbury *et al.* 1999). Centrosome maturation is critical for cell division to occur and is regulated by several kinases including *polo* kinase and *aurora* kinase. Centrosome maturation begins with centriole duplication, which occurs in G_1 and is triggered by CDK2/cyclin E and CDK2/cyclin D activity. Elongation of the centriole occurs throughout S phase so that by prophase, the cell has two pairs of centrioles within the pericentriolar material (reviewed by Blagden and Glover 2003). Polo kinase is involved in recruiting γ-tubulin and in activating the Asp protein, abnormal spindles gene product (Blagden and Glover 2003). The Aurora kinase is also involved in centrosome maturation. This **protein kinase** appears to be required for correct spindle pole structure and bipolarity of the spindle (Glover *et al.* 1995), and appears to be essential in the duplication/separation stage of the centriole cycle (Geit and al. 2002). Survivin has been implicated in the regulation of the mitotic spindle and in the preservation of cell viability, due in large part to its expression during cell division in a cell cycle-dependent manner and localisation to the mitotic apparatus (Altieri 2001; Reed and Bischoff 2000). Cyclin B1/cdc2 activity during mitosis plays a critical role in survivin expression and function in cell viability (O'Connor *et al.* 2002).

2.3 Programmed cell death

Apoptosis is an active, energy-dependent process in which the cell participates in its own destruction. Morphologic features of apoptosis include cell shrinkage, nuclear chromatin condensation, and the formation of pedunculated protuberances on the cell surface known as apoptotic bodies (Kerr *et al.* 1972; Reed 1999), a process that results in the degradation of genomic DNA by endonucleases (Martin and Green 1995). The molecular cascade of apoptosis is characterised by the early release of mitochondrial cytochrome C, activation of 'apoptotic protease activating factor' (Apaf-1), activation of **caspase** 9, and subsequent cleavage of downstream or 'effector' caspases in a self-amplifying cascade. Effector caspases finally degrade a number of cellular proteins, such as poly-adenosine $5'$-diphosphate-ribosyl polymerase (PARP), laminin and β-actin (see Fig. 6.3.) (Kaufmann *et al.* 1993; Lazebnik *et al.* 1995) The biochemical cascade of apoptosis is subject to regulation at several levels.

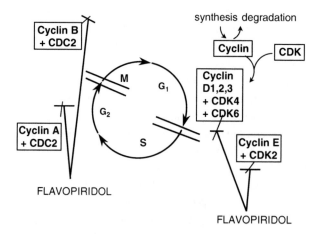

Fig. 6.3 Flavopiridol cell cycle-effects. Flavopiridol is a pan-CDK inhibitor of CDK2, CDK4, and CDK6 at nanomolar concentrations resulting in cell-cycle arrest at both the G_1/S transition and the G_2/M transition.

Members of the Bcl-2 family of proteins may be either anti-apoptotic in nature (Bcl-2, Bcl-XL, Bcl-W, Mcl-1, A1/Bfi-1), or pro-apoptotic, acting to enhance apoptosis (BAD, Bax, Bak, and others). Bcl-2 or Bcl-XL bind and inhibit Apaf-1 and consequently prevent the activation of caspases. In the presence of excess Bax, however, Bcl-2 is displaced from Apaf-1 allowing caspase cleavage and activation. Bax further promotes apoptosis by mediating the release of cytochrome C from **mitochondria**. Caspases, themselves are subject to regulation. A number of inhibitors of apoptosis protein (IAP), or caspase inhibitors, have been identified (Reed 1999).

The failure of many chemotherapeutic agents reflects an inability of these drugs to induce apoptosis. Indeed, neoplastic cells have acquired a number of cellular adaptations and mutations, which act as survival factors, thus preventing the induction of apoptosis. For example, tumour cells with a mutation in the **p53** gene have shown resistance to undergo apoptosis in the presence of chemotherapy (Lowe et al. 1993). Other examples of tumour resistance to the induction of apoptosis is the overexpression of Bcl-2 (Eliopoulos et al. 1995), Bcl-x$_L$ (Datta et al. 1995; Ibardo et al. 1996), and the induction of NfκB activity (Gajewski and Thompson 1996; Jarvis and Grant 1999).

The cell cycle and apoptosis are intimately related, as evidenced by the central role of p53, both in cell cycle arrest and in the induction of apoptosis. p53 induction by DNA damage causes arrest in both the G$_1$ and G$_2$ phases of the cell cycle (El-Diery et al. 1994; Levine 1997). G$_1$ arrest is due primarily to the induction of p21, whereas the arrest in G$_2$ is due to the induction of both p21 and 14–3–3σ, a protein that normally sequesters cyclinB/cdc2 complexes in the nucleus (Bunz et al. 1999; Chan et al. 2000). p53 is also critical in the induction of apoptosis by activating the transcription of multiple apoptosis-associated genes(Clarke et al. 1994; Yu et al. 1999). Another example of this intimate relationship is demonstrated in human colon cancer cell lines that differ only in their p21 checkpoint status. Cells with **wild type** p21, when irradiated with gamma-radiation, undergo a cell cycle growth arrest followed by clonogenic survival; whereas cells lacking p21, when irradiated with gamma-radiation, do not undergo a cell cycle growth arrest and proceed to apoptosis (Waldman 1997). Cells that undergo a growth arrest may be protected from apoptosis and may therefore be ultimately resistant to the cytotoxic agent.

3   The cell cycle as a target for cancer therapeutics

The rationale for targeting the cell cycle, and in particular the CDKs, in anticancer therapy lies in the frequency of their perturbations in human malignancy and the observation that cell cycle arrest by CDK inhibition would induce apoptosis. Most tumour suppressor genes and **oncogenes** are components of signal **transduction** pathways that control several cellular functions including cell cycle entry and exit (Harper and Elledge 1996; Hartwell and Kastan 1994). In contrast to normal cells, tumour cells are unable to stop at predetermined points of the cell cycle because of loss of checkpoint integrity. This can be due to inactivation of critical CDKIs, or to overexpression of cyclins. For example, p16 is an INK4 gene that is particularly sensitive to epigenetic silencing by hypermethylation of its **promoter** region, which results in inhibition of transcription and loss of gene expression. When this occurs, uncontrolled proliferation can result. Accordingly, loss of p16 function has been associated with a multitude of malignancies including melanoma, lung, breast, and color-ectal tumours (Shahjehan *et al.* 2001). Similarly, overexpression of cyclin D1 has been associated with the development and progression of breast cancer (Buckley *et al.* 1993; Sutherland and Musgrove 2002). Thus, targeting CDKs would re-capitulate cell cycle checkpoints, which would necessarily limit a tumour cell's ability to cycle, and this may then facilitate the induction of apoptosis (Chen *et al.* 1999).

This rationale led to the development of CDK inhibitors as novel anti-tumour agents. These compounds can inhibit CDKs by direct effects that target the catalytic CDK subunit, or by indirect means that target regulatory pathways that govern CDK activity (Senderowicz 2002). Several small molecule CDK inihibitors are currently in development, as described below.

3.1 Flavopiridol

Flavopiridol is a novel anti-neoplastic agent that originally was noted for its ability to inhibit the activity of a number of protein kinases. Flavopiridol is now best classified as a CDKI because of its considerable affinity for CDKs and its ability to induce cell cycle arrest in a number of cell lines (Carlson *et al.* 1996; Losiewicz *et al.* 1994). It has been shown to bind to and directly inhibit CDK1 (cyclin B1-cdc2 kinase), CDK2, CDK4, and CDK6 (see Fig. 6.3).

Flavopiridol administration has been associated with the selective induction of apoptotic cell death, particularly in haematopoietic cell lines (Byrd *et al.* 1998; Konig *et al.* 1997). This induction of apoptosis may be mediated by an early activation of the MAPK protein kinase family of proteins (MEK, p38, and JNK), leading to activation of caspases (Cartee *et al.* 2001). Cell cycle arrest and the induction of apoptosis have been also demonstrated in squamous head and neck cell lines and other pre-clinical models (Bible and Kaufmann 1996; Schrump *et al.* 1998). The apoptotic effect appears to be independent of p53 and is associated with the depletion of cyclin D1 (Carlson *et al.* 1999). **Xenograft** studies have confirmed these *in vitro* results (Drees *et al.* 1997;

Patel *et al.* 1998), leading to single-agent clinical evaluation. The initial schedule of administration, based on the pre-clinical data, was a 72-h continuous infusion schedule administered every 2 weeks, resulting in nanomolar peak flavopiridol concentrations (Senderowicz *et al.* 1998; Thomas *et al.* 2002). To date, flavopiridol has demonstrated no significant clinical activity as a single agent in non-small cell lung cancer, gastric cancer, colorectal cancer, melanoma, renal cell cancer, or lymphoma (Bennett *et al.* 1999; Burdette-Radoux *et al.* 2002; Lin *et al.* 2002; Schwartz *et al.* 2001; Shapiro *et al.* 2001; Stadler 2000).

3.2 UCN-01

UCN-01 (7-hydroxystaurosporine) is a staurosporine analogue isolated from the culture broth of *Streptomyces* species, and is a selective inhibitor of protein kinase C (Takahashi *et al.* 1989). UCN-01 is associated with a G_1/S cell cycle arrest (Kawakami *et al.* 1996), associated with the induction of p21CIP/Waf1,

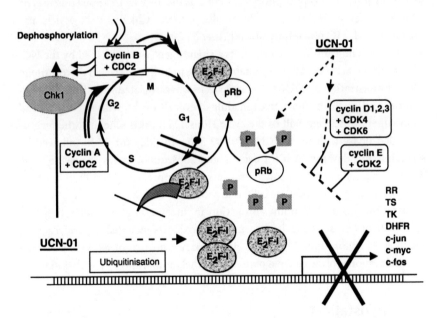

Fig. 6.4 UCN-01 cell cycle effects. UCN-01 has cell-cycle effects at both the G_1/S and G_2/M transition. At G_1/S, UCN-01 hypophorphorylates Rb and causes the destruction of free E2F-1 by ubiquitinisation and targeting for proteosome degradation. The net effect is an arrest in G_1 and a significant reduction in early S-phase proteins, including ribonucleotide reductase and TS. At the G_2/M transition, through inhibition of Chk1, UCN-01 increases the activity of Cyclin B/CDC2 resulting in a G_2-checkpoint abrogation and a pre-mature entry into M.

dephosphorylation of CDK2 (Akiyama *et al.* 1997), and with the resultant dephosphorylation of the retinoblastoma gene product (pRb) (Akiyama *et al.* 1997; Kawakami *et al.* 1996). Hypophosphorylated pRb remains tightly bound to E2F-1, thereby preventing cell cycle progression into S phase (Fan and Steer 1996). Additionally, UCN-01 causes the degradation of E2F-1 by targeting the transcription factor for proteosome degradation by ubiquitinisation (see Fig. 6.4) (Hsueh *et al.* 1998).

UCN-01 also abrogates the G_2 checkpoint. It inhibits the Chk1 kinase, which is involved in the regulation of Cdc25C and 14-3-3 proteins in response to DNA damage (Busby *et al.* 2000; Graves *et al.* 2000). The 14-3-3 protein binds to Cdc25C and prevents this phosphatase from entering the nucleus where it dephosphorylates Cdc2. This dephosphorylation activates the cyclin B/Cdc2 kinase and allows cells to progress towards mitosis. The phosphorylation of Cdc25C on serine 216 by Chk1 prevents 14-3-3 protein binding, thereby allowing Cdc25C to enter the nucleus and dephosphorylate Cdc2. UCN-01 inhibits this phosphorylation of Cdc25C by Chk1 kinase (Busby *et al.* 2000; Graves *et al.* 2000). UCN-01 also inhibits Chk2 kinase, which also regulates Cdc25C phosphorylation (Yu *et al.* 2002).

The first clinical trial of UCN-01 as a single agent was published by the NCI (Sausville *et al.* 2001). Due to protein binding to human α-1-acid glycoprotein, the administration of UCN-01 every 2 weeks was associated with drug accumulation, leading to an alternative schedule of every 4 weeks, with the second and subsequent doses one-half of the cycle 1 dose. With this schedule, the recommended phase II dose of UCN-01 is 42.5 mg/m^2/day for 72 h, followed by 42.5 mg/m^2/day for 36 h for cycle 2 and subsequent cycles (Sausville *et al.* 2001). Free salivary drug concentrations were approximately 100 nM, which has been shown to modulate cell cycle processes. This was supported by demonstration of G_2 checkpoint abrogation in an *ex vivo* assay, suggesting that UCN-01 did in fact reach its target. Major toxicities included hyperglycaemia, nausea and vomiting. There was preliminary evidence of activity with one partial response observed in a patient with melanoma, and 19 patients demonstrating stable disease with a median duration of 5 months (Sausville *et al.* 2001).

3.3 Bryostatin-1

The bryostatins are macrocyclic lactones with a unique polyacetate backbone. Bryostatin-1 was isolated from the marine invertebrate *Bugula neritina* and first characterised after showing high activity against the murine P388 lymphocytic leukaemia. Currently there are 20 known natural bryostatins, distinguished by their substituents at C7 and C20 (Mutter and Wills 2000).

The main binding sites in bryostatins include the C_1, C_{19} and C_{26} oxygen atoms (Wender *et al.* 1988).

Bryostatin-1 has a unique mechanism of action in that, like phorbol esters, it can be a potent activator of PKC (Kraft *et al.* 1986). Short-term exposure of tumour cells to bryostatin-1 induces PKC activation and autophosphorylation, followed by translocation of the enzyme to the cellular or nuclear membrane. However, despite sharing the same binding sites, phorbolesters have tumour-promoting properties, while bryostatin-1 has anti-neoplastic properties that, in fact, can inhibit phorbol ester-mediated tumour promotion (Hennings *et al.* 1987). Prolonged exposure of tumour cells to bryostatin-1 induces PKC inhibition by causing depletion from the cell (Isakov *et al.* 1993), probably through ubiquitin-mediated proteasomal degradation (Lee *et al.* 1996).

Bryostatin-1 affects the activity of certain cell cycle regulatory proteins, although the resulting effects on apoptosis are inconsistent. Bryostatin-1 produces transient induction of p21 and subsequent dephosphorylation and inactivation of CDK2 (Fig. 6.5). The degree of CDK2 dephosphorylation correlated with the inhibition of tumour cell growth (Asiedu *et al.* 1995). However, bryostatin-1 also interferes with the up-regulation of p21 produced by phorbol esters (Vrana *et al.* 1998). In U937 cells, pretreatment with deoxycytidine blocked bryostatin-mediated p21 induction, and enhanced apoptosis (Vrana *et al.* 1999). Bryostatin also decreased cyclin-B expression in tumour xenografts, resulting in the prevention of paclitaxel-mediated cdc2 kinase activation (Koutcher *et al.* 2000). The net effect is an arrest of cells in G_2.

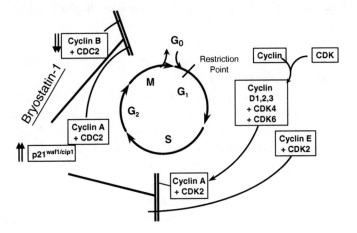

Fig. 6.5 Bryostatin-1 cell cycle effects. The cell cycle effects of bryostatin-1 primarily are in CDK2 inhibition, by the transient induction of p21 and by the decrease in cyclin B levels. The net result is a G_2 cell-cycle arrest.

Phase I studies of bryostatin have explored various infusion rates and dosing schedules (Philip *et al.* 1993; Prendiville *et al.* 1993), with dose-limiting toxicity being myalgia. The MTD remains $25\mu g/m^2$/week when bryostatin-1 is infused over 24-h (Jayson *et al.* 1995). The MTD of bryostatin, given as a 72-h continuous infusion every 2 weeks, was $120\mu g/m^2$. In contrast to shorter infusion durations, haematologic toxicity was uncommon (Varterasian *et al.* 1998). Limited single-agent activity was noted with bryostatin in patients with melanoma, ovarian cancer, and non-Hodgkin's lymphoma in a phase I trial (Jayson *et al.* 1995). However, single-agent phase II trials have not demonstrated significant activity, including trials in melanoma (Bedikian *et al.* 2001; Gonzalez *et al.* 1999; Propper *et al.* 1998), renal cell carcinoma (Pagliaro *et al.* 2000), colorectal cancer (Zonder *et al.* 2001), non-Hodgkin's lymphoma (Blackhall *et al.* 2001), and soft tissue sarcoma (Brockstein *et al.* 2001).

4 CDK inhibitors in combination therapy

4.1 Cell cycle mediated drug resistance: an emerging concept

The concept of tumour resistance to chemotherapy is based in part on the work of Luria and Delbruck, who found that bacteria spontaneously developed mutations that made them resistant to bacteriophage (DeVita 1997; Luria and Delbruck 1943). When applying this concept to cancer, Goldie and Coldman proposed that the probability that a given tumour will contain resistant clones at the time of diagnosis would be a function of the mutation rate of that cancer and the size of the tumour at diagnosis (Goldie and Coldman 1979, 1985). Even with low mutation rates of 1 in 10^6 mitoses, it would be virtually certain that drug-resistant mutants would populate the cells of a clinically detectable 1-cm tumour deposit (10^9 tumour cells) (DeVita 1997; Goldie and Coldman 1979, 1985).

In contrast, cell cycle mediated drug resistance is best described as a relative insensitivity to a chemotherapeutic agent due to the position of the cell in the cell cycle or, more precisely, due to the activation of cell cycle checkpoints, that interrupt cell cycle progression to allow time for repair. This is a recently recognised mechanism of resistance to cytotoxic chemotherapy. In combination chemotherapy, for example, one chemotherapeutic agent can impact the cell cycle such that the next chemotherapeutic agent given immediately in sequence becomes less effective (Shah and Schwartz 2001). Cell cycle mediated drug resistance limits the efficacy of many standard cytotoxic drugs and can be overcome by the appropriately scheduled administration of novel CDKIs. Below, we provide pre-clinical evidence of cell cycle mediated drug resistance and how it is overcome by CDKIs, and the initial clinical evaluation of CDKIs in combination chemotherapy.

To understand the role a cell cycle modulator may play in combination therapy, one must first understand the cell cycle effects of the cytotoxic agent. The cellular response to DNA damage is the activation of cell cycle checkpoints that serve as natural surveillance mechanisms for DNA integrity. Different cytotoxic agents are more effective in certain points during the cell cycle, and may elicit different cell cycle checkpoint responses. Below, we describe the cell cycle effects of taxanes, camptothecins, and gemcitabine as model cytotoxic chemotherapeutic classes, and then provide the pre-clinical and clinical data that support the use of CDK inhibitors to modulate their cytotoxicity in an effort to overcome cell cycle mediated drug resistance.

5 Combinations of CDK inhibitors with taxanes

5.1 Taxane cell cycle effects

The taxanes act by stabilising microtubules, thereby causing a G_2/M arrest followed by apoptosis. Unlike other known mitotic spindle inhibitors (vinca alkaloids, colchicine, and podophyllotoxin), which inhibit tubulin polymerisation, taxanes markedly enhance microtubule assembly and disrupt the transition through mitosis. The two primary taxanes in clinical use today are paclitaxel (Taxol®) and docetaxel (Taxotere®), however significantly more pre-clinical and clinical information has been presented with paclitaxel.

Paclitaxel promotes microtubule assembly and stabilises tubulin polymer formation (Schiff et al. 1979), thereby interrupting the dynamic cellular re-organisation necessary for mitosis (Schiff and Horwitz 1981), and resulting in a G_2/M arrest. (Schiff and Horwitz 1980) Paclitaxel is also associated with down-regulation of CDK4 (Yoo et al. 1998) with concomitant G_1/S arrest. The primary effect of paclitaxel is to interfere with the assembly of the mitotic spindle, resulting in the failure of chromosomes to segregate (Long and Fairchild 1994). As a microtubule promoter, paclitaxel shifts the equilibrium in favour of the microtubule and thus decreases the concentration of tubulin necessary for subsequent assembly (Brown et al. 1991). Mitosis is initiated by the activation of the cyclin B1-CDK1 complex (also called cyclin B1-cdc2 kinase), and as mitosis progresses, cyclin B is destroyed by ubiquitin-mediated proteolysis. Cyclin B and Cdc2 kinase activity are closely related to paclitaxel function. Expression of cyclin B and the activation of CDK1 occur coincidentally with paclitaxel-induced apoptosis (Donaldson et al. 1994a; Ling et al. 1998), and destruction of cyclin B1 can be inhibited by paclitaxel (Clute and

Pines 1999). Furthermore, a dominant negative mutant of p34cdc2 blocks paclitaxel-induced apoptosis (Yu *et al.* 1998).

Although cytotoxicity is maximal at G_2/M and minimal at G_1/S (Donaldson *et al.* 1994b), paclitaxel may induce apoptosis by other mechanisms as well. In particular, paclitaxel exposure is also associated with hyperphosphorylation of bcl-2 and phosphorylation of c-Raf-1 (Blagosklonny 1997; Johnson and Walker 1999), steps necessary for apoptosis.

5.2 Combinations with flavopiridol and bryostatin with taxanes: laboratory evaluation

The combination of each of these agents (flavopiridol or bryostatin-1) with taxanes demonstrates the concept of cell cycle mediated drug resistance. Flavopiridol was examined in combination with paclitaxel in various sequences in the MKN-74 human gastric cancer cell line, as well as the human breast cancer cell line MCF-7, which are both **heterozygous** for p53 (Motwani *et al.* 1999). Cell cycle mediated resistance was demonstrated when flavopiridol exposure was followed by paclitaxel. Flavopiridol's multiple cell cycle effects (including the inhibition of CDK4, CDK6, and CDK2 at G_1, and the inhibition of cyclin B1-cdc2 kinase activity at G_2; Motwani *et al.* 1999), creates a cell cycle arrest. This prevents cells from entering M phase, the phase during which paclitaxel is most active, and leads to a significant reduction in paclitaxel sensitivity in culture (Motwani *et al.* 1999). Similar results were reproduced in *in vitro* and *in vivo* combination studies with docetaxel (Motwani *et al.* 2003).

In a mouse mammary tumour xenograft system, treatment with bryostatin-1 followed by paclitaxel demonstrated bryostatin-1 mediated suppression of cyclin B1, and an associated decrease in cyclin B1-cdc2 kinase activity. This resulted in a significant reduction in paclitaxel sensitivity. In the mouse xenograft system, bryostatin-1 followed by paclitaxel was associated with a significant decrease in tumour doubling time as compared to paclitaxel alone (9.3 ± 1.9 days vs. 22.7 ± 2.5 days, $P<0.001$) (Kaubisch *et al.* 1999; Koutcher *et al.* 2000). Therefore, when either flavopiridol or bryostatin-1 is given first, as a consequence of cell cycle mediated drug resistance, sensitivity to the taxane is markedly reduced. In the case of flavopiridol, cells are arrested in the cell cycle and are insensitive to paclitaxel, which asserts its activity as cells enter M phase. In the case of bryostatin-1, cyclin B1-cdc2 kinase activity is reduced, resulting in cells arresting in G_2, as the cyclin B1-cdc2 kinase is associated with the activity of the spindle-assembly checkpoint (Clute and Pines 1999), and is required to initiate entry into M phase (Grana and Reddy 1995). Koutcher *et al.* demonstrated the G_2 cell cycle arrest *in vitro*: treatment of human MKN-74 gastric cancer cells with bryostatin-1 followed by paclitaxel, resulted in a decrease in cells entering M phase (23% vs. 56% with paclitaxel alone), and a concomitant increase in cells in G_2 (69% vs. 21% with paclitaxel alone) (Koutcher *et al.* 2000). As fewer cells enter M phase, the net effect is a significant decrease in paclitaxel sensitivity.

Cell cycle mediated drug resistance may be overcome by appropriate sequencing of the drug combination. The reverse sequence of paclitaxel followed by flavopiridol is associated with an increased induction of apoptosis (Bible and Kaufmann 1997; Motwani *et al.* 1999). This sequence is associated with an accelerated exit of cells from mitosis; an event that may be critical for the sequence-dependent enhancement of paclitaxel-induced apoptosis by flavopiridol. In the case of paclitaxel followed by bryostatin-1, there is decreased tumour metabolism and blood flow (Koutcher *et al.* 2000), which may impact on tumour growth. The increased sensitivity to paclitaxel when followed by bryostatin-1 may be explained in part by Bcl-2: Bax, the heterodimer pair that is closely associated with mitochondrial dysfunction and the initiation of apoptosis. Loss of the Bcl-2 phosphorylation loop domain (Wang *et al.* 1999a), and ectopic expression of Bcl-x_L (Schmitt *et al.* 1998), can protect human leukemia cells (U937) from paclitaxel-mediated apoptosis. Administration of bryostatin-1 following paclitaxel can overcome paclitaxel resistance in U937 cells ectopically expressing Bcl-x_L (Wang *et al.* 1999b), and is associated with an increase in the pro-apoptotic factor, Bax, with resultant increased sequence dependent apoptosis (Wang *et al.* 1998).

5.3 Taxane combinations with flavopiridol and bryostatin: clinical evaluation

The sequential combination of paclitaxel followed by flavopiridol has been evaluated in a phase I study (Schwartz 2001). The clinical results are remarkable for major responses in patients with chemotherapy refractory malignancies (i.e. prostate and esophagus), including patients who have received prior paclitaxel therapy. In particular, five of seven patients with oesophageal cancer responded to the combination treatment, three of whom received prior paclitaxel therapy (Schwartz *et al.* 2001). In this clinical trial, there was no effect of flavopiridol on paclitaxel pharmacokinetics. In a trial combining paclitaxel and bryostatin, patients were treated with a weekly dose of paclitaxel 80 mg/m^2 followed 24-h later with increasing doses bryostatin-1. Two partial responses were demonstrated, with 9/27 patients demonstrating stable disease, including a patient with metastatic pancreatic carcinoma, whose disease remained radiographically stable for 15 months. Again, we found no pharma-cokinetic effects on paclitaxel by bryostatin-1.

6 Combination of CDK inhibitors with camptothecins

6.1 Camptothecin cell cycle effects

Camptothecins induce their primary cytotoxicity during the period of DNA synthesis. These agents form a class of chemotherapeutic drugs derived from the Chinese tree *Camptotheca acuminata*. They are alkaloids that are potent inhibitors of the nuclear enzyme topoisomerase I (Slichenmeyer *et al.* 1993), an enzyme that functions primarily in the S phase of the cell cycle. In fact, cells in S phase are 100 to 1000 times more sensitive to camptothecin than cells in G_1 or G_2 (Li *et al.* 1972). Topoisomerase I induces transient single-stranded breaks of DNA, relieving torsional strain and permitting DNA unwinding ahead of the replication fork during S phase. Camptothecins stabilise the 'cleavable com-plex' between topoisomerase I and DNA. When these cleavable complexes collide with the moving DNA replication fork, double-stranded DNA breaks occur leading to cell death (Creemers *et al.* 1994). This apoptotic cell death is mediated by caspase activation, and inhibition of this caspase activation shifts the cells from apoptosis to transient G_1 arrest followed by cell necrosis (Sane and Bertrand 1999). Camptothecin treatment is associated with a G_2 cell cycle arrest (Tsao *et al.* 1992) at low concentrations, and an S-phase arrest at higher concentrations (Kohn *et al.* 2002). This arrest is p53 independent and is regulated via the ATM/ATR kinases, which are activated by DNA damage during S phase, with subsequent phosphorylation of Chk1 (Zhou *et al.* 2002). Apoptosis from short bolus exposure to camptothecin is not associated with changes in bcl-2, bax, p53, or p21 acutely, however prolonged exposure (greater than 72 h) is associated with increased expression of Bax (Weller *et al.* 1997). Finally, camptothecin treatment is associated with the transient and unscheduled stimulation of cyclin B1-cdc2 kinase activity prior to apoptosis in HL60 cells (Shimizu *et al.* 1995). The clinically important members of this class of chemotherapeutic agents include irinotecan and topotecan.

6.2 Irinotecan and flavopiridol

Cell cycle mediated drug resistance has been demonstrated in the human colon cancer cell line, HCT-116 (with an intact p53-p21 axis), both with irinotecan alone and with the combination of flavopiridol and irinotecan. The p21 gene is transcriptionally activated by p53 and is responsible for the p53-dependent checkpoint that results in a G_1 and G_2 arrest following DNA damage (Motwani *et al.* 2001). Treatment of human colon cancer HCT-116 cells with SN-38 alone (the active metabolite of irinotecan) is associated with an induction of p21, and a concomitant G_2 arrest, thereby rendering these cells resistant to SN-38 (and therefore to irinotecan), which is 1000 times more effective in S phase (Li *et al.* 1972). This cell cycle mediated drug resistance was demonstrated in culture by QFM analysis, where SN-38 exposure to HCT-116 cells resulted in only $1 \pm 1\%$ cell death (Motwani *et al.* 2001).

As a CDK inhibitor, flavopiridol itself induces a G_1 and G_2 cell cycle arrest: therefore, when flavopiridol precedes irinotecan, cell cycle mediated drug resistance should again be demonstrated. When HCT-116 cells were exposed to the drug sequence of flavopiridol followed by SN-38, QFM analysis demonstrated only $15\% \pm 2\%$ cell death. However, this cell cycle mediated resistance was again overcome by appropriate drug sequencing: SN-38 $\rightarrow$ flavopiridol resulted in significantly increased HCT-116 cell death at $44 \pm 2\%$ ($P<0.001$) (Motwani *et al.* 2001). This sequence (SN-38 $\rightarrow$ flavopiridol) demonstrated significant induction of apoptosis, as evidenced by PARP cleavage, caspase-3 activation, and DNA laddering.

The augmentation of the irinotecan's anti-tumour effect was also demonstrated in HCT-116 xenografts (Motwani *et al.* 2001). HCT-116 tumour implants were treated with irinotecan, flavopiridol, and irinotecan followed by flavopiridol separated by varying intervals from 2 to 24-h. In these experiments, the greatest tumour regression (the percent decrease in tumour volume) and cures were observed if the interval between irinotecan and flavopiridol was at least 7 to 16 h. Two weeks after the end of treatment (day 30), there was a $40 \pm 25\%$ regression of the tumour in mice treated with irinotecan alone; whereas in mice treated with CPT-11 followed by 7 or 16 h flavopiridol, the tumour regression was $86 \pm 9\%$ or $82 \pm 5\%$, respectively. The difference between the areas under the volume–time curve of CPT-11 alone and CPT-11 followed by flavopiridol after 7 or 16 h were statistically significant ($P = 0.0002$ and $P = 0.0005$, respectively). The cure rates for irinotecan followed by 7 or 16 h flavopiridol was 30% (3 of 10) or 29% (2 of 7), respectively. This was in contrast to CPT-11 alone or CPT-11 followed by flavopiridol at 4 h, where no cures were found (Motwani *et al.* 2001).

6.3 Clinical evaluation of irinotecan and flavopiridol

The combination of irinotecan followed by flavopiridol is being examined in a phase I clinical trial with a 7-h interval prior to the administration of flavopiridol (Shah *et al.* 2002). This trial represents the first evaluation of flavopiridol as a 1-h infusion given weekly. Pharmacokinetic studies demonstrated weekly flavopiridol Cmax ranged from $2.04 \pm 0.60\,\mu M$ (flavopiridol dose level 50 mg/m^2) to $2.89 \pm 0.62\,\mu M$ (flavopiridol dose level 70 mg/m^2), exceeding the nanomolar concentrations necessary to enhance irinotecan-induced apoptosis *in vitro*. Pooled cycle 1 flavopiridol AUC (2.29 μM/h) was significantly lower than pooled cycle 2 flavopiridol AUC (3.10 μM/h) with $P = 0.0078$, suggesting an increase in flavopiridol metabolism when preceded by irinotecan.

Preliminary anti-tumour efficacy was observed. Several patients with stable disease, and one minor response patient with colorectal cancer who progressed on prior irinotecan therapy, were noted. This has led to a phase II clinical trial in colorectal cancer. Additionally, investigators observed two patients with adrenocortical cancer who both had an extended duration of stable disease, with minor responses in lung and liver metastases (average time on study over 10 months). Prolonged disease stabilisation was noted in several patients with hepatocellular cancer, leading to a phase II evaluation of irinotecan → flavopiridol in this disease as well (Shah *et al.* 2002).

6.4 Irinotecan and UCN-01

Several reports have suggested that UCN-01 selectively potentiates the cytotoxicity of DNA-damaging agents in cells that lack functional p53 (Shao *et al.* 1997; Wang *et al.* 1996). The general interpretation is that p53-deficient cells are unable to arrest in G_1 following genotoxic stress and therefore rely more on the G_2 checkpoint for survival. However, it has been shown that p53 is also critical for the maintenance of the G_2 DNA damage checkpoint (Bunz *et al.* 1998). Therefore, it has been hypothesised that pharmacological disruption of the Chk1-dependent pathway using UCN-01 may selectively sensitise cells lacking p53 (p53 null) to genotoxic triggers. Laboratory studies now indicate that sequential treatment with SN-38 followed by UCN-01 markedly enhanced the induction of apoptosis in 23% of p53 null cells but in only 2% of cells with intact p53 (Tse and Schwartz 2004). When the ability of UCN-01 to abrogate the G_2 checkpoint induced by SN-38 was compared between the two HCT-116 cell lines using bi-parameter flow cytometry, treatment with SN-38 alone for 24-h resulted in a G_2 arrest and loss of MPM-2 labelling, a mitotic marker, in both cell lines. However, UCN-01 resulted in marked abrogation of the G_2/M checkpoint in p53-null cells over that seen in parental cells as 43 $\pm$ 3 % of the G_2-arrested p53-null cells were at mitosis 9 h following UCN-01 addition, compared with a peak **mitotic index** of only 11 $\pm$ 4% at 9 h in parental HCT116 cells (Tse and Schwartz 2004). This combination has been shown to prolong survival in a pre-clinical liver metastasis model of human colon cancer cells (Cai *et al.* 2004). The clinical combination of sequential CPT-11 and UCN-01 is now being tested in a phase I clinical trial for patients with advanced solid tumours at the Washington University School of Medicine (St. Louis, MO, USA).

7 Combination with CDK inhibitors with gemcitabine

7.1 Gemcitabine cell cycle effects

Gemcitabine (difluorodeoxycytidine; dFdC) is an agent with promising anti-tumour activity in a variety of solid tumours, with activity in pancreas, bladder, and lung cancer. Gemcitabine is an S phase active drug. It is a nucleoside analogue of cytidine, and is phosphorylated inside cells leading to the diphosphate (dFdCDP) and triphosphate (dfdCTP) derivatives. The diphosphate derivative inhibits DNA synthesis indirectly through inhibition of ribonucleotide reductase (Huang and Plunkett 1995a). This inhibits *de novo* synthesis of DNA, thereby self-potentiating gemcitabine activity by decreasing intracellular concentrations of normal deoxynucleotide triphosphates. The tri-phosphate derivative of gemcitabine is incorporated into DNA by replication synthesis in the cytidine sites of the growing DNA strand (Huang and Plunkett 1995a; Plunkett *et al.* 1995). Once incorporated into the DNA strand, an additional natural nucleoside is added, masking dFd-CTP and preventing DNA repair by $3'$-$5'$-exonuclease activity. DNA polymerases are unable to proceed, leading to a process termed 'masked DNA chain termination' (Plunkett *et al.* 1995).

As might be anticipated, given gemcitabine's mechanism of action, cell cycle analysis of gemcitabine's effects reveal a G_1/S phase arrest or delay (Cappella *et al.* 2001; Huang and Plunkett 1995b). However, unlike an immediate induction of apoptosis seen in CEM leukemic cells (Huang and Plunkett 1995b), the induction of apoptosis seen in an epithelial ovarian cell line was delayed by 24–48 h (Cappella *et al.* 2001). The authors suggest that, following release from a gemcitabine-induced G_1/S-phase arrest, recycling cells experience subsequent blocks at G_2/M and G_1 again. There is a competition between recovery and apoptotic pathways that determines whether the majority of cells survive or die. The molecular determinants of this decision are, as yet, unidentified. However, p53 may play a critical role in this determination of cell cycle arrest versus programmed cell death. This is supported by the observation that loss of p53 function leads to loss of cell cycle control and alterations in the apoptotic cascade, conferring resistance to gemcitabine (Galmarini *et al.* 2002).

The observation that gemcitabine-treated cells are most sensitive to subsequent induction of programmed cell death upon resuming an initial G_1/S- phase arrest, also has important implications with regard to combination therapies. This is demonstrated *in vivo* where potentiation with other cytotoxic drugs is seen with a 24-h interval and coincides with the presence of recycled cells (Cappella *et al.* 2001). This observation may additionally have important implications when considering combinations with CDKIs.

7.2 Gemcitabine and flavopiridol

Flavopiridol was found to potentiate gemcitabine-induced apoptosis in a sequence-dependent manner in several epithelial gastrointestinal cell lines (Jung *et al.* 2001). Cells were treated with gemcitabine, flavopiridol, and their combination in varying sequences and schedules. In pancreas, human gastric and colon cancer cell lines, maximal anti-tumour effect was observed with the combination of gemcitabine followed by flavopiridol. This was demonstrated by the induction of apoptosis as assessed by QFM analysis, PARP cleavage, and cytochrome c release, and by colony formation assays (Jung *et al.* 2001). The reverse sequence of flavopiridol followed by gemcitabine demonstrated no additional anti-tumour efficacy over that of flavopiridol or gemcitabine alone. This sequence dependence is due to a G_1/S arrest induced by flavopiridol, as demonstrated by a significant reduction of incorporation of [^{3}H]Thd into DNA (Jung *et al.* 2001). The synergy was associated with a reduction in RNA and protein levels of the M2 subunit of the early S-phase protein, ribonucleotide reductase.

Ribonucleotide reductase consists of two subunits, M1 and M2. The M2 subunit is primarily involved with ribonucleotide reductase activity during S phase, and has been correlated with DNA synthesis and the invasive potential of cancer cells (Zhou *et al.* 1998). Increased ribonucleotide reductase activity expands the deoxynucleotide triphosphate pool, thereby competitively inhibiting the incorporation of dFdCTP into the DNA. This expanded pool of deoxynucleotide triphosphates also down-regulates the activity of deoxycytidine kinase, reducing the phosphorylation of gemcitabine, further reducing gemcitabine's efficacy (Goan *et al.* 1999). Jung *et al.* demonstrated that the addition of flavopiridol is associated with a reduction in the M2 subunit of ribonucleotide reductase, thereby potentiating gemcitabine's anti-tumour activity (Jung *et al.* 2001).

The S-phase delay induced by gemcitabine may also play an important role in flavopiridol's ability to potentiate gemcitabine's activity (Cappella *et al.* 2001; Matranga and Shapiro 2002). Flow cytometry studies demonstrate that the cells at risk for programmed cell death are those in the S-phase population, following a G_1/S arrest. In a specific, sequence and schedule dependent manner, the subsequent delayed administration of flavopiridol is observed to induce maximal apoptosis (Matranga and Shapiro 2002). Based on these pre-clinical results, the NCI is now sponsoring a phase I clinical trial combining gemcitabine with flavopiridol in a sequence-dependent manner.

7.3 Gemcitabine and UCN-01

Cell cycle arrest plays a critical role in resistance to nucleoside analogues, such as cytarabine, fludarabine, and gemcitabine. For example, when primary leukaemic cells in the marrow are exposed to cytarabine, a substantial portion of the cells undergo a cell cycle arrest, with resultant termination of DNA synthesis, and accumulation in S phase. Decreasing DNA synthesis results in less cytotoxicity of the nucleoside analogue, and resultant protection from cell death (Banker *et al.* 1998; Shi *et al.* 2001). *In vitro*, UCN-01 has demonstrated an enhancement of the anti-tumour efficacy of these analogues, perhaps through G_2 cell cycle checkpoint abrogation (Monks *et al.* 2000). However, a recent study that confirms the UCN-01-mediated enhancement of apoptosis by gemcitabine, addresses this question of overcoming the cell cycle arrest with UCN-01 more closely. Shi *et al.* elegantly demonstrate that gemcitabine increases the percentage of cells arrested in S phase with a significant reduction in DNA synthesis. Subsequent exposure to UCN-01 demonstrated no reactivation of DNA synthesis, but rather an increase in nucleosomal DNA fragmentation, activation of caspase-3, and induction of apoptosis (Shi *et al.* 2001). Therefore, it appears that the augmentation of apoptosis by UCN-01 may not require cells to proceed through the S-phase arrest induced by nucleoside analogues, such as gemcitabine. The combination of gemcitabine and UCN-01 is now being tested in a phase I clinical trial for patients with advanced solid tumours (Mayo Clinic, Rochester, Minn., USA)

8 Other cell cycle active drugs in clinical development

Flavopiridol, UCN-01 and bryostatin-1 are agents that have cell cycle effects. A clear understanding of these effects is critical before these drugs can be effectively combined with chemotherapy, especially when the chemotherapeutic agents themselves can affect the cycle. This understanding will be critical, not only for these agents, but for all new therapies that target the cell cycle. The agent CYC202 (R-roscovitine, Cyclacel, Ltd) is a potent inhibitor of CDK2 with an IC50 of 100 nM (McClue *et al.* 2002a, 2002b). It is one of a growing list of CDK inhibitors currently under clinical development that are orally bioavailable. It has been shown to have single-agent *in vitro* and *in vivo* activity against a broad range of tumour cell types (Maier *et al.* 2003). Intraperitoneal injections of CYC202 have been shown to reduce tumour growth of Lovo human colon tumour xenografts and oral administration to nude mice has had a comparable effect on the growth of human uterine xenograft MESSA-DX5. Studies with this agent in combination with chemotherapy have not been reported. CYC202 is now completing phase I clinical trials in Europe (Benson *et al.* 2002). Preliminary results have been reported in abstract form with an oral starting dose of 100 mg twice daily for 7 days on an every 21-day cycle. No toxicities were reported (Benson *et al.* 2002).

Other CDK inhibitors in clinical trial include BMS-387032, an N-acyl-2-aminothiazole analogue (Jones *et al.* 2003; Shapiro *et al.* 2003). This agent is reported to be a selective inhibitor of CDK2/cyclin E with an IC50 of 48 nM. It induces cell cycle arrest and induces apoptosis in a large panel of tumour cell lines. In combination with chemotherapy it provides additive or synergistic effects. Preliminary clinical results have been reported from two single-agent phase I clinical trials in which BMS-387032 was administered as a either a 1-h or a 24-h infusion every 3 weeks. In both trials fatigue was the most common side-effect. Other toxicities included nausea, vomiting, diarrhoea, and constipation (Jones *et al.* 2003; Shapiro *et al.* 2003). E7070 is a synthetic sulphonamide that targets the G_1-phase of the cell cycle by depleting cyclin E, inducing p53 and p21, and inhibiting cdc2 phosphorylation (Terret *et al.* 2003; Van Kesteren *et al.* 2002). A phase II trial administering E7070 as a 1-h infusion every 3 weeks in patients with advanced head and neck cancers was associated with limited clinical activity (Haddad *et al.* 2003). However, post-treatment biopsies from selected patients on the clinical trial indicated inhibition of Rb phosphorylation suggesting that more frequent administration of drug may be required to sustain this effect. The imidazopyridines are also a novel class of CDK inhibitors with particular specificity for CDK2 (Byth *et al.* 2003). One such compound (AstraZeneca-Compound 1) has been shown to enhance both gemcitabine and cisplatin-induced apoptosis (Cai *et al.* 2004). This effect was sequence (chemotherapy followed by the CDK inhibitor) and E2F-1 dependent. A series of pyrido[2,3-d]pyrimidine-7-ones have also been reported by Pfizer Global Research to have a relative selectivity for CDK4 (Vanderwel *et al.* 2004). Clinical trials with these classes of compounds by Astra-Zeneca and Pfizer, both as oral agents in patients with advanced solid tumours, are now under way. It remains to be determined whether such specificity offers any advantage over a CDKI, such as flavopiridol, which is a pan-CDK inhibitor. In fact, recent studies have indicated that selectively inhibiting CDK2 or CDK4 may not be sufficient to induce cell cycle arrest (Kozar *et al.* 2004; Malumbres *et al.* 2004; Tetsu and McCormick 2003). Rather, growth inhibition may be best achieved when multiple CDKs are inhibited concurrently. In view of the redundancy of these pathways at both the G_1/S checkpoint, the concept of less CDK specificity for a CDKI, rather than more specificity, may in fact make the most sense for drug development.

9 Future directions

Cell cycle perturbations are commonly observed in human malignancies. Additional targets involving the cell cycle and mitosis are presently being evaluated as well. Polo-kinase 1 and Aurora 2 are attractive novel targets attacking the mitotic machinery and intimately related to the G_2/M transition checkpoint (Vankayalapati *et al.* 2003). These proteins are overexpressed in a variety of malignanicies, including colon cancer (Takahashi *et al.* 2003), pancreatic cancer, and non-Hodgkins lymphoma (Hamada *et al.* 2003), and may provide additional options for cancer patients in the future.

Presently, CDKIs have demonstrated limited clinical activity as single agents in advanced solid tumours. The reason for this is unclear. Many of these single-agent clinical trials have focused on flavopiridol. However, it has only become recently apparent that this drug is highly protein-bound and this may have a significant impact on the biological activity of the drug. In order to achieve biologically active, nanomolar concentrations of flavopiridol (100–300 nM), it is necessary to achieve 2–3 µM in the plasma of patients. Preliminary clinical data now indicate that achieving such plasma levels of flavopiridol in patients is possible without significant toxicity provided the drug is administered over 1 h (Shah *et al.* 2002). More recent data now indicate that, not only is it important to achieve these peak levels, but these levels should be maintained for several hours thereafter, in order to maximise the pro-apoptotic effects of flavopiridol. This theoretical approach has been recently applied to the treatment of patients with refractory chronic lymphocytic leukaemia (CLL). In this study, patients with CLL were treated with flavopiridol for 30 min followed by a 4-h continuous infusion of the drug. This resulted in profound tumour lysis and a dramatic anticancer effect (Lin *et al.* 2004). These results indicate that with pharmacokinetic modelling it may be possible to make flavopiridol an active single-gent drug, at least in haematological malignancies. Whether this applies to solid tumours as well, remains to be tested.

However, it is the combination of CDKIs with standard cytotoxic agents that is emerging as an alternative approach to anticancer therapy. This approach exploits the cell cycle perturbations of malignancy. Pre-clinical studies demonstrate the concept of cell cycle mediated drug resistance, and suggest that the combination of standard cytotoxic agents with CDKIs will require thoughtful sequencing and scheduling. The importance of drug sequence is not limited to this class of targeted drugs. In fact, any targeted drug that has the capabilities of inhibiting the cell cycle can antagonise the effects of chemotherapy. For example, geftinib (ZD1839, Iressa) is an inhibitor of the epidermal growth factor (EGF)-receptor. However, it also causes tumour cells to arrest at the G_1 phase of the cell cycle. In view of potential cell cycle interaction, such an effect by Iressa on the cell cycle could attenuate subsequent therapy with any M-phase specific drug such as paclitaxel. This assertion has recently been tested. Continuous treatment with gefitinib significantly attenuated the effect of paclitaxel in mice bearing breast and lung cancer xenografts. These laboratory results are sufficient to explain the basis for the negative clinical results from the large randomised phase III trial comparing continuous daily administration of gefitinib in combination with paclitaxel and carboplatin to chemotherapy alone in the treatment of metastatic lung cancer. With this in mind, an understanding of the cell cycle remains critical for the development of each targeted therapy before it enters clinical trial in combination with chemotherapy. Sequence is critical. In addition, dosing and schedule of drug must also be taken into account. As indicated from the pre-clinical studies with gefitinib, chronic dosing with low levels of drug will only result in protracted cell cycle arrest. In contrast, short-pulse dosing will activate pathways responsible for the induction of apoptosis and inhibit those pathways that prevent apoptosis (Solit et al. 2003). This hypothesis is also supported by studies with flavopiridol. Thus, current clinical trials with flavopiridol in solid tumours are developing flavopiridol schedules that can achieve 2–3 μM of the drug in patients plasma (Shah et al. 2002). Even with 80–90% protein binding of the drug, this should result in free plasma levels that are more than sufficient to activate the pathways that enhance chemotherapy induced apoptosis. In view of this, there are presently several clinical investigations underway examining the combination of a standard cytotoxic with a novel CDKI, with particular attention to sequence, dose and scheduling. Although phase-II evaluation of these combination studies will provide initial evidence of anti-tumour activity, definitive phase-III studies will be needed to establish this class of agents in the care of patients with cancer.

References

Akiyama T, Yoshida T, Tsujita T, et al. (1997) G1 phase accumulation induced by UCN-01 is associated with dephosphorylation of Rb and CDK2 proteins as well as the induction of

CDK inhibitor p21/CIP/WAF1/Sdi1 in p53-mutated human epidermoid carcinoma A431 cells. *Cancer Res*, **57**, 1495–501.

Altieri DC (2001) The molecular basis and potential role of survivin in cancer diagnosis and therapy. *Trends Mol Med*, **7**, 542–47.

Anderson SSL (2000) Spindle assembly and the art of regulating microtubule dynamics by MAPs and stathmin/Op18. *Trends Cell Biol*, **10**, 261–67.

Asiedu C, Biggs J, Lilly M and Kraft M (1995) Inhibition of leukemic cell growth by the protein kinase C activator bryostatin-1 correlates with the dephosphorylation of cyclin-dependent kinase 2. *Cancer Res*, **55**, 3716–30.

Banker DE, Groudine M, Willman CL, Norwood T and Appelbaum FR (1998) Cell cycle perturbations in acute myeloid leukemia samples following in vitro exposures to therapeutic agents. *Leuk Res*, **22**, 221–39.

Bedikian AY, Plager C, Stewart J.R *et al.* (2001) Phase II evaluation of bryostatin-1 in metastatic melanoma. *Melanoma Res*, **11**, 183–8.

Bennett P, Mani S, O'Reilly S *et al.* (1999) Phase II trial of flavopiridol in metastatic colorectal cancer: preliminary results. *Proc Am Soc Clin Oncol*, **18**, abs 1065.

Benson C, Raynaud F, O'Donnell A *et al.* (2002) Pharmacokinetics (PK) of the oral cyclin dependent kinase inhibitor CYC202 (R-roscovitine) in patients with cancer. *Amer Assoc Cancer Res*, **43**, abs 273.

Bible KC and Kaufmann SH (1996) Flavopiridol: a cytotoxic flavone that induces cell death in noncycling A549 human lung carcinoma cells. *Cancer Research*, **56**, 4856–61.

Bible KC and Kaufmann SH (1997) Cytotoxic synergy between flavopiridol (NSC 649890, L86-8275) and various antineoplastic agents: the importance of Sequence of administration. *Cancer Research*, **57**, 3375–80.

Blackhall FH, Ranson M, Radford JA et al. (2001) A phase II trial of bryostatin 1 in patients with non-Hodgkin's lymphoma. *Br J Cancer*, **84**, 249–54.

Blagden SP and Glover DM (2003) Polar expeditions—provisioning the centrosome for mitosis. *Nature Cell Biol*, **5**, 505–11.

Blagosklonny MV, Giannakakou P, el-Deiry WS *et al.* (1997) Raf-1/bcl-2 phosphorylation: a step from microtubule damage to cell death *Cancer Res*, **57**, 130–5.

Brockstein B, Samuels, Humerickhouse R *et al.* (2001) Phase II studies of bryostatin-1 in patients with advanced sarcoma and advanced head and neck cancer. *Invest New Drugs*, **19**, 249–54.

Brown T, Havlin K, Weiss G *et al.* (1991) A phase I trial of taxol given by a 6-hour intravenous infusion. *Journal of Clinical Oncology*, **9**, 1261–7.

Buckley M, Sweeney KJ, Hamilton JA *et al.* (1993) Expression and amplification of cyclin genes in human breast cancer. *Oncogene*, **8**.

Bunz F, Dutriaux A, Lengauer C *et al.* (1998) Requirement for p53 and p21 to sustain G2 arrest after DNA damage. *Science*, **282**, 1497–501.

Bunz F, Hwang PM, Torrance C *et al.* (1999) Disruption of p53 in human cancer cells alters the responses to therapeutic agents. *J Clin Invest*, **104**, 263–69.

Burdette-Radoux S, Tozer RG, Lohmann R *et al.* (2002) NCIC CTG phase II study of flavopiridol in patients with previously untreated metastatic malignant melanoma. *Proc Amer Soc Clin Onc*, **21**, abs 1382.

Busby EC, Leistritz DF, Abraham RT, Karnitz LM and Sarkaria JN (2000) The radiosensitizing agent 7-hydroxystaurosporine (UCN-01) inhibits the DNA damage checkpoint kinase hChk1. *Cancer Res*, **60**, 2108–12.

Byrd JC, Shinn C, Waselenko JK *et al.* (1998) Flavopiridol induces apoptosis in chronic lymphocytic leukemia cells via activation of caspase-3 without evidence of bcl-2 modulation or dependence of functional p53. *Blood*, **92**, 3804–16.

Byth K, Geh C, Forder C *et al.* (2003) Novel cell cycle inhibitors: Characterization in tumour cell lines and normal cycling cells. *Am Assoc Cancer Res*, **44**, abs 714.

Cai D, Byth K and Shapiro G (2004) A novel CDK inhibitor induces cell cycle blockade, E2F-1 dependent apoptosis, and cytotoxic synergy with DNA damaging agents. *Proc Am Assoc Cancer Res*, **45**, 190.

Cai SR, Fracasso PM, Garbow JR, Piwnica-Worms H and H. M (2004) Irinotecan plus UCN-01 combination therapy significantly increased liver metastasis apoptosis and prolonger survival in preclin liver metastatic model. *Proc Am Assoc Cancer Res*, **45**.

Cappella P, Tomasoni D, Faretta M *et al.* (2001) Cell cycle effects of gemcitabine. *Int J. Cancer*, **93**, 401–8.

Carlson BA, Pearlstein RA, Naik RG, Sedlacek HH, Sausville EA and Worland PJ (1996) Inhibition of CDK2, CDK4 and CDK7 by flavopiridol and structural anologs. *Proc Am Assoc Cancer Res*, **37**, 424.

Carlson B, Lahusen T, Singh S *et al.* (1999) Down-Regulation of Cyclin D1 by Transcriptional Repression in MCF-7 Human Breast Carcinoma Cells Induced by Flavopiridol. *Cancer Res*, **59**, 4634–41.

Cartee L, Wang Z, Decker RH, Chellappan SP, Fusaro G, Hirsch KG *et al.* (2001) The Cyclin-dependent Kinase Inhibitor (CDKI) Flavopiridol Disrupts Phorbol 12-Myristate 13-Acetate-induced Differentiation and CDKI Expression while Enhancing Apoptosis in Human Myeloid Leukemia. Cells *Cancer Res*, **61**, 2583–91.

Chan TA, Hwang PM, Hermeking J, Kinzler KW and Vogelstein B (2000) Cooperative effects of genes controling the G2/M checkpoint. *Genes & Devel*, **14**, 1584–88.

Chen Y-N, Sharma SK, Ramsey M *et al.* (1999) Selective killing of transformed cells by cyclin/cyclin-dependent kinase 2 antagonists. *Proc Natl Acad Sci*, **96**, 4325–29.

Clarke AR, Gledhill S, Hooper ML *et al.* (1994) p53 dependence of early apoptotic and proliferative responses within the mouse intestinal epithelium following gamma-irradiation. *Oncogene*, **9**, 1767–73.

Clute P and Pines J (1999) Temporal and spatial control of cyclin B1 destruction in metaphase. *Nature Cell Biol*, **1**, 82–6.

Creemers CJ, Lund B and Verweij J (1994) Topoisomerase I inhibitors: Topotecan and Irinotecan. *Cancer Treat Rev*, **20**, 73–96.

Datta R, Manome Y, Taneja N *et al.* (1995) Overexpression of Bcl-xl by cytotoxic drug exposure confers resistance to ionizing radiation-induced internucleosomal DNA fragmentation. *Cell Growth Differ*, **6**, 363–70.

DeVita VT (1997) In *Cancer: principles and practice of oncology* (ed., DeVita VT, H. S., Rosenberg SA.), pp. 333–47. Lippincott-Raven Publishers, Philadelphia PA.

Donaldson KL, Goolsby GL, Kiener PA and Wahl AF (1994a) Activation of p34cdc2 coincident with taxol-induced apoptosis. *Cell Growth & Differentiation*, **5**, 1041–50.

Donaldson KL, Goolsby GL and Wahl AF (1994b) Cytotoxicity of the anticancer agents cisplatin and taxol during cell proliferation and the cell cycle. *Int J Cancer*, **57**, 847–55.

Drees M, Dengler WA, Roth T *et al.* (1997) Flavopiridol (L86–8275): selective antitumour activity in vitro and activity in vivo for prostate carcinoma cells. *Clin Cancer Res*, **3**, 271–9.

El-Diery WS, Harper JW, O'Connor PM *et al.* (1994) Waf1/Cip1 is induced in p53-mediated G1 arrest and apoptosis. *Cancer Res*, **54**, 1169–74.

Eliopoulos AG, Kerr DJ, Herod J, Hodgkins L, Krajewski S, Reed JC et al. (1995) The control of apoptosis and drug resistance in ovarian cancer: influence of p53 and Bcl-2. Oncogene, 11, 1217–28.

Elledge SJ and Harper JW (1998) The role of protein stability in the cell cycle and cancer. Biochim Biophys Acta, 1377, M61–70.

Falck J, Mailand N, Syljuasen RG et al. (2001) The ATM-Chk2-Cdc25A checkpoint pathway gaurds against radioresistant DNA synthesis. Nature, 410, 842–47.

Fan G and Steer CJ (1996) The retinoblastoma gene product is a negative modulator of the apoptotic pathway Adv Enzyme Regul, 36, 283–303.

Ford HL and Pardee AB (1998) The S phase: beginning, middle, and end: a perspective. J Cell Biochem, 30(Suppl 31), 1–7.

Ford HL and Pardee AB (1999) Cancer and the cell cycle. J. Cell Biochem, 32(Suppl 33), 166–72.

Gajewski TF and Thompson CB (1996) Apoptosis meets signal transduction: elimination of a BAD influence. Cell, 87, 589–92.

Galmarini CM, Clarke ML, Falette N et al. (2002) Expression of non-functional p53 affects the sensitivity of cancer cells to gemcitabine. Int J Cancer, 97, 439–45.

Giet R, McLean D, Descamps L et al. (2002) Drosophila Aurora A kinase is required to localize D-TACC to centrosomes and to regulate astral microtubules. J Biol Chem, 156, 437–51.

Glover DM, Leibowitz MH, McLean DA and Perry H (1995) Mutations in aurora prevent centrosome separation leading to the formation of monopolar spindles. Cell, 81, 95–105.

Goan YG, Zhou BS, Hu E et al. (1999) Overexpression of ribonucleotide reductase as a mechanism of resistance to 2,2-difluorodeoxycytidine in human KB cancer cell line. Cancer Research, 59, 4204–7.

Goldie JH and Coldman AJ (1979) A mathematic model for relating the drug sensitivity of tumours to their spontaneous mutation rate. Cancer Treat Rep, 63, 1727–33.

Goldie JH and Coldman AJ (1985) A model for tumour response to chemotherapy: an integration of the stem cell and somatic mutation hypotheses. Cancer Invest, 3, 553–64.

Gonzalez R, Ebbinghaus S, Henthorn TK, Miller D and Kraft AS (1999) Treatment of patients with metastatic melanoma with bryostatin-1—a phase II study. Melanoma Res, 9, 599–606.

Grana X and Reddy EP (1995) Cell cycle control in mammalian cells: role of cyclins, cyclin dependent kinases (CDKs), growth suppressor genes and cyclin-dependent kinase inhibitors (CKIs). Oncogene, 11, 211–219.

Graves PR, Yu L, Schwarz JK, Gales J, Sausville EA, O'Connor PM et al. (2000) The Chk1 protein kinase and the Cdc25C regulatory pathways are targets of the anticancer agent UCN-01. J Biol Chem, 275, 5600–5.

Haddad RI, Shapiro GI, Weinstein L et al. (2003a) A phase II study of E7070 in patients with metastatic, recurrent, or refractory head and neck squamous cell carcinoma (HNSCC): Clinical activity and post-treatment modulation of Rb phosphorylation. Amer Soc Clin Onc, 22, abs 201.

Hamada M, Yakushijin Y, Ohtsuka M et al. (2003b) Aurora2/BTAK/STK15 is involved in cell cycle checkpoint and cell survival of aggressive non-Hodgkin's lymphoma. Br J Haematology, 121, 439–47.

Harper J and Elledge SJ (1996) Cdk inhibitors in devlopment and cancer. Curr Opin Genet & Develop, 6, 56–64.

Hartwell LH and Kastan MB (1994) Cell cycle control and cancer. *Science*, 266, 1821–8.

Hennings H, Blumberg PM, Pettit GR, Herald CL, Shores R and Yuspa S (1987) Bryostatin-1, an activator of protein kinase C inhibits tumour promotion by phorbol esters in Sencar mouse skin. *Carcinogenesis*, 9, 1343–6.

Hsueh CT, Kelsen D and Schwartz GK (1998) UCN-01 suppresses thymidylate synthase gene expression and enhances 5-fluorouracil-induced apoptosis in a sequence-dependent manner. *Clin Cancer Res*, 4, 2201–6.

Huang P and Plunkett W (1995a) Induction of apoptosis by gemcitabine. *Semin Oncol*, 22, 19–25.

Huang P and Plunkett W (1995b) Fludarabine- and gemcitabine-induced apoptosis: incorporation of analogs into DNA is a critical event. *Cancer Chemother Pharmacol*, 36, 181–8.

Ibardo AM, Huang Y, Fang G and Bhalla K (1996) Bcl-xl overexpression inhibits taxol-induced yama protease activity and apoptosis. *Cell Growth Differ*, 7, 1087–94.

Isakov N, Galron D, Mustelin T, Pettit GR and Altman A (1993) Inhibition of phorbol ester-induced T cell proliferation by bryostatin is associated with rapid degradation of protein kinase C. *J Immunol*, 150, 1195–204.

Jarvis WD and Grant S (1999) Protein kinase C targeting in antineoplastic treatment strategies. *Invest New Drugs*, 17, 227–40.

Jayson GC, Crowther D, Prendiville J, McGown A, Scheid C *et al.* (1995) A phase I trial of bryostatin 1 in patients with advanced malignancy using a 24-hour intravenous infusion. *Br J Cancer*, 72, 461–8.

Johnson DG and Walker CL (1999) Cyclins and cell cycle checkpoints. *Ann Rev Pharmacol Toxicol*, 39, 295–312.

Jones SF, Burris HA, Kies M *et al.* (2003) A phase I study to determine the safety and pharmacokinetics (PK) of BMS-387032 given intravenously every three weeks in patients with metastatic refractory solid tumours. *Amer Soc Clin Onc*, 22, abs 199.

Jung CP, Motwani MV and Schwartz GK (2001) Flavopiridol increases sensitization to gemcitabine in human gastrointestinal cancer cell lines and correlates with down-regulation of ribonucleotide reductase M2 subunit. *Clin Cancer Res*, 7, 2527–36.

Kaldis P, Russo AA, Chou HS, Pavletich NP and Solomon MJ (1998) Human and yeast CDK-activating kinases (CAKs) display distinct substrate specificities. *Mol Biol Cell*, 9, 2545–60.

Kaubisch A, Kelsen DP, Saltz L *et al.* (1999) A phase I trial of weekly sequential bryostatin (Bryo) and paclitaxel in patients with advanced solid tumours. *Proc Amer Soc Clin Oncol*, 18, abs 639.

Kaufmann SH, Desnoyers S, Ottaviano Y, Davidson NE and Poirier GG (1993) Specific proteolytic cleavage of poly (ADP-ribose) polymerase: An early marker of chemotherapy-induced apoptosis. *Cancer Res*, 53, 3976–85.

Kawakami K, Futami H, Takahara J and Yamaguchi K (1996) UCN-01, 7-hydroxylstaurosporine, inhibits kinase activity of cyclin-dependent kinases and reduces the phosphorylation of the retinoblastoma susceptibility gene product in A549 human lung cancer cell line. *Biochem Biophys Res Commun*, 219, 778–83.

Kerr JFR, Wyllie AH and Currie AR (1972) Apoptosis: a basic biological phenomenon with wide ranging implications in tissue kinetics. *Br J Cancer*, 26, 239–57.

Kohn EA, Ruth ND, Brown MK *et al.* (2002) Abrogation of the S phase DNA damage checkpoint results in S phase progression of premature mitosis depending on the concentration of 7-Hydroxystaurosporine and the kinetics of Cdc25C activation. *J Biol Chem*, 277, 26553–64.

Konig A, Schwartz GK, Mohammad RM *et al.* (1997) The novel cyclin-dependent kinase inhibitor flavopiridol downregulates Bcl-2 and induces growth arrest and apoptosis in chronic B-cell leukemia cell lines. *Blood*, 90, 4307–12.

Koutcher JA, Motwani M, Dyke JP, Ballon D, H.Y. H and Schwartz GK (2000) The in vitro effect of bryostatin-1 on paclitaxel-induced tumour growth, mitotic entry, and blood flow. *Clin Cancer Res*, 6, 1498–507.

Kozar K, Ciemerych M, Rebel VI *et al.* (2004) Mouse Development and Cell Proliferation in the Absence of D-Cyclins. *Cell*, 118, 477–491.

Kraft AS, Smith JB and Berkow RL (1986) Bryostatin, an activator of the calcium phospholipid-dependent protein kinase, blocks phorbol ester-induced differentiation of human promyelocytic leukemia cells HL-60. *Proc Natl Acad Sci USA*, 83, 1334–8.

Lazebnik YA, Takahashi A., Moir RD *et al.* (1995) Studies of the lamin proteinase reveal multiple parallel biochemical pathways during apoptotic execution. *Proc Natl Acad Sci USA*, 92, 9042–6.

Lee HW, Smith L, Pettit GR, Vinitsky A and Smith JB (1996) Ubiquitination of protein kinase C-alpha and degradation by the proteasome. *J Biol Chem*, 271, 20973–6.

Levine AJ (1997) p53, the cellular gatekeeper for growth and division. *Cell*, 88, 323–31.

Li LH, Fraser TJ, Olin EJ and Bhuyan BK (1972) Action of camptothecin on mammalian cells in culture. *Cancer Res*, 32, 2643–50.

Lin TS, Howard OM, Neuberg DS *et al.* (2002) Seventy-two hour continuous infusion flavopiridol in relapsed and refractory mantle cell lymphoma. *Leuk Lymphoma*, 43, 793–7.

Lin T, Dalton JT, Wu B *et al.* (2004) Flavopiridol given as a 30 minute intravenous (IV) bolus followed by 4-hr continous IV infusion results in clinical activity and tumour lysis in refractory chronic lymphocytic leukemia. *Proc Am Soc Clin Oncol*, 23, abs 6564.

Ling YH, Yank Y, Consoli U, Tornos C, Andreeff M and Perez-Soler R (1998) Accumulation of cyclin B1, activation of cyclin B1-dependent kinase and induction of programmed cell death in human epidermoid carcinoma KB cells treated with Taxol. *Int J. Cancer*, 75, 925–32.

Long BH and Fairchild CR (1994) Paclitaxel inhibits progression of mitotic cells to G1 phase by interference with spindle formation without affecting other microtubule functions during anaphase and telephase. *Cancer Res*, 54, 4355–61.

Losiewicz MD, Carlson BA, Kaur G, Sausville EA and Worland PJ (1994) Potent inhibition of cdc2 kinase activity by the flavonoid L86–8275. *Biochem Biophys Biophys Res Commun*, 201, 589–95.

Lowe SW, Ruley HE, Jact T and Housman DE (1993) p53-Dependent apoptosis modulates the cytotoxicity of anticancer agents. *Cell*, 74, 957–67.

Luria SE and Delbruck M (1943) Mutations of bacteria from virus sensitivity to virus resistance. *Genetics*, 28, 491.

Maier A, Kelter G, Gianella-Borradori A and Fiebig H (2003) Antitumour activity of CYC202, a cyclin-dependent kinase inhibitor, in human tumour xenografts in vitro. *Amer Assoc Cancer Res*, 44, abs 713.

Malumbres M and Barbacid M (2001) To cycle or not to cycle: a critical decision in cancer. *Nat Cancer Rev*, 1, 222–31.

Malumbres M, Sotillo R and Santamary D *et al.* (2004) Mammalian Cells Cycle without the D-TypeCyclin-Dependent Kinases Cdk4 and Cdk6. *Cell*, 118, 477–91.

Martin SJ and Green DR (1995) Protease activation during apoptosis. Death by a thousand cuts? *Cell*, **82**, 349–52.

Matranga CB and Shapiro GI (2002) Selective sensitization of transformed cells to flavopiridol-induced apoptosis following recruitment to S phase. *Cancer Research*, **62**, 1707–17.

McClue SJ, Blake D, Clarke AR *et al.* (2002a) In vitro and in vivo antitumour properties of the cyclin dependent kinase inhibitor CYC202 (R-roscovitine). *Int J. Cancer*, **102**, 463–8.

McClue SJ, Fischer P, Blake D *et al.* (2002b) Studies on the mechanism of action of CYC202 (R-roscovitine). *Am Assoc Cancer Res*, **43**, abs 666.

Monks A, Harris ED, Vaigro-Wolff A *et al.* (2000) UCN-01 enhances the in vitro toxicity of clinical agents in human tumour cell lines. *Invest New Drugs*, **18**, 95–107.

Motwani M, Delohery TM and Schwartz GK (1999) Sequential dependent enhancement of caspase activation and apoptosis by flavopiridol on paclitaxel-treated human gastric and breast cancer cells. *Clinical Cancer Research*, **5**, 1876–83.

Motwani M, Jung C, Sirotnak FM, She Y, Shah MA, Gonen M and Schwartz GK (2001) Augmentation of apoptosis and tumour regressions by flavopiridol in the presence of CPT-11 in HCT116 colon cancer monolayers and xenografts. *Clin Cancer Res*, **7**, 4209–19.

Motwani MV, Rizzo C, Sirotnak F *et al.* (2003) Flavopiridol enhances the effect of docetaxel in vitro and in vivo in human gastric cancer cells. *Mol Cancer Ther*, **2**, 549–55.

Mutter R and Wills M (2000) Chemistry and clinical biology of the bryostatins. *Bioorg Med Chem*, **8**, 1841–60.

Nicklas RB (1997) How cells get the right chromosome. *Science*, **275**, 632–37.

O'Connor DS, Wall NR, Porter ACG and Altieri DC (2002) A p34cdc2 survival checkpoint in cancer. *Cancer Cell*, **2**, 43–54.

Pagliaro L, Daliani D, Amato R, Tu SM, Jones D *et al.* (2000) A phase II trial of bryostatin-1 for patients with metastatic renal cell carcinoma. *Cancer*, **89**, 615–8.

Pardee AB (1974) A restriction point control for normal animal cell proliferation. *Proc Natl Acad Sci USA*, **71**, 1286–90.

Patel V, Senderowicz AM, Pinto D *et al.* (1998) Flavopiridol, a Novel Cyclin-dependent Kinase Inhibitor, Suppresses the Growth of Head and Neck Squamous Cell Carcinomas by Inducing Apoptosis. *J Clin Invest*, **102**, 1674–81.

Philip PA, Rea D, Thavasu P *et al.* (1993) Phase I study of bryostatin 1: assessment of interleukin 6 and tumour necrosis factor alpha induction *in vivo*. The Cancer Research Campaign Phase I Committee. *J Natl Cancer Inst*, **85**, 1812–8.

Plunkett W, Huang P, Xu Y *et al.* (1995) Gemcitabine: metabolism, mechanisms of action and self-potentiation. *Semin Oncol*, **22**(4)(Suppl 11), 3–10.

Prendiville J, Crowther D, Thatcher N *et al.* (1993) A phase I study of intravenous bryostatin 1 in patients with advanced cancer. *Br J Cancer*, **68**, 418–24.

Propper D, Macaulay V, O'Bryne KJ *et al.* (1998) A phase II study of bryostatin 1 in metastatic malignant melanoma. *Br J Cancer*, **78**, 1337–41.

Reed JC (1999) Dysregulation of apoptosis in cancer. *J Clin Oncol*, **117**, 2941–53.

Reed JC and Bischoff JR (2000) Ringing chromosomes through cell division-and survivin' the experience. *Cell*, **102**, 545–48.

Rudner AD and Murray AW (1996) The spindle assembly checkpoint. *Curr Opin Cell Biol*, **8**, 773–80.

Salisbury JL, Whitehead CM, Lingle WL and Barrett SL (1999) Centrosomes and cancer. *Biol Cell*, **91**, 451–60.

Sane AT and Bertrand R (1999) Caspase inhibition in camptothecin-treated U-937 cells is coupled with a shift from apoptosis to transient G1 arrest followed by necrotic cell death. *Cancer Res*, **59**, 3565–9.

Sausville EA, Arbuck S, Messmann R *et al.* (2001) Phase I trial of 72-hour continuous infusion of UCN-01 in patients with refractory neoplasms. *J Clin Oncol*, **19**, 2319–33.

Schiff PB, Fant J and Horwitz SB (1979) Promotion of microtubule assembly in vitro by taxol. *Nature*, **277**, 665–7.

Schiff PB and Horwitz SB (1980) Taxol stabilizes microtubules in mouse fibroblast cells. *Proc Natl Acad Sci USA*, **77**, 1561–5.

Schiff PB and Horwitz SB (1981) Taxol assembles tubulin in the absence of exogenous guanosine 5$'$-triphosphate or microtubule-associated proteins. *Biochemistry*, **20**, 3247–52.

Schmitt E, Cimoli G, Steyaert A and Bertrand R (1998) Bcl-xL modulates apoptosis induced by anticancer drugs and delays DEVDase and DNA fragmentation-promoting activities. *Exper Cell Res*, **240**, 107–21.

Schrump DS, Mathews W, Chen GA *et al.* (1998) Flavopiridol mediates cell cycle arrest and apoptosis in esophageal cancer cell lines. *Clin Cancer Res*, **4**, 2885–90.

Schwartz GK, Ilson D, Saltz L *et al.* (2001) Phase II study of the cyclin-dependent kinase inhibitor flavopiridol administered to patients with advanced gastric carcinoma. *J Clin Oncol*, **19**, 1985–92.

Senderowicz AM (2002) In *Cancer chemotherapy and biological response modifiers, annual 20* (ed., Giaccone G, Schilsky R and Sondel P), pp.169–88. Elsevier Science.

Senderowicz AM, Headlee D, Stinson SF *et al.* (1998) Phase I trial of continuous infusion flavopiridol, a novel cyclin-dependent kinase inhibitor, in patients with refractory neoplasms. *J Clin Oncol*, **16**, 2986–99.

Shah MA, Kortmansky J, Gonen M *et al.* (2002) A phase I/pharmacologic study of weekly sequential irinotecan (CPT) and flavopiridol. *Proc. Am Soc Clin Oncol*, **21**, abs 373.

Shah MA and Schwartz GK (2001) Cell Cycle mediated drug resistance: An emerging concept in cancer therapy. *Clinical Cancer Research*, **7**, 2168–81.

Shahjehan WA, Laird P and DeMeester T (2001) DNA methylation: an alternative pathway to cancer. *Ann Surg*, **234**, 10–20.

Shao RG, Cao CX, Shimizu T, O'Connor PM, Kohn KW and Pommier Y (1997) Abrogation of an S phase checkpoint and potentiation of camptothecin cytotoxicity by 7-hydroxystaurosporine (UCN-01) in human cancer cell lines, possibly influenced by p53 function. *Cancer Res*, **57**, 4029–35.

Shapiro GI, Patterson A, Lynch C *et al.* (2001) A phase II trial of the cyclin-dependent kinase inhibitor flavopiridol in patients with previously untreated stage IV non-small cell lung cancer. *Clin Cancer Res*, **7**, 1590–9.

Shapiro GI, Lewis N, Bai S *et al.* (2003) A phase I study to determine the safety and pharmacokinetics (PK) of BMS-387032 with a 24-hour infusion given every three weeks in patients with metastatic refractory solid tumours. *Am Soc Clin Onc*, **22**, abs 200.

Sherr CJ (2000) The Pezcoller Lecture: cancer cell cycles revisited. *Cancer Res*, **60**, 3689–95.

Sherr CJ and Roberts JM (1999) CDK inhibitors: positive and negative regulators of G1-phase progression. *Genes Dev*, **13**, 1501–12.

Shi Z, Azuma A, Sampath D, Li Y-X, Huang P and Plunkett W (2001) S phase arrest by nucleoside analogues and abrogation of survival without cell cycle progression by 7-hydroxystaurosporine. *Cancer Res.*, **61**, 1065–72.

Shimizu T, O'Connor PM, Kohn KW and Pommier Y (1995) Unscheduled activation of cyclin B1/cdc2 kinase in human promyelocytic leukemia cell line HL60 cells ungroing apoptosis induced by DNA damage. *Cancer Res*, 55, 228–31.

Slichenmeyer WJ, Rowinsky EK, Donehower RC and Kaufmann SC (1993) The current status of camptothecin analogues as antitumour agents. *JNCI*, 85, 271–91.

Solit DB, She Y, Moasser MM *et al.* (2003) Pulsatile administration of the EGF receptor inhibitor Iressa (ZD1839) is significantly more effective than continuous dosing for sensitizing tumours to Taxol. *Am Assoc Cancer Res*, 44(2), abs 83.

Stadler WM, Vogelzang N, Amato R *et al.* (2000) Flavopiridol, a novel cyclin-dependent kinase inhibitor, in metastatic renal cancer: a University of Chicago phase II consortium study. *J Clin Oncol*, 18, 371–75.

Sutherland R and Musgrove E (2002) Cyclin D1 and mammary carcinoma: new insights from transgenic mouse models *Breast Cancer Res*, 4, 14–7.

Takahashi I, Saitoh Y and Yoshida M (1989) UCN-01 and UCN-02, new selective inhibitors of protein kinase C. Purification, physico-chemical properties, structural determination and biological activities. *J Antibiotics*, 42, 571–6.

Takahashi T, Sano B, Nagata T *et al.* (2003) Polo-like kinase 1 (PLK1) is overexpressed in primary colorectal cancers. *Cancer Sci.*, 94, 148–52.

Terret C, Zanetta S, Roche H *et al.* (2003) A phase I clinical and pharmacokinetic study of E7070, a novel sulfonamide given as a 5-day continuous infusion repeated every 3 weeks in patients with solid tumours. *Eur J Cancer*, 39, 1097–104.

Tetsu O and McCormick F (2003) Proliferation of cancer cells despite CDK2 inhibition. *Cancer Cell*, 3, 233–45.

Thomas JP, Tutsch KD, Cleary JF *et al.* (2002) Phase I clinical and pharmacokinetic trial of cyclin-dependent kinase inhibitor flavopiridol. *Cancer Chemother Pharmacol*, 50, 465–72.

Tsao YP, D'Apra P and Liu LF (1992) The involvement of active DNA synthesis in camptothecin-induced G2 arrest: altered regulation of p34cdc2/cyclin B. *Cancer Res*, 52, 1823–29.

Tse A and Schwartz G (2004) Potentiation of cytotoxicity of topoisomerase I poison in human colon carcinoma cells by concurrent and sequential treatment with the checkpoint inhibitor 7-hydroxystaurosporine involves disparate mechanisms resulting in different pharmacological endpoints. *Cancer Res*, 64, 6635–44.

Van Kesteren C, Beijnen JH and Schellens JH (2002) E7070: a novel synthetic sulfonamide targeting the cell cycle progression for the treatment of cancer. *Anticancer Drugs*, 13, 989–97.

Vanderwel S, Harvey, PJ, Sheehan, DJ *et al.* (2004) Highly selective inhibition of CDK4 with pyrido[2,3-d]pyrimidine-7-ones. *Proc Am Assoc Cancer Res*, 45, 190, abs 828.

Vankayalapati H, Bearss DJ, Saldanha JW *et al.* (2003) Targeting aurora2 kinase in oncogenesis: a structural bioinformatics approach to target validation and rational drug design. *Mol Cancer Ther*, 2, 283–94.

Varterasian ML, Mohammad RM, Eilender DS *et al.* (1998) Phase I study of bryostatin 1 in patients with relapsed non-Hodgkin's lymphoma and chronic lymphocytic leukemia. *J Clin Oncol*, 16, 56–62.

Vrana JA, Saunders AM, Chellappan SP and Grant S (1998) Divergent effects of bryostatin 1 and phorbol myristate acetate on cell cycle arrest and maturation in human myelomonocytic leukemia cells (U937). *Differentiation*, 63, 33–42.

Vrana JA, Kramer LB, Saunders AM *et al.* (1999) Inhibition of protein kinase C activator-mediated induction of p21cip1 and p27kip1 by deoxycytidine analogs in human leukemia cells: relationship to apoptosis and differentiation. *Biochem Pharmacol*, **58**, 121–31.

Waldman T (1997) Cell cycle arrest versus cell death in cancer therapy. *Nat Med*, **3**, 1034–36.

Wang Q, Fan S, Eastman A, Worland PJ, Sausville EA and O'Connor PM (1996) UCN-01: a potent abrogator of G2 checkpoint function in cancer cells with disrupted p53. *J Natl Cancer Inst*, **88**, 956–65.

Wang S, Guo C, Castillo A, Dent P and Grant S (1998) Effect of Bryostatin-1 on Taxol-induced Apoptosis and Cytotoxicity in Human Leukemia Cells (U937). *Biochemical Pharmacology*, **56**, 635–44.

Wang S, Wang Z, Boise L, Dent P and Grant S (1999a) Loss of the bcl-2 phosphorylation loop domain increases resistance of human leukemia cells (U937) to paclitaxel-mediated mitochondrial dysfunction and apoptosis. *Biochem Biophys Res Commun*, **259**, 67–72.

Wang S, Wang Z, Boise LH, Dent P and S G (1999b) Bryostatin-1 enhances paclitaxel induced mitochondrial dysfunction and apoptosis in human leukemia cells (U937) ectopically expressing Bcl-xl. *Leukemia*, **13**, 1564–73.

Weller M, Winter S, Schmidt C *et al.* (1997) Topisomerase-I inhibitors for human malignant glioma: differential modulation of p53, p21, bax, and bcl-2 expression and of CD95-mediated apoptosis by camptothecin and beta-lapachone. *Int J Cancer*, **73**, 707–714.

Wender PA, Cribbs CM, Koehler KF *et al.* (1988) Modeling of the bryostatins to the phorbol ester pharmacophore on protein kinase C. *Proc Natl Acad Sci USA*, **85**, 7197–201.

Xu B, Kim S-T and Kastan MB (2001) Involvement of BRCA1 in S phase and G2-phase checkpoints after ionizing radiation. *Mol Cell Biol*, **21**, 3445–50.

Yoo YD, Park JD, Choi JY *et al.* (1998) CDK4 down-regulation induced by paclitaxel is associated with G1 arrest in gastric cancer cells. *Clin Cancer Res*, **4**, 3063–8.

Yu D, Jing T, Liu B *et al.* (1998) Overexpression of ErbB2 blocks taxol-induced apoptosis by upregulation of p21Cip1 which inhibits p34Cdc2 kinase. *Mol Cell*, **2**, 581–91.

Yu J, Zhang L, Hwang PM *et al.* (1999) Identification and classification of p53-regulated genes. *Proc Natl Acad Sci USA*, **96**, 14517–22.

Yu Q, Rose JH, Zhang H *et al.* (2002) UCN-01 inhibits p53 up-regulation and abrogates gamma-radiation-induced G2-M Checkpoint independently of p53 by targeting both of the checkpoint kinases, Chk2 and Chk1. *Cancer Res*, **62**, 5743–48.

Zhou BS and Elledge SJ (2000) The DNA damage response: putting checkpoints in perspective. *Nature*, **408**, 433–39.

Zhou BS, Tsai P, Ker R *et al.* (1998) Overexpression of transfected human ribonucleotide reductase M2 subunit in human cancer cells enhances their invasive potential. *Clin Exp Metastasis*, **16**, 43–9.

Zhou X, Wang X and Hu B (2002) An ATM-independent S phase checkpoint response involves Chk1 pathway. *Cancer Res*, **62**, 1598–1603.

Zonder JA, Shields AF, Zalupski M *et al.* (2001) A phase II trial of bryostatin 1 in the treatment of metastatic colorectal cancer. *Clin Cancer Res*, **7**, 38–42.

Chapter 7

Therapeutic monoclonal antibodies

Peter Borchmann and Andreas Engert

1 Humanisation of monoclonal antibodies

The therapeutic potential of **monoclonal antibodies** (mAbs) was realised a
long time before their structure had been explored. It was Paul Ehrlich in the
late nineteenth century who developed the idea of a targeted therapy against
malignant tumours. Still today, it is fascinating to read his Croonian lecture
or the Nobel Prize lecture given in 1908 (see *http://www.nobel.se/medicine/
laureates/1908/ehrlich-lecture.pdf*; Ehrlich 1900). It took some generations of
researchers to reveal the origin and structure of antibodies and then to produce
monoclonal antibodies with a defined specificity in significant amounts (Porter 1967; Edelman *et al.* 1968; Kohler and Milstein 1975). In 1975, Kohler and
Milstein published details of the **hybridoma** technology, which is the fusion of
an antigen-specific B-cell with an immortal cell-line, resulting in an immortal
clone producing the antigen-specific antibody (Kohler and Milstein 1975).
This was perhaps the last milestone discovery in medical sciences that was not
patented and thereby enabled the rapid development of thousands of antibodies and the definition of thousands of antigens. To obtain monoclonal
antibodies, mice are immunised in order to generate the antigen-specific
B-cells, thus the resulting antibodies are of murine origin. For many purposes,
including diagnostic procedures such as immunohistochemistry or fluorescence-
activated cell sorting (FACS), murine antibodies work very well. But
for therapeutic use, they present several obstacles that have to be overcome.
The first therapeutic approach was the 'tailored antibody', developed in the
early 1980s: single hybridoma cultures for single patients suffering from B-cell
lymphomas, so called 'anti-idiotype antibodies' (Miller *et al.* 1982). Early
clinical results were spectacular, but a tremendous effort had to be undertaken
before one of these patients could finally be treated. Early enthusiasm turned
into disappointment, when in 1994 the development of the anti-CD52

antibody alemtuzumab was halted due to unexpected toxicity and profound immunosuppression. Between 1975 and 1994, only one antibody had made its way into the clinic, the anti-CD3 antibody OKT3 (muromomab) (Wilde and Goa 1996). Since then, the situation has changed dramatically. At the time of writing, 17 antibodies are approved for various indications and with the anti-CD20 antibody rituximab in 1997, one of the commercially most successful drugs ever, has been introduced into the market (see Table 7.1).

The main reason for this change has been improved production technology based on molecular genetics associated with the humanisation of antibodies. As pointed out above, the hybridoma technology produced murine antibodies (or from other species such as rats, hamster, rabbits, monkeys). Since antibodies are large molecules (around 150 kDa), they are highly **immunogenic** in humans. Therefore, the infusion of murine antibodies causes the induction of human anti-mouse antibodies (HAMAs), which then either inactivate the therapeutic antibody and change the antibody's half-life or even lead to anaphylactic reactions (Chester and Hawkins 1995; Vose *et al.* 2000). In both cases, the clinical use of the antibodies are hampered. Thus, humanisation of antibodies was a critical step towards their clinical application.

A knowledge of the physiological structure and function of antibodies is essential for any **recombinant** production strategy (for anybody looking for a deeper insight, the following site is recommended http://www-immuno.path. cam.ac.uk/~mrc7/humanisation/index.html). An antibody is a large and flexible protein that has multiple regions with different functions (see Fig. 7.1). First, there are the **complementarity-determining regions (CDRs)**, which form a pocket that specifically binds an antigen. The CDRs are part of the variable region of the light chain as well as the heavy chain. Light and heavy chains differ by the number of their constant regions. There is only one constant region for the light chain, but three for the heavy chain. After enzymatic cleavage with papain, antibodies disintegrate into a binding and a non-binding fragment. Together with their variables regions, the first constant region of the heavy chain and the constant region of the light chain constitute the fragment antigen binding (**Fab**). So the main function of the constant region near the variable region is to stabilise the variable region. Although Fabs are small proteins of about 50 kDa, they can already induce an anti-Fab immune response. The second and third region of the heavy chain are also **Fc**, denoting fragment crystalline, because it precipitates after cleavage from the Fabs. The Fc fragment activates the **innate** and the **adaptive** immune system by binding to **complement** (complement dependent cytotoxicity, CDC) and to Fc-receptors (Fc-R) on immunocompetent cells, such as NK cells, T cells, and macrophages (**antibody-dependent cell-mediated cytotoxicity, ADCC**).

Table 7.1 Antibodies approved by the FDA

FDA approved	Product	Target	Type	Indication
1986	Muromomab (Orthoclone OKT3®)	CD3	Murine IgG2a	Transplant rejection
1994	Abciximab (ReoPro®)	GP IIb/IIIa	Chimeric Fab	Prevention of re-stenosis after PTCA
1997	Daclizumab (Zenapax®)	CD25	Humanised IgG1	Transplant rejection
1997	Rituximab (Rituxan®)	CD20	Chimeric IgG1	B-cell lymphoma
1998	Basiliximab (Simulect®)	CD25	Chimeric IgG1	Transplant rejection
1998 P	alivizumab (Synagis®)	RSV	Humanised IgG1	RSV bronchiolitis
1998	Infliximab (Remicade®)	TNF	Chimeric IgG1	Crohn's disease, rheumatoid arthritis
1998	Trastuzumab (Herceptin®)	HER2/neu	Humanised IgG1	Breast cancer
2000	Gemtuzumab (Mylotarg®)	CD33	Humanised IgG4-toxin-conjugate	Acute myeloid leukaemia
2001	Alemtuzumab (MabCampath®)	CD52	Humanised IgG1	Chronic lymphatic leukaemia
2002	90Y-ibritumomab (Zevalin®)	CD20	Murine IgG1-radionuclide-conjugate	B-cell lymphoma
2002	Adalimumab (Humira®)	TNF	Human IgG1	Rheumatoid arthritis
2003	Omalizumab (Xolair®)	IgE	Humanised IgG1	Asthma
2003	131I-tositumomab (Bexxar®)	CD20	Murine IgG1-radionuclide-conjugate	B-cell lymphoma
2003	Efalizumab (Raptiva®)	CD11a	Humanised IgG1	Psoriasis
2004	Bevacizumab (Avastin®)	VEGF	Humanised IgG1	Colorectal cancer
2004	Cetuximab (Erbitux®)	EGFR	Chimeric IgG1	Colorectal cancer

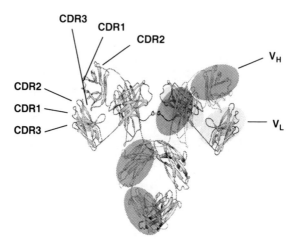

CDR = complementarity-determining region

Fig. 7.1 Antibody model.

There are different degrees of humanisation. First, one can replace, for example, the murine constant regions with human constant regions (see Fig. 7.2). The result is a **chimeric** antibody, still containing about a quarter of the original antibody. Chimeric antibodies can be immunogenic, but to a much lesser extent than their parent molecules (Hosono *et al.* 1992). Going one step further, the CDRs are engrafted into the framework of the variable region of a human antibody. The result is called a humanised antibody. It contains only about 3% of the foreign protein. At a quick glance, this seems to be an easy procedure, but often the construct loses affinity to the antigen and single amino acids have to be substituted to improve the binding properties. Finally, there are the so-called fully human antibodies. Fully human antibodies in clinical trials are obtained by immunising transgenic mice. In these mice, the **immunoglobulin**-encoding **DNA** sequences have been replaced with human sequences (Fishwild *et al.* 1996; Bruggemann and Taussig 1997; Vaughan *et al.* 1998; Tomizuka *et al.* 2000). Recombination and **somatic** hypermutation occur obviously correctly and thus these strains produce entirely human antibodies.

Although there is little doubt that chimeric human/mouse antibodies induce HAMA response to a much lesser extent than fully murine antibodies, it is currently unclear whether or not humanised or even human antibodies really confer any clinically significant advantage over chimeric antibodies (Clark 2000). It has to be considered that the human Ig framework sequences are obtained from plasma cells and have undergone somatic mutations.

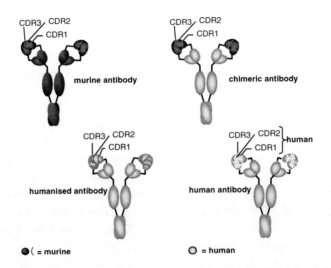

Fig. 7.2 Degrees of humanisation of monoclonal antibodies. Murine antibody indicated by momab for therapeutic antibodies, e.g. muromomab; human antibody (umab); chimeric antibody with human constant regions replacing mouse constant regions (ximab e.g. rituximab); humanised antibody with mouse complementarity-determining regions (CDR) engrafted into the framework of the variable region of the human antibody (zumab e.g. alemtuzumab).

So, even these human antibodies are not completely identical to the germ-line sequence. In addition, development of human anti-chimeric antibodies (HACAs) is no problem in the use of rituximab, the antibody for which by far the most extensive experience exists (Piro *et al.* 1999). Taken together, all approaches are basically suited to prevent an anti-antibody response in humans. But since this response is not predictable, clinical trials must investigate this question in each case anew. With regard to their effector functions, there should not be major differences. These will depend more on the subtype of the immunoglobulin (e.g. IgG1, IgG2, IgG3, or IgG4), which determines affinity to complement or the different types of FcRs thus affecting CDC and ADCC.

2 For haematological malignancies—rituximab, alemtuzumab

2.1 Rituximab

With the introduction of rituximab, a chimeric human/mouse monoclonal antibody directed against the CD20 antigen, the era of therapeutic antibodies had begun. The story of rituximab started in 1997, when the application of rituximab in the treatment of relapsed or refractory indolent CD20 positive B-cell non-Hodgkin's lymphoma (NHL) was endorsed by the US Food and

Drug Administration. More recently, rituximab has also been approved for the first-line treatment of aggressive NHL, when combined with standard chemotherapy, and for the first-line treatment of indolent NHL. Approval for the treatment of rheumatoid arthritis is expected to take place in the near future. To give an impression about the extent of use of this antibody, one can consider that in 2004 rituximab was sold for $1711.2 million. The rapidly increasing volume of data makes an overview difficult to give; more comprehensive information is summarised elsewhere (Boye *et al.* 2003).

Rituximab is a chimeric human/mouse antibody with human constant regions and mouse variable regions obtained from a murine anti-CD20 antibody (Fig. 7.3). CD20 is trans-membrane phosphoprotein with the following properties: (I) CD20 is expressed on the majority of B-cell lymphomas cells, but not on other human cells, (II) it is expressed on almost all B-lymphocytes excluding immature precursor cells (allowing reconstitution of the B-cell compartment after therapy) and plasma cells (allowing the ongoing production of immunoglobulins), (III) CD20 neither is shed into the plasma after binding of rituximab, nor is it internalised after antibody engagement, (IV) CD20 is essential in the **differentiation** and proliferation of B-lymphocytes, and (V) its binding results in **apoptosis** of the malignant cells due to calcium influx.

2.1.1 Indolent and follicular lymphoma

The efficacy and safety of rituximab, given as a single agent in relapsed indolent and follicular lymphoma, were established in an international multi-centre trial. A total of 166 patients received four weekly doses of $375 \, \mathrm{mg/m^2}$. In this trial, the mean serum half-life after the first infusion was shorter than

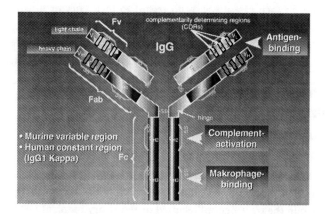

Fig. 7.3 Rituximab structure.

after the fourth infusion (76.3 versus 205.8 h) indicating a saturation of compartments. The overall response rate (ORR) was 48%, including (McLaughlin *et al.* 1998) 6% complete responses (CR) and 42% partial responses (PR). Overall, only 13% of patients had no response or progressive disease. Median time to progression (TTP) was 13.2 months for responders and duration of response (DR) was 11.6 months. Flu-like adverse events such as fever, chills, nausea, and aches were mainly associated with the first infusion and were typically modest. No haematological toxicity was observed apart from a nearly complete elimination of B-lymphocytes in 86% of patients. Importantly, no significant changes were observed in serum immunoglobulin levels and serious infections were not a significant problem. Overall, it was very well-tolerated, especially when compared with conventional chemotherapy. The overall response rates are still good, 43%, if patients with bulky disease (>10 cm) are being treated (Davis *et al.* 1999). This is especially noteworthy, because for some reason antibodies are believed to be ineffective in larger tumour masses. First, they may be captured by the outer cell layers of the tumour, so they cannot penetrate into the tumour. Second, the intratumoral pressure is increased making it difficult for these large molecules to reach their target against this gradient.

Recently, rituximab has also been shown to improve the response rate and to double the time to progression when combined with conventional chemotherapy (cyclophosphamide, vincristine, prednisone, COP) in the first-line treatment of indolent NHL from 15 to 32 months (Marcus *et al.* 2005). The combination of rituximab and chemotherapy was first shown to act synergistically in pre-clinical studies (Demidem *et al.* 1997). Rituximab can sensitise resistant malignant cells to the effect of **cytotoxic** agents. Thus, a large number of different clinical trials has been initiated evaluating the combination of rituximab and various chemotherapeutics (summarised in Table 7.2). When combined with the doxorubicin-containing regimen CHOP, response rates of >90% are achieved and the median duration of response is very long, 63.3 months (Hainsworth 2002).

Retreatment with rituximab is feasible and safe. Although there is a modest loss of activity, overall response rates are still around 40% and the duration of response is not shortened (Davis *et al.* 2000). This is in contrast to conventional chemotherapy, where development of resistance frequently occurs. This is due to the fact that the selection of CD20 negative lymphoma cells is rarely observed. Currently, maintenance therapy with rituximab after induction of a remission is being tested (Hainsworth *et al.* 2002, 2005). Rituximab is applied every 6 months at standard dose (four weekly doses of $375 \, \text{mg/m}^2$). Though final results are still pending, results obtained so far indicate a prolonged

Table 7.2 Clinical studies using rituximab combined with chemotherapy in indolent and follicular NHL

Histology	n	Schedule	Response	Reference
foll. NHL (67% relapsed, 33% untreated)	40	7×375 mg/m² R + 6 cycles flu	CR 82.5% PR 7.5%	Czuczman et al. (2002)
indol. NHL (77.5% untreated, 22.5% pretreated)	40	6×375 mg/m² R + 6 cycles CHOP	CR 55% PR 40% 7/8 pts became bcl-2 negative	Czuczman et al. (2004)
indol. NHL (untreated, all were bcl-2 positive in PB and/or BM)	128	Pts who were in CR/PR after CHOP, but still bcl-2 positive by PCR were eligible for a standard dose* of R (77 pts received R)	74% became bcl-2 negative after R	Rambaldi et al. (2002)
indol. NHL (relapsed or untreated)	16	4×FND+ standard dose* R; for pts with PR after the 1. cycle: 2× FND +2 × 375 mg/m²R	at the end of the whole treatment program: CR/CRu 81% PR 12.5% 8/12 pts became bcl-2 negative	Vitolo et al. (2001)
l-g/foll. NHL (relapsed or refractory)	43	Two arms: A: FCM day 1–3 B: FCM day 1–3, R one day before FCM	A: CR 21% PR 47% B: CR 35% PR 60%	Hiddemann et al. (2001)
indol. NHL (pretreated)	10	day 1: 1×375 mg/m² R day 2: cyclophosphamide day 1–7: decadron; cycles were repeated every 4 weeks till a maximum response (median 6 cycles)	CR 40% PR 60%	Patel et al. (2001)
indol. NHL (untreated)	19	4–6 cycles flu/ mitoxantrone + standard dose* R	CR 53% PR 42%	Gregory et al. (2001)

(continued)

Table 7.2 (*continued*) Clinical studies using rituximab combined with chemotherapy in indolent and follicular NHL

indol. NHL (relapsed)	20	day 1–3: bendamustine day 1: mitoxantrone week 2–5: standard dose* R; followed by a maximum of 5 courses of bendamustine/mitoxantrone	CR 35% PR 60%	Weide et al. (2002)
indol. NHL (pretreated)	25	day 1–3: flu + bendamustine week 2–5: standard dose* R; followed by a maximum of 4 courses of flu/bendamustine	CR 28% CR 48%	Kirchner et al. (2001)
indol. NHL	124	Two arms: A: 8× MCP B: 8× MCP + standard dose* R	CR 40% PR 41% (evaluation has to be continued)	Herold et al. (2001)

*4×375 mg /m² R weekly; R = rituximab; l-g = low-grade; foll. = follicular; ORR = overall response rate; CR = complete response; PR = partial response; m = months; indol. = indolent; pts = patients; flu = fludarabine; CHOP = cyclophosphamide, doxorubicin, vincristine, prednisone; PB = peripheral blood; BM = bone marrow; FND = fludarabine, mitoxantrone, dexamethasone; MCP = mitoxantrone, chlorambucil, prednisone; TTP = time to progression; DR = duration of response.

relapse-free interval (34 months) and an improved response rate compared with retreatment in case of relapse only.

In summary, rituximab has been introduced as a single agent in the second-line treatment of indolent follicular B-cell lymphomas, followed by its approval for the first-line treatment in combination with a polychemotherapy regimen, and first clinical data support its use as a maintenance therapy, at least. Thus, this antibody has become, within a very short time, an important part of indolent B-cell lymphoma therapy. This is surprising, taking into account that the single agent ORR is only around 50%. But its superior toxicity profile compared with that of conventional chemotherapy, as well as its completely different mechanism of action, make this drug highly attractive for both patients and doctors. Nevertheless, data showing a survival benefit for patients treated with rituximab are not yet available.

2.1.2 Diffuse large B-cell NHL

As a single-agent, rituximab shows an ORR of about 30% in relapsed diffuse large B-cell NHL (Coiffier *et al.* 1998). Response duration is short and treatment can be recommended only for palliative reasons. But in combination with the standard chemotherapy regimen for the first-line treatment (R-CHOP), results of the conventional therapy could be substantially improved. In a large, prospectively randomised multicentre trial in previously untreated patients with aggressive NHL, CHOP alone was compared with R–CHOP (Coiffier *et al.* 2002). This study involved 399 elderly patients (aged 60–80 years) with diffuse large B-cell lymphoma (stage II–IV). With a median follow-up of 24 months, R-CHOP led to significantly more CRs (76% versus 63%), an improved 2-year event-free survival (EFS) (57% versus 38%, $P<0.001$) and overall survival (OS) (70% versus 57%, $P = 0.007$) compared with CHOP alone (Fig. 7.4). This study showed a significant benefit of the combined immunochemotherapy in high- and low-risk patients. A major factor affecting the response to conventional chemotherapy is the BCL-2 expression of the tumour cells, an anti-apoptotic protein expressed in about two-thirds of all patients. Analysis of the patients in this trial showed that rituximab was able to overcome this resistance to chemotherapy in BCL-2 positive tumours. In BCL-2 negative tumours, the addition of rituximab had no benefit (Mounier *et al.* 2003). There was no major difference between the two arms in terms of toxicity or severe infections.

Thus, this 'proof of concept' study showed that the addition of rituximab to conventional CHOP is associated with superior results without adding toxicity, and therefore R-CHOP is the new standard for patients with aggressive NHL. Results were confirmed in other investigations, as well as in patients younger

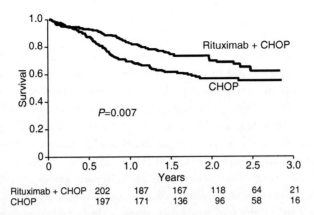

	0	0.5	1.0	1.5	2.0	2.5	3.0
Rituximab + CHOP	202	187	167	118	64	21	
CHOP		197	171	136	96	58	16

Fig. 7.4 Rituximab ± CHOP (cyclophosphamide, doxorubicin, vincristine and prednisone). Overall survival for previously untreated aggressive non-Hodgkin's lymphoma (Coiffier *et al.* 2002).

than 60 years. In addition, a large international study (MInT) has been halted in 2004 due to the superiority of the rituximab-containing arm in a CHOP-like chemotherapy in previously untreated younger patients with aggressive NHL. To summarise, adding rituximab to CHOP has become the new gold standard first-line treatment of diffuse large B-cell NHL. This is especially noteworthy since CHOP had been the standard of care for 25 years and numerous studies had failed to improve on this schedule (Fisher *et al.* 1993).

2.1.3 Other indications

CLL In chronic lymphocytic leukaemia, rituximab is not as active as a single agent as in other indolent B-cell NHL. One reason might be the lower density of CD20 expression of CLL cells. Response rates in the pivotal trial were only 13%. In combination with chemotherapy (fludarabine plus cyclophosphamide) though, response rates in untreated patients are extremely high, 95% including 70% CR (Keating *et al.* 2005). Also, in relapsed patients, the ORR is between 70% and 90% (Schulz *et al.* 2002; Wierda *et al.* 2005). It should be noted, however, that these numbers are the results of uncontrolled phase II trials, and no data concerning overall survival have been presented so far.

Waldenström's macroglobulinaemia In Waldenström's macroglobulinaemia, lymphoplasmocytic NHL in the WHO classification of malignant lymphoma, rituximab is active as a single agent in first-line therapy, as well as in relapsed patients, with response rates of around 50% (Dimopoulos *et al.* 2002). As in the other indolent B-cell lymphomas, combination with chemotherapy might be useful, but no data are currently available.

Auto-immune diseases Since all antibody-mediated auto-immune diseases might be influenced by B-cell depletion, rituximab obviously might be effective in this indication. Promising case reports had been published from the beginning on a broad variety of auto-immune diseases, but the first larger number of patients treated within a clinical study were published for refractory chronic idiopathic thrombocytopenia. In these patients, rituximab had an ORR of 52% including durable remissions (Stasi *et al.* 2001). Rituximab has also shown activity in smaller uncontrolled studies against systemic lupus erythematosus and pemphigus vulgaris (Herrmann *et al.* 2003).

A real breakthrough though was a large phase III study evaluating rituximab's efficacy in active rheumatoid arthritis despite methotrexate treatment. A single course of two infusions of rituximab, alone or in combination with either cyclophosphamide or continued methotrexate, provided significant improvement in disease symptoms at both weeks 24 and 48 (Edwards *et al.* 2004). Thus, **immunotherapy** with rituximab has been introduced successfully into the treatment of auto-immune diseases and more clinical studies are ongoing.

2.2 Alemtuzumab

Alemtuzumab (Campath) is a humanised rat-IgG1 antibody binding to CD52, an antigen with unknown function found on >95% of peripheral blood lymphocytes and monocytes and to a smaller extent on granulocytes. In addition, it is expressed in the male genital tract. Alemtuzumab is the final product of a long-lasting development period, starting more than two decades ago. Initially developed as a rat IgM-antibody, the antibody was administered to individual lymphoma patients. Results were disappointing: the antibody produced only transient depletion of blood lymphocytes, but had no effect on solid tumour masses or bone marrow (Dyer *et al.* 1989). Its IgM-**isotype** allowed complement activation but did not mediate any antibody-dependent cytotoxicity (ADCC). The molecule was therefore further engineered resulting in a rat IgG2b antibody activating human Fc-receptors and thereby inducing ADCC. However, due to its murine structure it induced the development of human anti-mouse antibodies (**HAMA**), which then neutralised the antibody after repeated administration. In 1988, the antibody was humanised and the first results in patients with advanced B-cell lymphoma were promising enough to warrant further studies. The antibody was primarily tested in auto-immune diseases, but toxicity was unacceptable, including a high number of serious infections. Finally, in the late 1990s, alemtuzumab proved its effectiveness in fludarabine-refractory B-CLL and was then approved in this indication in the year 2000. The results of this study (Rai *et al.* 2002) showed an ORR of 33% with a median time to progression of 9 months in responding patients. The T-cell depletion resulted in serious infectious complications in 10% of all patients, though prophylactic medication was applied. In particular cytomegalovirus (CMV) reactivation occurs frequently and must therefore be monitored until T-cell recovery. Clinical research is now focused on combined treatment with conventional chemotherapy. Very promising phase II studies have been published in combination with fludarabine reporting an ORR of 85% including molecular remissions (Elter *et al.* 2004). Data on overall survival are still pending.

3 For solid tumours—cetuximab, bevacizumab, trastuzumab

3.1 Cetuximab

Cetuximab (C225, Erbitux) is a chimeric monoclonal antibody that binds to the extracellular domain of the epidermal growth factor receptor (EGFR) to block **ligand** binding, which results in inhibition of autophosphorylation of EGFR. EGFR is expressed in a large number of solid tumours and its expression correlates with a poor outcome (see Chapter 4). EGFR-binding by cetuximab results in cell-cycle arrest, and increased expression of pro-apoptotic proteins or decreased expression of anti-apoptotic proteins. Furthermore, cetuximab decreases the production of vascular endothelial growth factor and basic fibroblast growth factor in orthotopic tumour models. Pre-clinical studies revealed synergism between cetuximab and a number of chemotherapeutic agents, including cisplatin and paclitaxel, in a wide variety of cell lines. Cetuximab appears to be synergistic with radiation treatment as well.

Clinical development focused on colorectal cancer. In patients with metastatic colon cancer refractory to treatment with irinotecan, single agent cetuximab showed a modest response rate of 10.8% with a short median TTP of 1.5 months. Combination with irinotecan increased the response rate to 22.9% and median TTP to 4.1 months (Cunningham *et al.* 2004). Based on these data, cetuximab received FDA approval in 2004 for the treatment of metastasised colorectal cancer in combination with irinotecan in patients refractory to irinotecan chemotherapy or as a single-agent treatment in patients intolerant to irinotecan-based chemotherapy. However, approval is based on response rates only and not on improvement of disease-related symptoms or prolongation of overall survival. In contrast, cetuximab treatment can cause an acneiform rash that in some instances necessitates dose reduction or delay. This rash seems to correlate with the tumour response to treatment. Other EGFR inhibitors, such as the small molecule erlotinib, also cause this skin reaction (Perez-Soler 2003).

Other indications for cetuximab are currently being tested. One of the most promising is non-small-cell lung cancer where the addition of cetuximab to cisplatin/vinorelbine in inoperable patients increased response rates from 20% to 32% in a randomised phase II trial including 86 patients (Rosell *et al.* 2004). Cetuximab has also been extensively investigated in patients with head and neck cancer (HNC). A phase III study recruited 121 patients with untreated HNC metastatic disease to compare cisplatin and cetuximab combination therapy with cisplatin alone. The response rate was higher in the combination treatment group: 23% versus 9%. However, there was no significant difference in time to tumour progression (4.1 versus 3.4 months) or overall median survival (9.2 versus 8.0 months) (Burtness *et al.* 2002). Another phase II study has shown some single-agent activity of cetuximab in platinum-refractory HNC patients and further phase III studies are underway (Trigo *et al.* 2004).

3.2 Bevacizumab

Any tumour growth depends on the tumour's supply of oxygen and nutrients. Therefore, malignant tumours induce their own blood vessel supply by the secretion of vascular endothelial growth factor (VEGF). This finding had been recognised as early as 1939 (Ide *et al.* 1939). Targeting tumour vasculature has since become an attractive approach. Advantages of this approach include the applicability to different tumour types, a low toxicity against normal tissue, and the excellent accessibility of the target structure to the antibody. Based on this rationale, the humanised anti-VEGF antibody bevacizumab was developed. In a pre-clinical animal model, this antibody dramatically changed the growth characteristics of a rhabdomyosarcoma cell line from being a rapidly growing malignancy to a dormant microcolony (Borgstrom *et al.* 1996).

Bevacizumab also was primarily developed for the treatment of colorectal cancer. In a large multicentre phase III trial ($n = 813$), the addition of bevacizumab (every two weeks) to irinotecan/5-fluorouracil bolus was compared with chemotherapy alone in the first-line treatment of metastasised colorectal cancer (Hurwitz *et al.* 2004). Overall survival was prolonged significantly from 15.6 to 20.3 months. Accordingly, response rates improved from 35% to 45%. Based on these results, bevacizumab was approved for the first-line treatment of metastasised colorectal cancer in combination with a 5-fluorouracil-based chemotherapy regimen in 2004.

Bevacizumab has also shown activity in advanced renal cancer. This tumour is characterised by a high VEGF expression and has a highly vascular histologic appearance. Bevacizumab prolonged the time to progression significantly by the factor 2.5, but overall survival was not influenced (Yang *et al.* 2003). Further development explores the combination not only with conventional chemotherapy, but also with EGFR inhibitors in different solid tumours. Some pre-clinical results suggest the use of bevacizumab in a minimal residual disease setting, therefore, phase III studies for the **adjuvant** treatment of colorectal cancer are underway.

3.3 **Trastuzumab**

The human epidermal growth factor receptor 2 (HER2, also referred to as HER2/neu or c-erbB-2) is a **proto-oncogene** that encodes a transmembrane protein with tyrosine kinase activity. HER2/neu is found on numerous epithelial tissues and overexpressed on 20–30% of breast cancer specimens (Slamon *et al.* 1989). Overexpression of HER2 correlates with hormone receptor negativity, a reduced sensitivity to hormone therapy and to chemotherapy, resulting in worse survival. Thus, HER2 is part of the oncogenesis in a subset of breast cancer patients and HER2/neu-status has to be assessed by immunohistochemistry before treatment. As a consequence of this overexpression, the chimeric anti-HER2/neu antibody trastuzumab was developed (human IgG1). The exact mechanism of action has not been fully elucidated, but several factors have been shown to contribute to its activity: HER2/neu-down-regulation, inhibition of the formation of HER2/neu heterodimers, induction of p27, and cell-cycle arrest in the G_1 phase, cleavage inhibition of HER2/neu, induction of ADCC and CDC. Pre-clinical studies revealed synergism with various different cytotoxic agents including carboplatin, 4-hydroxycyclophosphamide, docetaxel, and vinorelbine (Pegram *et al.* 2004). Recent research has revealed synergism between HER2/neu and HER1 (human epidermal growth factor receptor 1) (Moulder *et al.* 2001).

Clinical studies have been initiated in metastatic breast cancer patients with an international open-label study including 222 patients with HER2-overexpressing metastatic breast cancer that had progressed after one or two chemotherapy regimens (Cobleigh *et al.* 1999). Patients were treated with trastuzumab single-agent therapy with a loading dose of 4 mg/kg followed by weekly doses of 2 mg/kg. The overall response rate was 15% (CR 4%, PR 11%) with a median duration of response of 9.1 months. The results of this trial led to approval of trastuzumab as single-agent therapy in second-line treatment for HER2-positive breast cancer in 2000. Trastuzumab shows comparable results in first line therapy with an ORR of 26% in metastatic breast cancer (Vogel *et al.* 2002).

Based on the pre-clinical results, a large number of combination therapies had been initiated. In the largest comparative trial, 469 patients were randomly assigned to receive either standard chemotherapy or standard chemotherapy plus trastuzumab (Slamon *et al.* 2001). Patients without prior anthracycline therapy were treated with a combination of the anthracycline doxorubicin or epirubicin and the alkylating agent cyclophosphamide (AC or EC, 138 women) alone or with trastuzumab (143 women). Patients previously treated with an anthracycline were treated with paclitaxel alone (96 women) or paclitaxel plus trastuzumab (92 women). Overall, 118 patients in the chemotherapy/trastuzumab groups responded (50%) compared with only 74 responses in the chemotherapy groups (32%). Furthermore, addition of trastuzumab to chemotherapy prolonged the median survival by 4.8 months (from 20.3 to 25.1 months). However, the combination of anthracyclines and trastuzumab revealed an unpredicted side-effect of trastuzumab, which is cardiotoxicity. As a single agent, trastuzumab is generally very well-tolerated besides the transient and transfusion related reaction as seen with other antibodies. Cardiac-adverse events occur in about 7% of all patients. In combination with anthracyclines this number increases to 28%. Review of clinical data revealed the following risk factors for the development of cardiotoxicity: anthracycline pretreatment, history of cardiac disease, irradiation of the left chest and age. In patients with these risk factors, advantages and disadvantages of trastuzumab treatment must be carefully considered. Other combinations with conventional chemotherapy have been tested in the clinical setting as well and are highly active as reviewed elsewhere (Montemuro *et al.* 2004). In particular the combination with vinorelbine shows promising activity.

In summary, trastuzumab certainly has benefit for the subset of metastatic breast cancer patients overexpressing HER2/neu. Combination with conventional chemotherapy is synergistic, not only in the laboratory, but also in the clinical setting. Future development will include the evaluation of trastuzumab's use in other epithelial neoplasias, as well as its combination with small molecules inhibiting other growth factors (Langer *et al.* 2004).

References

Borgstrom P, Hillan KJ, Sriramarao P, Ferrara N (1996) Complete inhibition of angiogenesis and growth of microtumors by anti-vascular endothelial growth factor neutralizing antibody: novel concepts of angiostatic therapy from intravital videomicroscopy. *Cancer Res*; 56: 4032–9.

Boye J, Elter T, Engert A (2003) An overview of the current clinical use of the anti-CD20 monoclonal antibody rituximab. *Ann Oncol*; 14: 520–35.

Bruggemann M, Taussig MJ (1997) Production of human antibody repertoires in transgenic mice. *Curr Opin Biotechnol*; 8: 455–8.

Burtness BA, Li Y, Flood W, Mattar BI, Forastiere AA (2002) Phase III trial comparing cisplatin (C) + placebo (P) to C+ anti-epidermal growth factor antibody (EGF-R) C225 in patients (pts) with metastatic/recurrent head & neck cancer (HNC). *Proc Am Soc Clin Oncol*; 21: 901.

Chester KA, Hawkins RE (1995) Clinical issues in antibody design. *Trends Biotechnol*; 13: 294–300.

Clark M (2000) Antibody humanization: a case of the 'Emperor's new clothes'? *Immunol Today*; 21: 397–402.

Cobleigh MA, Vogel CL, Tripathy D, Robert NJ, Scholl S, Fehrenbacher L et al. (1999) Multinational study of the efficacy and safety of humanized anti-HER2 monoclonal antibody in women who have HER2-overexpressing metastatic breast cancer that has progressed after chemotherapy for metastatic disease. *J Clin Oncol*; 17: 2639–48.

Coiffier B, Haioun C, Ketterer N, Engert A, Tilly H, Ma D et al. (1998) Rituximab (anti-CD20 monoclonal antibody) for the treatment of patients with relapsing or refractory aggressive lymphoma: a multicenter phase II study. *Blood*; 92: 1927–32.

Coiffier B, Lepage E, Briere J, Herbrecht R, Tilly H, Bouabdallah R et al. (2002) CHOP chemotherapy plus rituximab compared with CHOP alone in elderly patients with diffuse large-B-cell lymphoma. *N Engl J Med*; 346: 235–42.

Cunningham D, Humblet Y, Siena S, Khayat D, Bleiberg H, Santoro A et al. (2004) Cetuximab monotherapy and cetuximab plus irinotecan in irinotecan-refractory metastatic colorectal cancer. *N Engl J Med*; 351: 337–45.

Czuczman MS, Fallon A, Mohr A, Stewart C, Bernstein ZP, McCarthy P et al. (2002) Rituximab in combination with CHOP or fludarabine in low-grade lymphoma. *Semin Oncol*; 29: 36–40.

Czuczman MS, Weaver R, Alkuzweny B, Berlfein J, Grillo-Lopez AJ (2004) Prolonged clinical and molecular remission in patients with low-grade or follicular non-Hodgkin's lymphoma treated with rituximab plus CHOP chemotherapy: 9-year follow-up. *J Clin Oncol*; 22: 4711–6.

Davis TA, White CA, Grillo-Lopez AJ, Velasquez WS, Link B, Maloney DG et al. (1999) Single-agent monoclonal antibody efficacy in bulky non-Hodgkin's lymphoma: results of a phase II trial of rituximab. *J Clin Oncol*; 17: 1851–7.

Davis TA, Grillo-Lopez AJ, White CA, McLaughlin P, Czuczman MS, Link BK et al. (2000) Rituximab anti-CD20 monoclonal antibody therapy in non-Hodgkin's lymphoma: safety and efficacy of re-treatment. *J Clin Oncol*; 18: 3135–43.

Demidem A, Lam T, Alas S, Hariharan K, Hanna N, Bonavida B (1997) Chimeric anti-CD20 (IDEC-C2B8) monoclonal antibody sensitizes a B cell lymphoma cell line to cell killing by cytotoxic drugs. *Cancer Biother Radiopharm*; 12: 177–86.

Dimopoulos MA, Zervas C, Zomas A, Kiamouris C, Viniou NA, Grigoraki V et al. (2002) Treatment of Waldenstrom's macroglobulinemia with rituximab. *J Clin Oncol*; 20: 2327–33.

Dyer MJ, Hale G, Hayhoe FG, Waldmann H (1989) Effects of CAMPATH-1 antibodies in vivo in patients with lymphoid malignancies: influence of antibody isotype. *Blood*; 73: 1431–9.

Edelman GM, Gall WE, Waxdal MJ, Konigsberg WH (1968) The covalent structure of a human gamma G-immunoglobulin. I. Isolation and characterization of the whole molecule, the polypeptide chains, and the tryptic fragments. *Biochemistry*; 7: 1950–8.

Edwards JC, Szczepanski L, Szechinski J, Filipowicz-Sosnowska A, Emery P, Close DR et al. (2004) Efficacy of B-cell-targeted therapy with rituximab in patients with rheumatoid arthritis. *N Engl J Med*; 350: 2572–81.

Elter T, Borchmann P, Schulz H, Reiser M, Trelle S, Staib P et al. (2004) FluCam—a New, 4-Weekly Combination of Fludarabine and Alemtuzumab for Patients with Relapsed Chronic Lymphocytic Leukemia. *Blood*; 104: 2517.

Ehrlich P (1900) On immunitiy with special reference to cell life. *Proc. R. Soc;* **66**: 424–48.

Fisher RI, Gaynor ER, Dahlberg S, Oken MM, Grogan TM, Mize EM *et al.* (1993) Comparison of a standard regimen (CHOP) with three intensive chemotherapy regimens for advanced non-Hodgkin's lymphoma. *N Engl J Med;* **328**: 1002–6.

Fishwild DM, O'Donnell SL, Bengoechea T, Hudson DV, Harding F, Bernhard SL *et al.* (1996) High-avidity human IgG kappa monoclonal antibodies from a novel strain of minilocus transgenic mice. *Nat Biotechnol;* **14**: 845–51.

Guddat LW, Shan L, Fan ZC, Andersen KN, Rosauer R, Linthicum DS *et al.* (1995) Intramolecular signaling upon complexation. *Faseb J;* **9**: 101–6.

Gregory SA, Venugopal P, Adler SS, O'Brien TM, O'Donnell KF, Yunus F (2001) Safety and efficacy of fludarabine and mitoxantrone with rituximab consolidation in untreated advanced low grade non-Hodgkin's lymphoma (LG-NHL) (Abstract 2534). *Blood;* **98**: 605a.

Hainsworth JD (2002) Rituximab as first-line and maintenance therapy for patients with indolent non-Hodgkin's lymphoma: interim follow-up of a multicenter phase II trial. *Semin Oncol;* **29**: 25–9.

Hainsworth JD, Litchy S, Burris HA, 3rd, Scullin DC, Jr, Corso SW, Yardley DA *et al.* (2002) Rituximab as first-line and maintenance therapy for patients with indolent non-hodgkin's lymphoma. *J Clin Oncol;* **20**: 4261–7.

Hainsworth JD, Litchy S, Shaffer DW, Lackey VL, Grimaldi M, Greco FA (2005) Maximizing therapeutic benefit of rituximab: maintenance therapy versus re-treatment at progression in patients with indolent non-Hodgkin's lymphoma–a randomized phase II trial of the Minnie Pearl Cancer Research Network. *J Clin Oncol;* **23**: 1088–95.

Herold M, Fiedler F, Pasold R, Knauf WU, Freund M, Naumann R *et al.* (2001) Efficacy and toxicity of rituximab plus mitoxantrone, chrorambucil, prednisolone (MCP) versus MCP alone in advanced indolent NHL—interim results of a clinical phase III study of the East German study group hematology/oncology (OSHO) (Abstract 2521). *Blood;* **98**: 601a.

Herrmann G, Hunzelmann N, Engert A (2003) Treatment of pemphigus vulgaris with anti-CD20 monoclonal antibody (rituximab). *Br J Dermatol;* **148**: 602–3.

Hiddemann W, Forstpointner R, Fiedler F, Gramatzki M, Dörken B, Illiger H-J *et al.* (2001) Combined immunotherapy (R-FCM) is superior to a fludarabine-containing chemotherapy (FCM) alone in recurrent indolent lymphoma—results of a prospective randomized comparison of the German Low Grade Lymphoma Study Group (Abstract 349). *Onkologe;* **24**: 90.

Hosono M, Endo K, Sakahara H, Watanabe Y, Saga T, Nakai T *et al.* (1992) Human/mouse chimeric antibodies show low reactivity with human anti-murine antibodies (HAMA). *Br J Cancer;* **65**: 197–200.

Hurwitz H, Fehrenbacher L, Novotny W, Cartwright T, Hainsworth J, Heim W *et al.* (2004) Bevacizumab plus irinotecan, fluorouracil, and leucovorin for metastatic colorectal cancer. *N Engl J Med;* **350**: 2335–42.

Ide AG, Baker NH, Warren SL (1939) Vascularization of the Brown Pearce rabbit epithelioma transplant as seen in the transparent ear chamber. *Am J Roentgenol;* **42**: 891–9.

Keating MJ, O'Brien S, Albitar M, Lerner S, Plunkett W, Giles F *et al.* (2005) Early results of a chemoimmunotherapy regimen of fludarabine, cyclophosphamide, and rituximab as initial therapy for chronic lymphocytic leukemia. *J Clin Oncol;* **23**: 4079–88.

Kirchner HH, Gaede B, Steinhauer EU, Panagiotou P, Sosada M (2001) Chemoimmunotherapy with Fludarabine, Bendamustine and Rituximab for Relapsed Low Grade Malignant Non-Hodgkin's Lymphoma (Abstract 568). *Blood*; 98: 135a.

Kohler G, Milstein C (1975) Continuous cultures of fused cells secreting antibody of predefined specificity. *Nature*; 256: 495–7.

Langer CJ, Stephenson P, Thor A, Vangel M, Johnson DH (2004) Trastuzumab in the treatment of advanced non-small-cell lung cancer: is there a role? Focus on Eastern Cooperative Oncology Group study 2598. *J Clin Oncol*; 22: 1180–7.

Marcus R, Imrie K, Belch A, Cunningham D, Flores E, Catalano J et al. (2005) CVP chemotherapy plus rituximab compared with CVP as first-line treatment for advanced follicular lymphoma. *Blood*; 105: 1417–23.

McLaughlin P, Grillo-Lopez AJ, Link BK, Levy R, Czuczman MS, Williams ME et al. (1998) Rituximab chimeric anti-CD20 monoclonal antibody therapy for relapsed indolent lymphoma: half of patients respond to a four-dose treatment program. *J Clin Oncol*; 16: 2825–33.

Miller RA, Maloney DG, Warnke R, Levy R (1982) Treatment of B-cell lymphoma with monoclonal anti-idiotype antibody. *N Engl J Med*; 306: 517–22.

Montemurro F, Valabrega G, Aglietta M (2004) Trastuzumab-based combination therapy for breast cancer. Expert *Opin Pharmacother*; 5: 81–96.

Moulder SL, Yakes FM, Muthuswamy SK, Bianco R, Simpson JF, Arteaga CL (2001) Epidermal growth factor receptor (HER1) tyrosine kinase inhibitor ZD1839 (Iressa) inhibits HER2/neu (erbB2)-overexpressing breast cancer cells in vitro and in vivo. *Cancer Res*; 61: 8887–95.

Mounier N, Briere J, Gisselbrecht C, Emile JF, Lederlin P, Sebban C et al. (2003) Rituximab plus CHOP (R-CHOP) overcomes bcl-2–associated resistance to chemotherapy in elderly patients with diffuse large B-cell lymphoma (DLBCL). *Blood*; 101: 4279–84.

Patel D, Gupta NK, Mehrotra B, Russo L, Driscoll N, Gor A et al. (2001) Rituximab, Cyclophosphamide and Decadron (RCD) Combination is an Effective Salvage Regimen for Previously Treated Low Grade Lymphoma. *J Clin Oncol*; 20: abs 2665.

Pegram MD, Konecny GE, O'Callaghan C, Beryt M, Pietras R, Slamon DJ (2004) Rational combinations of trastuzumab with chemotherapeutic drugs used in the treatment of breast cancer. *J Natl Cancer Inst*; 96: 739–49.

Perez-Soler R (2003) Can rash associated with HER1/EGFR inhibition be used as a marker of treatment outcome? *Oncology (Huntingt)*; 17: 23–8.

Piro LD, White CA, Grillo-Lopez AJ, Janakiraman N, Saven A, Beck TM et al. (1999) Extended Rituximab (anti-CD20 monoclonal antibody) therapy for relapsed or refractory low-grade or follicular non-Hodgkin's lymphoma. *Ann Oncol*; 10: 655–61.

Porter RR (1967) The structure of antibodies. The basic pattern of the principal class of molecules that neutralize antigens (foreign substances in the body) is four cross-linked chains. This pattern is modified so that antibodies can fit different antigens. *Sci Am*; 217: 81–7.

Rai KR, Freter CE, Mercier RJ, Cooper MR, Mitchell BS, Stadtmauer EA et al. (2002) Alemtuzumab in previously treated chronic lymphocytic leukemia patients who also had received fludarabine. *J Clin Oncol*; 20: 3891–7.

Rambaldi A, Lazzari M, Manzoni C, Carlotti E, Arcaini L, Baccarani M et al. (2002) Monitoring of minimal residual disease after CHOP and rituximab in previously untreated patients with follicular lymphoma. *Blood*; 99: 856–62.

Rosell R, Daniel C, Ramlau R, Szczesna A, Constenla M, Mennecier B *et al.* (2004) Randomized phase II study of cetuximab in combination with cisplatin (C) and vinorelbine (V) vs. CV alone in the first-line treatment of patients (pts) with epidermal growth factor receptor (EGFR)-expressing advanced non-small-cell lung cancer (NSCLC). *J Clin Oncol*; 7012.

Schulz H, Klein SK, Rehwald U, Reiser M, Hinke A, Knauf WU *et al.* (2002) Phase 2 study of a combined immunochemotherapy using rituximab and fludarabine in patients with chronic lymphocytic leukemia. *Blood*; **100**: 3115–20.

Slamon DJ, Godolphin W, Jones LA, Holt JA, Wong SG, Keith DE *et al.* (1989) Studies of the HER-2/neu proto-oncogene in human breast and ovarian cancer. *Science*; **244**: 707–12.

Slamon DJ, Leyland-Jones B, Shak S, Fuchs H, Paton V, Bajamonde A *et al.* (2001) Use of chemotherapy plus a monoclonal antibody against HER2 for metastatic breast cancer that overexpresses HER2. *N Engl J Med*; **344**: 783–92.

Stasi R, Pagano A, Stipa E, Amadori S (2001) Rituximab chimeric anti-CD20 monoclonal antibody treatment for adults with chronic idiopathic thrombocytopenic purpura. *Blood*; **98**: 952–7.

Tomizuka K, Shinohara T, Yoshida H, Uejima H, Ohguma A, Tanaka S *et al.* (2000) Double trans-chromosomic mice: maintenance of two individual human chromosome fragments containing Ig heavy and kappa loci and expression of fully human antibodies. *Proc Natl Acad Sci USA*; **97**: 722–7.

Trigo J, Hitt R, Koralewski P, Diaz-Rubio E, Rolland F, Knecht R *et al.* (2004) Cetuximab monotherapy is active in patients (pts) with platinum-refractory recurrent/metastatic squamous cell carcinoma of the head and neck (SCCHN): Results of a phase II study. *J Clin Oncol*; **22**: 5502.

Vaughan TJ, Osbourn JK, Tempest PR (1998) Human antibodies by design. *Nat Biotechnol*; **16**: 535–9.

Vitolo U, Boccomini C, Astolfi M, Bertini M, Botto B, Calvi R *et al.* (2001) Chemoimmunotherapy with Fludarabine + Mitoxantrone + Dexamethasone (FND) and rituximab in Indolent Non-Hodgkin's Lymphoma (NHL): a pilot study to evaluate feasability, safety, clinical and molecular response (Abstract 4739 A). *Blood*; **98**: 252b.

Vogel CL, Cobleigh MA, Tripathy D, Gutheil JC, Harris LN, Fehrenbacher L *et al.* (2002) Efficacy and safety of trastuzumab as a single agent in first-line treatment of HER2-overexpressing metastatic breast cancer. *J Clin Oncol*; **20**: 719–26.

Vose JM, Wahl RL, Saleh M, Rohatiner AZ, Knox SJ, Radford JA *et al.* (2000) Multicenter phase II study of iodine-131 tositumomab for chemotherapy-relapsed/refractory low-grade and transformed low-grade B-cell non-Hodgkin's lymphomas. *J Clin Oncol*; **18**: 1316–23.

Weide R, Heymanns J, Gores A, Koppler H (2002) Bendamustine mitoxantrone and rituximab (BMR): a new effective regimen for refractory or relapsed indolent lymphomas. *Leuk Lymphoma*; **43**: 327–31.

Wierda W, O'Brien S, Wen S, Faderl S, Garcia-Manero G, Thomas D *et al.* (2005) Chemoimmunotherapy with fludarabine, cyclophosphamide, and rituximab for relapsed and refractory chronic lymphocytic leukemia. *J Clin Oncol*; **23**: 4070–8.

Wilde MI, Goa KL (1996) Muromonab CD3: a reappraisal of its pharmacology and use as prophylaxis of solid organ transplant rejection. *Drugs*; **51**: 865–94.

Yang JC, Haworth L, Sherry RM, Hwu P, Schwartzentruber DJ, Topalian SL *et al.* (2003) A randomized trial of bevacizumab, an anti-vascular endothelial growth factor antibody, for metastatic renal cancer. *N Engl J Med*; **349**: 427–34.

Chapter 8

Antibody-directed enzyme prodrug therapy (ADEPT)

Surinder K. Sharma, Kenneth D. Bagshawe, and Richard H. J. Begent

1 Development of monoclonal antibodies

Conventional cancer chemotherapeutic agents lack selectivity and in the past effort has mainly been focused on high-dose systemic chemotherapy, which tried to balance minimal adverse effects to normal tissues with maximal anti-tumour activity. To achieve selectivity, the focus since the 1960s has been to search for substances that differentiate malignant tumours from normal tissue. These biochemical factors that characterise specific types of cancer are known as **tumour-associated antigens** or tumour markers. The most widely studied tumour-associated antigen is carcinoembryonic antigen or CEA (Gold and Freedman 1975) that is overexpressed in almost all cancers of the colon and several others. Although the tumour-associated antigens are not specific for cancer, they are sufficiently overexpressed in many cancers to allow localisation of antibodies directed against them (Begent *et al.* 1980; Goldenberg *et al.* 1978; Mach *et al.* 1974) and targeted cancer therapy has emerged as a novel approach in the treatment of both haematological and solid tumours (Carter 2001; Stern and Herrmann 2005).

In the early studies, antibodies used were in the form of purified immune sera from animals such as rabbit and sheep. However, with the advent of **hybridoma** technology (Kohler and Milstein 1975), where fusing an antibody-producing cell with a malignant cell conferred the property of immortality on the antibody-producing cell and all the antibodies produced by that cell are identical, the so-called **monoclonal antibodies** (mAbs) capable of binding to specific tumour antigens were produced.

The first monoclonal antibodies directed at tumour antigens were of murine origin. One of the disadvantage of these antibodies was that most patients developed human anti-mouse antibodies or **HAMA** leading to allergic reactions and reduced efficacy (Reilly *et al.* 1995). However, advances in **DNA** technology led to production of monoclonal **chimeric** antibodies (Jones *et al.* 1984) from two different species, in which the constant regions are of human origin as well as humanised antibodies where the **complementarity-determining region** is from a non-human source and then fully humanised antibodies (Winter and Harris 1993). The recent development of phage technology (Winter *et al.* 1994) and antibody engineering allow creation of antibodies with required characteristics for specific purposes and methods to produce fully human antibodies (reviewed in: Osbourn *et al.* 2003).

As part of the response to infectious organisms, the production of antibodies contributes to their elimination, but it was soon found that antibodies alone had little capacity to delay the progress of carcinomas. In the past decade it has, however, been found that naked antibodies to a particular marker on lymphocytes make a substantial contribution to the control of many forms of lymphoma (Byrd *et al.* 1999; Maloney *et al.* 1994)and used in conjunction with conventional chemotherapy the prognosis in Hodgkins and non-Hodgkins lymphoma has been greatly improved (Davis *et al.* 2000; Maloney *et al.* 1997). Also, the recent success of monoclonal antibodies, such as rituximab, a chimeric IgG1 monoclonal antibody against the CD20 antigen for the treatment of non-Hodgkin lymphoma, and transtuzumab for breast cancer, have further advanced the use of monoclonal antibodies for cancer therapy (Carter 2001; Stern and Herrmann 2005).

However, the lack of obvious benefit from antibodies directed at most solid tumours resulted in many attempts to arm antibodies with various cell-killing agents. Most of these studies were done in nude mice xenografted with human tumours. Although these are perhaps not perfect models for studying the growth and response to therapy of human cancers, they have proved invaluable. Several therapeutic approaches have been explored by linking antibodies to target radionuclides (Lane *et al.* 1994), toxins (Pastan and Kreitman 2002), and **cytotoxic** drugs (Hamann *et al.* 2002; Payne 2003; Saleh *et al.* 2000; Tolcher *et al.* 2003).

One of the disadvantages of the antibody–drug conjugates approach was that an antibody could carry only a limited number of cytotoxic drugs without losing its capacity to bind to its tumour marker. Also that antibodies, being large molecules, could only penetrate a limited distance into tumours (Pedley *et al.* 1993). In order to get round these problems highly potent toxins were attached to antibodies. There was evidence that a single molecule of a toxin such as ricin (Thorpe *et al.* 1982) could kill a cell. Early attempts with toxin-armed antibodies resulted in damage to blood vessels resulting in a vascular leak syndrome (Vitetta *et al.* 1991). However, the main obstacle to both the cytotoxic and to the toxin-armed antibodies is due to the phenomenon of heterogeneity in tumour-marker expression, so that a significant proportion of a population of carcinoma cells do not express the marker (Edwards 1985) and are therefore not exposed to the action of the cytotoxic drug or toxin. It is interesting that marker expression by lymphomas is more uniform than on carcinomas and this may contribute to their success in those malignancies. Therefore, effective therapy depended on approaches that took account of this heterogeneity in marker expression. The most obvious way to kill both marker and non-marker expressing cells was to use antibodies that were radiolabelled with an isotope such as iodine-131, although several other radionuclides have also been used. Non-marker expressing cells would be hit by the 'cross-fire' of the isotope attached to marker expressing cells. In order to deliver a cell-killing dose of radiolabelled antibody, quite large amounts of radioactivity are required and normal tissues, particularly bone marrow, are irradiated while the radiolabelled antibody is circulating. Radiolabelled antibody therapy is highly effective in treating lymphoma but the greater radioresistance and more disorganised blood flow of common cancers make them a target in which it seems unlikely that radiolabelled antibodies will provide a therapeutic able to destroy established tumours. However, there is a prospect of success in combination with antivascular drugs (Pedley *et al.* 1991, 1999, 2001)

2 Principles of ADEPT

Most cytotoxic agents have effects, not only on dividing cancer cells but also on normal dividing cells. Although different cytotoxic drugs have different patterns of normal tissue toxicity, these effects are dose-limiting in all cases and time is required for normal tissue recovery. The cancer cells that have not been killed by a cycle of chemotherapy proliferate during the normal tissue recovery phase and hence the development of drug resistance.

By the mid-1980s, consideration of these issues made it clear that avoidance of normal tissue toxicity was a key element for progress. It was known that certain drugs that were not cytotoxic as given became cytotoxic in the body through the action of particular enzymes. The widely used drug cyclophosphamide is an example of such a prodrug that is converted by enzymes in the liver into a cytotoxic drug. Ideally, if there was an enzyme that occurred exclusively in cancers it would probably be possible to make a non-toxic prodrug that would be converted at tumour sites into a cell-killing agent. A single molecule of an enzyme can convert many prodrug molecules into active drug and therefore a high dose of a drug would be generated there.

Capecitabine, activated by thymidine phosporylase, present in many tumours with hypoxic areas is an example but to date has only shown modest benefit compared the equivalent active drug, fluorouracil given systemically (Han *et al.* 2005; Quinney *et al.* 2005).

The fact that there was a mass of clinical evidence that monoclonal antibodies directed at tumour markers localised at tumour sites (Begent 1985; Goldman *et al.* 1985) posed the question whether they could deliver an enzyme to tumours. It was desirable that the enzyme should not be one that occurred elsewhere in the human body so as to avoid any action in normal tissues. In addition, the enzyme should be able to convert a large number of prodrug molecules rapidly into cytototoxic molecules. Bacterial enzymes tend to have better turnover rates than those of human origin. As for the prodrug, it was necessary that this should be non-toxic and that the drug generated from it should be very toxic because this differential would determine how much of the prodrug could be given. It was also clear at the outset that the active drug should decay quickly, i. e. have a short half-life, so that it would not escape from the tumour and affect normal tissues. Constructing such a system that became known as **antibody-directed enzyme prodrug therapy (ADEPT)** required a multidisciplinary approach.

The aim of ADEPT (see Fig. 8.1) is to generate a potent cytotoxic drug selectively within tumours from its non-toxic precursor by a targeted enzyme not normally present in the body (Bagshawe 1987; Bagshawe *et al.* 1988; Senter

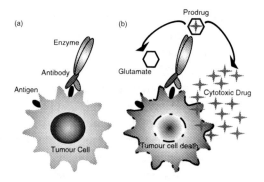

Fig. 8.1 Diagramatic representation of the ADEPT principle. (a) An antibody–enzyme construct is injected IV and allowed to localise to tumour sites. After enzyme activity clearance from circulation, a glutamated mustard based non-toxic prodrug is given. (b) The enzyme cleaves the glutamate moiety to generate the active cytotoxic drug. The drug is generated extracellularly and being a small molecule, can diffuse throughout the tumour mass to kill antigen-positive tumour cells, as well as the near by antigen-negative cells, thereby giving a 'bystander' effect.

et al. 1988). Higher concentration of drug at tumour sites may be obtained by this method than by direct administration of drug alone, as the enzyme provides an amplification effect. Another advantage of ADEPT approach is that the drug is generated extracellularly and, being a small molecule, can diffuse throughout the tumour mass and can kill cells that do not express the tumour marker as well as those that do (Cheng *et al.* 1999).

The bacterial enzyme carboxypeptidase G2 (CPG2), which had been isolated from a *Pseudomonas* spp. (Sherwood *et al.* 1985) was utilised in our studies. CPG2 catalyses the hydrolytic cleavage of reduced and non-reduced folates to pteroates and glutamic acid. Because CPG2 was a bacterial enzyme, it was realised that it would evoke an immune response in the mouse and in patients but it was expected that, in time, antibody molecules would be humanised and would be made to have enzymatic action (so-called abzymes) and would eventually replace bacterial enzymes in this role (Bagshawe 1989). The requirements for the **prodrug**-drug system were considered. It seemed desirable to avoid drugs that would be excluded by the known methods of drug resistance, such as gene amplification and exclusion by the P-glycoprotein exclusion pump, and there was evidence that alkylating agents were less susceptible to drug resistance mechanisms (Frei, III *et al.* 1988) than many other cytotoxic agents. Therefore the first prodrug (CMDA) for this purpose was a simple alkylating agent with a glutamic acid attachment (Springer *et al.* 1990). The glutamic acid was expected to act by withdrawing electrons from the business end of the alkylating agent and so make it non-toxic. The CPG2 would cleave the glutamic acid moiety at tumour sites.

3 Antibody–enzyme/prodrug systems in ADEPT

Numerous pre-clinical studies of enzyme/prodrug systems have been described since the ADEPT approach was first proposed (Bagshawe 1987). These utilised endogenous and non-endogenous enzymes to activate both novel and prodrugs of clinically used chemotherapeutic agents (Bagshawe *et al.* 2004; Senter & Springer 2001). The enzymes utilised in ADEPT systems can be divided into three main categories:

mammalian enzymes including human enzymes;
non-mammalian enzymes with mammalian homologue;
non-mammalian enzymes that have no mammalian homologue.

3.1 Mammalian enzymes including human enzymes

These include alkaline phosphatase, β-glucuronidase, and carboxypeptidase A. One of the earliest studies in ADEPT utilised alkaline phosphatase conjugated to a monoclonal antibody for conversion of etoposide phosphate prodrug to etoposide. This resulted in effective therapy of the human colon carcinoma **xenograft**, H3347 in nude mice (Senter *et al.* 1988). Human β-glucuronidase fused to an anti-CEA antibody was one of the first human enzymes to be used in the ADEPT system (Bosslet *et al.* 1994). This fusion protein was used to catalyse a doxorubicin glucuronide prodrug to result in anti-tumour effects in human colon carcinoma xenografts.

The human enzymes have the potential advantage of being less **immunogenic** than non-mammalian enzymes but endogenous enzymes capable of non-specific prodrug activation may compromise specificity. However, specificity can be achieved by mutating the human enzyme such that it retains the catalytic activity for a prodrug that is not a substrate for the endogenous enzyme but is activated only by the mutated enzyme. Such an approach was used for human pancreatic carboxypeptidase A, which has been mutated to activate prodrugs of methotrexate (Smith *et al.* 1997) to give cytotoxic effects *in vitro*. However, it did not give encouraging results *in vivo*.

An alternative approach is to use antibodies as catalysts (Shabat *et al.* 1999; Wentworth *et al.* 1996). Although the potential of catalytic antibodies (abzymes) was anticipated in an early description of ADEPT (Bagshawe 1989), and although catalytic antibodies have been found to activate several prodrugs, they mostly remained too inefficient to compete with naturally occurring enzymes and major progress in developing efficient catalytic antibodies has only recently been described (Rader *et al.* 2003; Shabat *et al.* 1999; Shamis, Lode, & Shabat 2004; Sinha *et al.* 2004).

3.2 Non-mammalian enzymes with mammalian homologue

This class of enzymes includes bacterial β-glucuronidase and nitroreductase. These are potentially usable as the bacterial glucuronidase has a higher turnover rate at ph 6.8 than its human counterpart and the nitroreductase has a different substrate specificity from the human enzyme (Bignami *et al.* 1992b; Houba *et al.* 1996). However, both these are potentially immunogenic in humans.

3.3 Non-mammalian enzymes with no human homologue

This category includes enzymes such as penicillin G-amidase, β-lactamase, and cytosine deaminase and carboxypeptidase G2. These enzymes having no human analogue and offer an advantage in terms of specificity, as prodrugs designed to be substrates are not activated by endogenous enzymes. However, the disadvantage is in terms of **immunogenicity**.

Many studies have been carried out using this class of enzymes. The monoclonal antibody-enzyme conjugate, L6-penicillin G amidase in combination with the prodrug, N-($4'$-hydroxyphenylacetyl)palytoxin shows marked cytotoxicity to a panel of carcinoma and lymphoma cell lines (Bignami *et al.* 1992). β-lactamase conjugated to monoclonal antibodies has been used to activate cephalosporin prodrugs of nitrogen mustard (Alexander *et al.* 1991), vinblastine, and doxorubicin to achieve regression in colon carcinoma xenografts (Meyer *et al.* 1993, 1995) and growth delay in a number of other xenograft models.

Antibody–cytosine deaminase conjugates mediated conversion of 5-fluorocytosine to 5-fluouracil resulted in a 17-fold increase in 5FU concentration within tumours compared to systemic administration of 5FU (Wallace *et al.* 1994).

3.3.1 Studies with CPG2

We have utilised the bacterial enzyme carboxypeptidase G2 for our extensive studies in ADEPT. The first model chosen for testing the ADEPT approach (Bagshawe *et al.* 1988) was a choriocarcinoma xenograft growing in nude mice that had proved resistant to conventional chemotherapy both in the mouse model and the clinic.

CPG2 was chemically conjugated to a monoclonal antibody directed against human chorionic gonadotrophin (hCG) (Searle *et al.* 1986). It was found that radiolabelled anti-hCG-CPG2 constructs localised in the choriocarcinoma xenografts just as well as radiolabelled anti-hCG antibodies, whether intact antibodies or F(ab)2 fragments were used (Melton *et al.* 1990). In mice with tumours of about $1\,cm^3$, when the antibody–enzyme constructs were followed, 48 h later, by three doses of CMDA, all the tumours shrank and most of the tumours were eliminated and did not come back (Springer *et al.* 1991).

The next system to be tested was based on human colon carcinoma xenografts (LS174T) with CEA as the target antigen and the CPG2 enzyme was attached to F(ab)2 anti CEA antibodies. This localised in radiolabelled form in the LS174T xenografts (Sharma *et al.* 1990). When the antibody–enzyme constructs were followed at 48 h by the same doses of the prodrug as used in the choriocarcinoma model, all the mice died from drug-induced toxicity. The difference between the two model systems was that the choriocarcinoma xenograft released into the blood a large amount of hCG, the target antigen, whereas there was no detectable CEA in the blood of the colon carcinoma model. Although the hCG in the blood of the choriocarcinoma model did not prevent the antibody–enzyme construct from localising in the tumour, it accelerated clearance of the enzyme from the blood, presumably through immune complex formation. In the colon model the enzyme still in the blood when the prodrug was given released active drug and caused fatal toxicity. The experiment was repeated with a longer interval between antibody–enzyme conjugate and prodrug but there were no significant tumour responses. The enzyme had cleared from the blood and from the tumour. These results indicated that the time window in which there is a concentration of enzyme in the tumour and no detectable enzyme in blood is critical to the success of ADEPT.

These problems had been anticipated and a mouse monoclonal antibody (SB43) directed at the enzyme was made. It was found that this antibody inactivated the enzyme and accelerated its clearance from blood (Sharma *et al.* 1990). With clearance of enzyme by SB43 it was possible to give the prodrug 24 h after the conjugate resulting in marked growth delay of the tumours (Sharma *et al.* 1991). In order for SB43 itself to clear quickly, it was galactosylated so that it was taken up readily by hepatic galactose receptors (Sharma *et al.* 1994a).

Other studies with the same ADEPT/prodrug system resulted in growth delay in a resistant ovarian cancer xenograft (Sharma *et al.* 1994b) and using a different antibody effected major regressions and cures in a human breast cancer xenograft model (Eccles *et al.* 1994).

These first agents had proved sufficiently effective to allow a pilot scale clinical trial since this might reveal unexpected problems. This was carried out on patients with terminal cancer of the colon or rectum who gave their full informed consent (Bagshawe *et al.* 1991). It was first necessary to carry out, on a minimal scale, a dose-escalation study with the prodrug by itself and this was done with only minimal toxicity.

A total of 17 patients received the antibody–enzyme conjugate followed by the galactosylates-clearing antibody SB43 before the prodrug was given (Bagshawe *et al.* 1995; Bagshawe and Begent 1996). There were many questions that needed to be answered relating to the dosage of the agents, the interval between them, and the method of the prodrug administration, such as whether it should be give by bolus injection or by slow infusion. The fact that the prodrug was soluble only in dimethyl sulphoxide (DMSO) did not make for easy administration and added to issues of toxicity. The antibody–enzyme conjugates were made in small batches and therefore potentially different from each other. It was recognised that the murine antibodies and the bacterial enzyme would provoke host–antibody responses and there was the question whether these could be delayed by the immunosuppressive agent cyclosporin. Blood enzyme levels were measured to avoid giving prodrug when it would be activated by enzyme in blood.

It was judged that eight patients were assessable and received adequate dosage of the conjugate and prodrugs (Bagshawe *et al.* 1995). Of these, four had greater than 50% reduction in all measurable tumours (partial response) and in one patient all but one tumour mass responding (mixed response). Two of three patients who received intravenous cyclosporin received three cycles of therapy. Patients who did not receive cyclosporin all developed antibodies to the murine **immunoglobulins** and the bacterial enzyme by 14 days, and those that received intravenous cyclosporine, by 21 days (Bagshawe and Sharma 1996). All patients developed marked but reversible myelotoxicity.

At first it appeared possible that the myelotoxicity resulted from the residual enzyme in blood. However, no enzyme activity in blood was detectable by the HPLC assay (Martin *et al.* 1997). The alternative explanation was that the cytotoxic drug was generated only at cancer sites but its half-life was so long as to allow it to escape into the blood from tumours.

A further small-scale clinical trial using the same agents but a lower dose of the antibody enzyme conjugate also resulted in responses and allowed biopsies of the liver metastases to be obtained in some patients (Napier *et al.* 2000). The tumour to enzyme activity ratio was found to be 10 000:1, making the drug half-life a key factor in the elimination of toxicity. These pilot-scale studies also confirmed the effectiveness of the antibody-based system for clearing enzyme activity from blood and the absence of any toxicity attributable to this component.

The lesson learned about the half-life of the CMDA drug led to the development of a new prodrug known as a bis-iodophenol (Springer *et al.* 1995). The drug generated from it has a half-life that is too short to measure. It is also an alkylating agent prodrug that is activated by the same CPG2 enzyme. Studies with this drug showed it to be highly potent in vivo (Blakey *et al.* 1996) and the mechanism of cell death to be **apoptosis** (Monks *et al.* 2001).

A further clinical trial was therefore carried out using the original antibody–enzyme conjugate and the new prodrug but without using the clearance system (Francis *et al.* 2002). In the absence of the clearing antibody, several days lapsed before blood enzyme levels fell to a level where the prodrug could be given. No responses occurred in these 27 patients, although DNA cross-links were demonstrated in tumour biopsy material of some patients (Webley *et al.* 2001).

These clinical studies showed the need for the development of an antibody–enzyme molecule that would encompass the characteristics of the three-phase ADEPT system but would be less complex. The possibility that such a two component system might work arose from the development of a fusion protein. The potential advantage of the fusion proteins is that these can be modified according to specific requirements of the system. The basic principle is to fuse the gene coding the antibody with that of the enzyme. The resulting product can be overexpressed in a suitable expression system. This has the advantage that the product is uniform and that it can be produced on a large scale. The fusion protein incorporates a high-affinity scFv anti-CEA antibody (MFE) (Chester *et al.* 2000) fused with CPG2 to give MFECP fusion protein (Michael *et al.* 1996). This was initially expressed in *Escherischia coli* and showed improved *in vivo* pharmacokinetics (Bhatia *et al.* 2000) compared to the chemical conjugate. However, the yield was too low to be used for a clinical trial. The fusion protein was subsequently expressed in *Pichia pastoris*, a yeast expression system to give high yields of the product, which is stable and glycosylated (Medzihradszky *et al.* 2004). *In vivo* studies in colon carcinoma xenografts showed this fusion protein to localise effectively in tumours and clear rapidly from blood via the liver, resulting in tumour to blood ratios of CPG2 activity 1400:1 within 6 h after injection. ADEPT with MFECP fusion protein in combination with the ZD2767P prodrug, showed significant anti-tumour effects in two human colon xenograft models without apparent toxicity (Sharma *et al.* 2005).

Following these studies, a single cycle ADEPT clinical trial with MFECP fusion protein in combination with the bis-iodo-phenol mustard prodrug (ZD2767P) has been carried out (Mayer *et al.* 2004b) to demonstrate safety and tolerability of the fusion protein. A repeated dose clinical study has recently been initiated.

4 Immunogenicity

As our initial studies utilised a bacterial enzyme conjugated to murine monoclonal antibodies, immune response to both components was expected and observed (Sharma *et al.* 1992). However, up to three cycles of treatment could be given under cover of an immunosuppressive agent, cyclosporine A (Bagshawe and Sharma 1996) during a 21-day period.

With our clinical studies of MFECP, the patient response to CPG2 has been much less frequent than with the chemical conjugates. The immunodominant **epitope** of CPG2 has been modified to reduce immunogenicity (Spencer *et al.* 2002). Mutations of the CM79-identified epitope or addition of a hexahistidine tag (His-tag) to the C-terminus of MFECP, which forms part of the epitope were effective in reducing the immunogenicity. Murine **immunisation** experiments with modified MFECP showed no significant antibody response to the CM79-identified epitope compared to A5CP, an unmodified version of CP chemically conjugated to an F(ab)2 antibody. Success of modification was also demonstrated in humans because patients treated with His-tagged MFECP had a significantly reduced antibody response to the CM79-identified epitope, compared to patients given A5CP. Moreover, the **polyclonal** antibody response to CP was delayed in both mice and patients given modified MFECP. This increases the prospect of repeated treatment with ADEPT for effective cancer. Further reductions in immunogenicity may be achievable by further engineering of **B cell** or T cell epitopes on CPG2 and by using a humanised version of the MFE23 antibody (Mayer *et al.* 2004a).

In summary, it is evident that numerous ADEPT systems have been studies at pre-clinical level but only one system has progressed to the clinical stage. The possibility that a two-component ADEPT system may work appears to be reasonable if prodrug could be given at the time when enzyme levels in tumour are optimal and no detectable level is present in blood. The half-life of drug is an important factor and optimum half-life needs to be defined. A non-immunogenic system for multi-cycle ADEPT should be investigated.

5 Obstacles to therapy

ADEPT has been shown to be highly effective in therapy of human colorectal, breast, ovarian carcinomas, and choriocarcinoma grown as xenografts in nude mice. In humans, there is evidence of highly selective localisation of enzyme to tumour, of prodrug activation, and of tumour response in some patients. Current clinical trials will elucidate whether the effects are sufficient for effective therapy using the latest generation of antibody–enzyme and prodrug molecules. If not, it is likely that the problem is one of degree of effect and it may be possible to overcome this with further advances in protein engineering of the antibody or enzyme or in new prodrugs. Immunogenicity of enzymes remains a problem but one that is yielding partially to re-engineering of antibody–enzyme molecules and may be addressed by adaptations of human enzymes to lose reactivity with their natural substrate, while gaining capacity to activate prodrug. The development process has been long but technology has advanced bringing new solutions to the original problems. The fundamental potential of ADEPT to deliver exquisite tumour selectivity with high potency of anti-tumour effect remains as attractive as ever and is still unattained by other treatments for common cancers.

References

Alexander, R.P., Beeley, N.R.A., O'Driscoll, M., O'Neill, F.P., Millican, T.A., Pratt, A. *et al.* (1991) Cephalosporin nitrogen-mustard carbamate prodrugs for ADEPT. *Tetrahed. Lett.* 32, 3269–72.

Bagshawe, K. D. (1987) Antibody directed enzymes revive anti-cancer prodrugs concept. *Br. J. Cancer*, **56**, 5, 531–2.

Bagshawe, K. D. (1989) The first Bagshawe lecture. Towards generating cytotoxic agents at cancer sites. *Br. J. Cancer*, **60**, 3, 275–81.

Bagshawe, K.D. and Begent, R.H.J. (1996) First clinical experience with ADEPT. *Adv. Drug Deliv. Rev.*, **22**, 365–7.

Bagshawe, K. D. & Sharma, S. K. (1996) Cyclosporine delays host immune response to antibody enzyme conjugate in ADEPT. *Transplant. Proc.*, **28**, 6, 3156–8.

Bagshawe, K. D., Springer, C. J., Searle, F., Antoniw, P., Sharma, S. K., Melton, R. G. *et al.* (1988) A cytotoxic agent can be generated selectively at cancer sites. *Br. J. Cancer*, **58**, 6, 700–3.

Bagshawe, K. D., Sharma, S. K., Springer, C. J., Antoniw, P., Boden, J. A., Rogers, G. T. *et al.* (1991) Antibody directed enzyme prodrug therapy (ADEPT): clinical report. *Dis. Markers*, **9**, 3–4, 233–8.

Bagshawe, K. D., Sharma, S. K., Springer, C. J., Antoniw, P. (1995) Antibody-directed enzyme prodrug therapy: a pilot scale clinical trial. *Tumor Targeting*, **1**, 17–29.

Bagshawe, K. D., Sharma, S. K., & Begent, R. H. (2004) Antibody-directed enzyme prodrug therapy (ADEPT) for cancer. *Expert. Opin. Biol. Ther.*, **4**, 11, 1777–89.

Begent, R. H. (1985) Recent advances in tumour imaging. Use of radiolabelled anti-tumour antibodies. *Biochim. Biophys. Acta*, **780**, 2, 151–66.

Begent, R. H., Searle, F., Stanway, G., Jewkes, R. F., Jones, B. E., Vernon, P. *et al.* (1980) Radioimmunolocalization of tumours by external scintigraphy after administration of 131I antibody to human chorionic gonadotrophin: preliminary communication. *J. R. Soc. Med.*, **73**, 9, 624–30.

Bhatia, J., Sharma, S. K., Chester, K. A., Pedley, R. B., Boden, R. W., Read, D. A. *et al.* (2000) Catalytic activity of an in vivo tumor targeted anti-CEA scFv::carboxypeptidase G2 fusion protein. *Int. J. Cancer*, **85**, 4, 571–7.

Bignami, G. S., Senter, P. D., Grothaus, P. G., Fischer, K. J., Humphreys, T., & Wallace, P. M. (1992) N-(4-hydroxyphenylacetyl)palytoxin: a palytoxin prodrug that can be activated by a monoclonal antibody-penicillin G amidase conjugate. *Cancer Res.*, **52**, 20, 5759–64.

Blakey, D. C., Burke, P. J., Davies, D. H., Dowell, R. I., East, S. J., Eckersley, K. P. *et al.* (1996) ZD2767, an improved system for antibody-directed enzyme prodrug therapy that results in tumor regressions in colorectal tumor xenografts. *Cancer Res.*, **56**, 14, 3287–92.

Bosslet, K., Czech, J., & Hoffmann, D. (1994) Tumor-selective prodrug activation by fusion protein-mediated catalysis. *Cancer Res.*, **54**, 8, 2151–9.

Byrd, J. C., Waselenko, J. K., Maneatis, T. J., Murphy, T., Ward, F. T., Monahan, B. P. *et al.* (1999) Rituximab therapy in hematologic malignancy patients with circulating blood tumor cells: association with increased infusion-related side effects and rapid blood tumor clearance. *J. Clin. Oncol.*, **17**, 3, 791–5.

Carter, P. (2001) Improving the efficacy of antibody-based cancer therapies. *Nat. Rev. Cancer*, **1**, 2, 118–29.

Cheng, T. L., Wei, S. L., Chen, B. M., Chern, J. W., Wu, M. F., Liu, P. W. *et al.* (1999) Bystander killing of tumour cells by antibody-targeted enzymatic activation of a glucuronide prodrug. *Br. J. Cancer*, **79**, 9–10, 1378–85.

Chester, K. A., Mayer, A., Bhatia, J., Robson, L., Spencer, D. I., Cooke, S. P. *et al.* (2000) Recombinant anti-carcinoembryonic antigen antibodies for targeting cancer. *Cancer Chemother. Pharmacol.*, **46**(Suppl), S8–12.

Davis, T. A., Grillo-Lopez, A. J., White, C. A., McLaughlin, P., Czuczman, M. S., Link, B. K. et al. (2000) Rituximab anti-CD20 monoclonal antibody therapy in non-Hodgkins lymphoma: safety and efficacy of re-treatment. *J. Clin. Oncol.*, **18**, 17, 3135–43.

Eccles, S. A., Court W. J., Box, G. A., Dean, C. J., Melton, R. G., & Springer, C. J. (1994) Regression of established breast carcinoma xenografts with antibody-directed enzyme prodrug therapy against c-erbB2 p185. *Cancer Res.*, **54**, 19, 5171–7.

Edwards, P. A. (1985) Heterogeneous expression of cell-surface antigens in normal epithelia and their tumours, revealed by monoclonal antibodies. *Br. J. Cancer*, **51**, 2, 149–60.

Francis, R. J., Sharma, S. K., Springer, C., Green, A. J., Hope-Stone, L. D., Sena, L. et al. (2002) A phase I trial of antibody directed enzyme prodrug therapy (ADEPT) in patients with advanced colorectal carcinoma or other CEA producing tumours. *Br. J. Cancer*, **87**, 6, 600–607.

Frei, E., III, Teicher, B. A., Holden, S. A., Cathcart, K. N., & Wang, Y. Y. (1988) Preclinical studies and clinical correlation of the effect of alkylating dose. *Cancer Res.*, **48**, 22, 6417–23.

Gold, P. & Freedman, S. O. (1975) Tests for carcinoembryonic antigen. Role in diagnosis and management of cancer. *JAMA*, **234**, 2, 190–2.

Goldenberg, D. M., Deland, F., Kim, E., Bennett, S., Primus, F. J., van, N. J., Jr. et al. (1978) Use of radiolabeled antibodies to carcinoembryonic antigen for the detection and localization of diverse cancers by external photoscanning. *N. Engl. J. Med.*, **298**, 25, 1384–6.

Goldman, A., Gordon, I., Pritchard, J., & Kemshead, J. (1985) A monoclonal antibody, UJ13A, used for radioimmunolocalisation of neuroblastoma in an animal model and patients. *Prog. Exp. Tumor Res.*, **29**, 85–92.

Hamann, P. R., Hinman, L. M., Hollander, I., Beyer, C. F., Lindh, D., Holcomb, R. et al. (2002) Gemtuzumab ozogamicin, a potent and selective anti-CD33 antibody-calicheamicin conjugate for treatment of acute myeloid leukemia. *Bioconjug. Chem.*, **13**, 1, 47–58.

Han, J. Y., Hong, E. K., Lee, S. Y., Yoon, S. M., Lee, D. H., & Lee, J. S. (2005) Thymidine phosphorylase expression in tumour cells and tumour response to capecitabine plus docetaxel chemotherapy in non-small cell lung cancer. *J. Clin. Pathol.*, **58**, 6, 650–4.

Houba, P. H., Leenders, R. G., Boven, E., Scheeren, J. W., Pinedo, H. M., & Haisma, H. J. (1996) Characterization of novel anthracycline prodrugs activated by human beta-glucuronidase for use in antibody-directed enzyme prodrug therapy. *Biochem. Pharmacol.*, **52**, 3, 455–63.

Jones, D., Fritschy, J., Garson, J., Nokes, T. J., Kemshead, J. T., & Hardisty, R. M. (1984) A monoclonal antibody binding to human medulloblastoma cells and to the platelet glycoprotein IIB-IIIA complex. *Br. J. Haematol.*, **57**, 4, 621–31.

Kohler, G. & Milstein, C. (1975) Continuous cultures of fused cells secreting antibody of predefined specificity. *Nature*, **256**, 5517, 495–7.

Lane, D. M., Eagle, K. F., Begent, R. H., Hope-Stone, L. D., Green, A. J., Casey, J. L. et al. (1994) Radioimmunotherapy of metastatic colorectal tumours with iodine-131-labelled antibody to carcinoembryonic antigen: phase I/II study with comparative biodistribution of intact and F(ab)2 antibodies. *Br. J. Cancer*, **70**, 3, 521–5.

Mach, J. P., Carrel, S., Merenda, C., Sordat, B., & Cerottini, J. C. (1974) *In vivo* localisation of radiolabelled antibodies to carcinoembryonic antigen in human colon carcinoma grafted into nude mice. *Nature*, **248**, 450, 704–6.

Maloney, D. G., Liles, T. M., Czerwinski, D. K., Waldichuk, C., Rosenberg, J., Grillo-Lopez, A. *et al.* (1994) Phase I clinical trial using escalating single-dose infusion of chimeric anti-CD20 monoclonal antibody (IDEC-C2B8) in patients with recurrent B-cell lymphoma. *Blood*, **84**, 8, 2457–2466.

Maloney, D. G., Grillo-Lopez, A. J., White, C. A., Bodkin, D., Schilder, R. J., Neidhart, J. A. *et al.* (1997) IDEC-C2B8 (Rituximab) anti-CD20 monoclonal antibody therapy in patients with relapsed low-grade non-Hodgkins lymphoma. *Blood*, **90**, 6, 2188–95.

Martin, J., Stribbling, S. M., Poon, G. K., Begent, R. H., Napier, M., Sharma, S. K. *et al.* (1997) Antibody-directed enzyme prodrug therapy: pharmacokinetics and plasma levels of prodrug and drug in a phase I clinical trial. *Cancer Chemother. Pharmacol.*, **40**, 3, 189–201.

Mayer, A., Sharma, S. K., Tolner, B., Minton, N. P., Purdy, D., Amlot, P. *et al.* (2004a) Modifying an immunogenic epitope on a therapeutic protein: a step towards an improved system for antibody-directed enzyme prodrug therapy (ADEPT). *Br. J. Cancer*, **90**, 12, 2402–10.

Mayer, A., Francis, R., Sharma, S. K., Sully C., Parker, S., Tolner, B. *et al.* (2004b) A Phase I/II trial of antibody directed enzyme prodrug therapy (ADEPT) with MFECP1 and ZD2767P. *Br. J. Cancer*, **91**(Suppl 1), S8.

Medzihradszky, K. F., Spencer, D. I., Sharma, S. K., Bhatia, J., Pedley, R. B., Read, D. A. *et al.* (2004) Glycoforms obtained by expression in Pichia pastoris improve cancer targeting potential of a recombinant antibody-enzyme fusion protein. *Glycobiology*, **14**, 1, 27–37.

Melton, R. G., Searle, F., Sherwood, R. F., Bagshawe, K. D., & Boden, J. A. (1990) The potential of carboxypeptidase G2: antibody conjugates as anti-tumour agents. II. In vivo localising and clearance properties in a choriocarcinoma model. *Br. J. Cancer*, **61**, 3, 420–4.

Meyer, D. L., Jungheim, L. N., Law, K. L., Mikolajczyk, S. D., Shepherd, T. A., Mackensen, D. G. *et al.* (1993) Site-specific prodrug activation by antibody-beta-lactamase conjugates: regression and long-term growth inhibition of human colon carcinoma xenograft models. *Cancer Res.*, **53**, 17, 3956–63.

Meyer, D. L., Law, K. L., Payne, J. K., Mikolajczyk, S. D., Zarrinmayeh, H., Jungheim, L. N. *et al.* (1995) Site-specific prodrug activation by antibody-beta-lactamase conjugates: preclinical investigation of the efficacy and toxicity of doxorubicin delivered by antibody directed catalysis. *Bioconjug. Chem.*, **6**, 4, 440–6.

Michael, N. P., Chester, K. A., Melton, R. G., Robson, L., Nicholas, W., Boden, J. A. *et al.* (1996) *In vitro* and *in vivo* characterisation of a recombinant carboxypeptidase G2:anti-CEA scFv fusion protein. *Immunotechnology.*, **2**, 1, 47–57.

Monks, N. R., Blakey, D. C., Curtin, N. J., East, S. J., Heuze, A., & Newell, D. R. (2001) Induction of apoptosis by the ADEPT agent ZD2767: comparison with the classical nitrogen mustard chlorambucil and a monofunctional ZD2767 analogue. *Br. J. Cancer*, **85**, 5, 764–71.

Napier, M. P., Sharma, S. K., Springer, C. J., Bagshawe, K. D., Green, A. J., Martin, J. *et al.* (2000) Antibody-directed enzyme prodrug therapy: efficacy and mechanism of action in colorectal carcinoma. *Clin. Cancer Res.*, **6**, 3, 765–72.

Osbourn, J., Jermutus, L., & Duncan, A. (2003) Current methods for the generation of human antibodies for the treatment of autoimmune diseases. *Drug Discov. Today*, **8**, 18, 845–51.

Pastan, I. & Kreitman, R. J. (2002) Immunotoxins in cancer therapy. *Curr. Opin. Investig. Drugs*, **3**, 7, 1089–91.

Payne, G. (2003) Progress in immunoconjugate cancer therapeutics. *Cancer Cell*, 3, 3, 207–12.

Pedley, R. B., Begent, R. H., Boden, J. A., Boden, R., Adam, T., & Bagshawe, K. D. (1991) The effect of radiosensitizers on radio-immunotherapy, using 131I-labelled anti-CEA antibodies in a human colonic xenograft model. *Int. J. Cancer*, 47, 4, 597–602.

Pedley, R. B., Boden, J. A., Boden, R., Dale, R., & Begent, R. H. (1993) Comparative radioimmunotherapy using intact or F(ab)2 fragments of 131I anti-CEA antibody in a colonic xenograft model. *Br. J. Cancer*, 68, 1, 69–73.

Pedley, R. B., Sharma, S. K., Boxer, G. M., Boden, R., Stribbling, S. M., Davies, L. *et al.* (1999) Enhancement of antibody-directed enzyme prodrug therapy in colorectal xenografts by an antivascular agent. *Cancer Res.*, 59, 16, 3998–4003.

Pedley, R. B., Hill, S. A., Boxer, G. M., Flynn, A. A., Boden, R., Watson, R. *et al.* (2001) Eradication of colorectal xenografts by combined radioimmunotherapy and combretastatin a-4 3-O-phosphate. *Cancer Res.*, 61, 12, 4716–22.

Quinney, S. K., Sanghani, S. P., Davis, W. I., Hurley, T. D., Sun, Z., Murry, D. J. *et al.* (2005) Hydrolysis of capecitabine to 5-deoxy-5-fluorocytidine by human carboxylesterases and inhibition by loperamide. *J. Pharmacol. Exp. Ther.*, 313, 3, 1011–6.

Rader, C., Turner, J. M., Heine, A., Shabat, D., Sinha, S. C., Wilson, I. A. *et al.* (2003) A humanized aldolase antibody for selective chemotherapy and adaptor immunotherapy. *J. Mol. Biol.*, 332, 4, 889–99.

Reilly, R. M., Sandhu, J., Alvarez-Diez, T. M., Gallinger, S., Kirsh, J., & Stern, H. (1995) Problems of delivery of monoclonal antibodies. Pharmaceutical and pharmacokinetic solutions. *Clin. Pharmacokinet.*, 28, 2, 126–42.

Saleh, M. N., Sugarman, S., Murray, J., Ostroff, J. B., Healey, D., Jones, D. *et al.* (2000) Phase I trial of the anti-Lewis Y drug immunoconjugate BR96-doxorubicin in patients with lewis Y-expressing epithelial tumors. *J. Clin. Oncol.*, 18, 11, 2282–92.

Searle, F., Bier, C., Buckley, R. G., Newman, S., Pedley, R. B., Bagshawe, K. D. *et al.* (1986) The potential of carboxypeptidase G2-antibody conjugates as anti-tumour agents. I. Preparation of antihuman chorionic gonadotrophin-carboxypeptidase G2 and cytotoxicity of the conjugate against JAR choriocarcinoma cells *in vitro*. *Br. J. Cancer*, 53, 3, 377–84.

Senter, P. D., Saulnier, M. G., Schreiber, G. J., Hirschberg, D. L., Brown, J. P., Hellstrom, I. *et al.* (1988) Anti-tumor effects of antibody-alkaline phosphatase conjugates in combination with etoposide phosphate. *Proc. Natl. Acad. Sci. U. S. A*, 85, 13, 4842–6.

Senter, P. D. & Springer, C. J. (2001) Selective activation of anticancer prodrugs by monoclonal antibody-enzyme conjugates. *Adv. Drug Deliv. Rev.*, 53, 3, 247–64.

Shabat, D., Rader, C., List, B., Lerner, R. A., & Barbas, C. F., III (1999) Multiple event activation of a generic prodrug trigger by antibody catalysis. *Proc. Natl. Acad. Sci. U. S. A*, 96, 12, 6925–30.

Shamis, M., Lode, H. N., & Shabat, D. (2004) Bioactivation of self-immolative dendritic prodrugs by catalytic antibody 38C2. *J. Am. Chem. Soc.*, 126, 6, 1726–31.

Sharma, S. K., Bagshawe, K. D., Burke, P. J., Boden, R. W., & Rogers, G. T. (1990) Inactivation and clearance of an anti-CEA carboxypeptidase G2 conjugate in blood after localisation in a xenograft model. *Br. J. Cancer*, 61, 5, 659–62.

Sharma, S. K., Bagshawe, K. D., Springer, C. J., Burke, P. J., Rogers, G. T., Boden, J. A. *et al.* (1991) Antibody directed enzyme prodrug therapy (ADEPT): a three phase system. *Dis. Markers*, 9, 3–4, 225–31.

Sharma, S. K., Bagshawe, K. D., Melton, R. G., & Sherwood, R. F. (1992) Human immune response to monoclonal antibody-enzyme conjugates in ADEPT pilot clinical trial. *Cell Biophys.*, 21, 1–3, 109–20.

Sharma, S. K., Bagshawe, K. D., Burke, P. J., Boden, J. A., Rogers, G. T., Springer, C. J. *et al.* (1994a) Galactosylated antibodies and antibody-enzyme conjugates in antibody-directed enzyme prodrug therapy. *Cancer*, 73, 3(Suppl), 1114–20.

Sharma, S. K., Boden, J. A., Springer, C. J., Burke, P. J., & Bagshawe, K. D. (1994b) Antibody-directed enzyme prodrug therapy (ADEPT). A three-phase study in ovarian tumor xenografts. *Cell Biophys.*, 24–25, 219–28.

Sharma, S. K., Pedley, R. B., Bhatia, J., Boxer, G. M., El Emir, E., Qureshi, U. *et al.* (2005) Sustained tumor regression of human colorectal cancer xenografts using a multifunctional mannosylated fusion protein in antibody-directed enzyme prodrug therapy. *Clin. Cancer Res.*, 11, 2 Pt 1, 814–25.

Sherwood, R. F., Melton, R. G., Alwan, S. M., & Hughes, P. (1985) Purification and properties of carboxypeptidase G2 from Pseudomonas sp. strain RS-16. Use of a novel triazine dye affinity method. *Eur. J. Biochem.*, 148, 3, 447–53.

Sinha, S. C., Li, L. S., Miller, G. P., Dutta, S., Rader, C., & Lerner, R. A. (2004) Prodrugs of dynemicin analogs for selective chemotherapy mediated by an aldolase catalytic Ab. *Proc. Natl. Acad. Sci. U. S. A*, 101, 9, 3095–9.

Smith, G. K., Banks, S., Blumenkopf, T. A., Cory, M., Humphreys, J., Laethem, R. M. *et al.* (1997) Toward antibody-directed enzyme prodrug therapy with the T268G mutant of human carboxypeptidase A1 and novel in vivo stable prodrugs of methotrexate. *J. Biol. Chem.*, 272, 25, 15804–15816.

Spencer, D. I., Robson, L., Purdy, D., Whitelegg, N. R., Michael, N. P., Bhatia, J. *et al.* (2002) A strategy for mapping and neutralizing conformational immunogenic sites on protein therapeutics. *Proteomics.*, 2, 3, 271–9.

Springer, C. J., Antoniw, P., Bagshawe, K. D., Searle, F., Bisset, G. M., & Jarman, M. (1990) Novel prodrugs which are activated to cytotoxic alkylating agents by carboxypeptidase G2. *J. Med. Chem.*, 33, 2, 677–81.

Springer, C. J., Bagshawe, K. D., Sharma, S. K., Searle, F., Boden, J. A., Antoniw, P. *et al.* (1991) Ablation of human choriocarcinoma xenografts in nude mice by antibody-directed enzyme prodrug therapy (ADEPT) with three novel compounds. *Eur. J. Cancer*, 27, 11, 1361–6.

Springer, C. J., Dowell, R., Burke, P. J., Hadley, E., Davis, D. H., Blakey, D. C. *et al.* (1995) Optimization of alkylating agent prodrugs derived from phenol and aniline mustards: a new clinical candidate prodrug (ZD2767) for antibody-directed enzyme prodrug therapy (ADEPT). *J. Med. Chem.*, 38, 26, 5051–65.

Stern, M. & Herrmann, R. (2005) Overview of monoclonal antibodies in cancer therapy: present and promise. *Crit Rev. Oncol. Hematol.*, 54, 1, 11–29.

Thorpe, P. E., Mason, D. W., Brown, A. N., Simmonds, S. J., Ross, W. C., Cumber, A. J. *et al.* (1982) Selective killing of malignant cells in a leukaemic rat bone marrow using an antibody-ricin conjugate. *Nature*, 297, 5867, 594–6.

Tolcher, A. W., Ochoa, L., Hammond, L. A., Patnaik, A., Edwards, T., Takimoto, C. *et al.* (2003) Cantuzumab mertansine, a maytansinoid immunoconjugate directed to the CanAg antigen: a phase I, pharmacokinetic, and biologic correlative study. *J. Clin. Oncol.*, 21, 2, 211–22.

Vitetta, E. S., Stone, M., Amlot, P., Fay, J., May, R., Till, M. *et al.* (1991) Phase I immunotoxin trial in patients with B-cell lymphoma. *Cancer Res.*, 51, 15, 4052–8.

Wallace, P. M., MacMaster, J. F., Smith, V. F., Kerr, D. E., Senter, P. D., & Cosand, W. L. (1994) Intratumoral generation of 5-fluorouracil mediated by an antibody-cytosine deaminase conjugate in combination with 5-fluorocytosine. *Cancer Res.*, **54**, 10, 2719–23.

Webley, S. D., Francis, R. J., Pedley, R. B., Sharma, S. K., Begent, R. H., Hartley, J. A. *et al.* (2001) Measurement of the critical DNA lesions produced by antibody-directed enzyme prodrug therapy (ADEPT) *in vitro, in vivo* and in clinical material. *Br. J. Cancer*, **84**, 12, 1671–6.

Wentworth, P., Datta, A., Blakey, D., Boyle, T., Partridge, L. J., & Blackburn, G. M. (1996) Toward antibody-directed abzyme prodrug therapy, ADAPT: carbamate prodrug activation by a catalytic antibody and its in vitro application to human tumor cell killing. *Proc. Natl. Acad. Sci. U. S. A*, **93**, 2, 799–803.

Winter, G., Griffiths, A. D., Hawkins, R. E., & Hoogenboom, H. R. (1994) Making antibodies by phage display technology. *Annu. Rev. Immunol.*, **12**, 433–55.

Winter, G. & Harris, W. J. (1993) Humanized antibodies. *Trends Pharmacol. Sci.*, **14**, 5, 139–43.

Chapter 9

Cytokines

Carla M.L. van Herpen, and Cornelis J.A. Punt
Department of Medical Oncology, Radboud University Medical
Centre Nijmegen, The Netherlands

1 Introduction

Cytokines are proteins secreted by the cells of **innate** and **adaptive immune**
system and mediate many of the functions of these cells. Cytokines are produced
in response to microbes and other antigens, for example, tumour antigens. They
stimulate the growth and **differentiation** of lymphocytes, and activate different
effector cells to eliminate microbes and other antigens. Of the many cytokines
that currently have been identified, granulocyte-macrophage colony-stimulating
factor (GM-CSF), interferon-α (IFNα), **interleukin**-2 (IL-2) and interleukin-12
(IL-12) are most advanced in their development in the treatment of cancer.

2 GM-CSF

GM-CSF is a cytokine secreted by activated **T cells**, monocytes, macrophages,
endothelial cells, smooth muscle cells, and bone marrow stromal cells. It is
produced and released after exposure to antigens or bacterial lipopolysa-
ccharides. GM-CSF potentiates the release of pro-inflammatory cytokines.
Haematopoietic cells are the primary target for GM-CSF. It stimulates the
proliferation and differentiation of committed progenitor cells to neutrophils,
eosinophils, and monocytes, and acts directly on megakaryocyte development.
Neutrophil function is enhanced with a decrease in **apoptosis**, and also
monocytes/macrophage function is upregulated (Groopman *et al.* 1989).
Furthermore, GM-CSF induces the proliferation, activation, and migration
of dendritic cells. Pre-clinical models have shown GM-CSF to be one of the
most potent immunomodulators when transfected into **autologous** or **allogeneic** tumour cells, with the induction of specific **CD4+** and **CD8+** T cells
mediated through **dendritic cell** stimulation. Comparative studies with other
cytokines in this setting have shown GM-CSF to be superior in terms of the
induction of systemic antitumour immunity as well as in the anti-tumour
response in established tumours.

2.1 Clinical results

GM-CSF is mainly used in neutropenic patients receiving cancer chemotherapy, or patients undergoing stem cell transplantation. The use of GM-CSF or G-CSF (granulocyte colony-stimulating factor) in neutropenic patients can be divided in primary prophylaxis in previously untreated patients and secondary prophylaxis in later chemotherapy cycles after febrile neutropenia has occurred in a prior cycle. It is well-established that the use of a CSF can reduce the incidence of febrile neutropenia by as much as 50%, but neither clinical benefit nor decreased mortality rates was shown in a number of prospective randomised controlled trials. The American Society of Clinical Oncology has made guidelines for the use of CSFs after chemotherapy (Ozer *et al.* 2000). The routine use of CSFs for primary prophylaxis is not recommended for most chemotherapy regimens. The use of CSFs for secondary prophylaxis is recommended only in patients with curable cancers. Its role in organ transplantation by improving resistance to bacterial infections is being investigated.

Because GM-CSF can generate mature and activate dendritic cells that are particularly well suited to capture dying cancer cells, GM-CSF-based tumour vaccines have been developed (Dranoff 2002). GM-CSF gene-modified tumour vaccines have been tested in cancer patients, with some evidence of immunological and clinical activity. Several phase I and II studies have been performed that showed induction of immunity without significant toxicity. Clinical efficacy was limited, responses were observed in a minority of patients with renal cell cancer (Wos *et al.* 1996). Given its immunostimulating properties, GM-CSF is frequently used as an **adjuvant** to cancer vaccines in early clinical studies (Ribas *et al.* 2003).

3 Interferon-α

Interferons are secreted by several cell types in response to a variety of stimuli such as viral infections, bacterial and cellular products, cytokines, and even chemicals. Interferons mediate their effects by binding and activating receptors with high specificity on cell surfaces. The effects of IFNα are pleiotropic, and include resistance to viral infections including promotion of apoptosis of virally infected cells, regulation of cell growth and differentiation, direct inhibition of tumour cell proliferation, and possibly inhibition of tumour neoangiogenesis (Williams 2000). Insight into the effect of IFNα on specific signal **transduction** pathways and the **transcription** genes involved in these pathways is increasing (Caraglia *et al.* 2005). Immunological effects include the augmentation of the lytic activity of natural killer (NK) cells, stimulation of memory T cells, and an increased expression of the Human Leukocyte Antibody (HLA) class I on tumour cells, regulation of T helper subsets and B cell functions. As a consequence the recognition and lysis of tumour cells by cytotoxic T-cells may be improved. The observation in a small number of patients that the addition of corticosteroids to IFNα does not seem to compromise response rates in renal cell cancer questions the immunological effects of IFNα in this tumour type (Fossa et al. 1992).

3.1 Clinical results

IFNα can be administered subcutaneously (s.c.), intramuscularly (IM) or intravenously (IV). The response rate is independent of the route of administration. The optimal schedule and dose-intensity have never been established in a randomised fashion. In the very low dose-range there is a dose–response relation. The minimal effective dosage is in the range of 20 to 40×10^6 units per week. Higher dosages give rise to more toxicity, but not to proven higher response rates. In the published studies, the frequency of administration varies between two times per week to daily and seems not to be a critical issue (De Mulder et al. 2004). The most frequently reported side-effects of IFNα are divided into acute and delayed symptoms. Acute symptoms consist of fever, chills, headache, and myalgia. Late symptoms are nausea, vomiting, fatigue, and anorexia. During treatment the acute side-effects tend to diminish. Neutropenia, neurotoxicity, depression, hyperthyroidism or hypothyroidism, and a rise in liver enzymes are observed less frequently.

Clinical efficacy of IFNα has been demonstrated in several tumour types, most notably in renal cell carcinoma, melanoma, Kaposi cell sarcoma, chronic myeloid leukaemia, hairy cell leukaemia, lymphoma, multiple myeloma, and neuro-endocrine tumours such as carcinoid. The results in renal cell carcinoma and melanoma will be shortly described.

3.1.1 Renal cell carcinoma

IFNa administered as single agent in advanced renal cell carcinoma gives a response rate between 8% and 26%. One-third of the responses are complete (CR). The median duration of a partial response (PR) is 10 months. In rare cases very long-lasting complete remissions are described. Also a stabilisation of disease occurring in approximately 30% of the patients can continue for a few months. Responses are most frequently seen in the lung and to a lesser degree in the lymph nodes. The median overall survival is approximately 13 months after treatment with IFNα.

Table 9.1 Randomised studies with IFNα in renal cell cancer (De Mulder *et al.* 2004; Aass *et al.* 2005)

Treatment	n	Response rate	Median PFS (months)	Median OS (months)	1-year OS
IFNα	167	14%	4[*]	8.5[*]	4[*]
MPA	168	2%	3	6	3
IFNα+ VBL	79	17%[*]	13 weeks[*]	68 weeks[*]	56%[*]
IFNα	81	3%	9 weeks	38 weeks	38%
IFNα+ CRA	139	12%	5	15	ns
IFNα	145	6%	5	15	
IFNα+ CRA	159	ns	5[*]	17[*]	ns
IFNα	161		3	13	
IFNα+ IL-2	140	21%[*]	20%[*a]	17	ns
IL-2	138	8%	15%	12	
IFNα	147	8%	12%	13	
IFNα+ TN	120	4%	ns	11[*]	50%[*]
IFNα− TN	121	4%		8	37%

Abbreviations: PFS = progression-free survival; OS = overall survival; MPA = medroxy-progesterone acetate; VBL = vinblastine; CRA = cis-retinoic acid; TN = tumour nephrectomy; ns = not stated.
[*] Statistically significant difference.
[a] At one year.

The number of randomised studies is limited (Table 9.1) (De Mulder *et al.* 2004). One study comparing treatment with IFNα with medroxy progesterone acetate revealed a significant improvement in the median and the 1-year survival for the IFNα-treated group. IFNα plus vinblastine showed a small but significant survival benefit over vinblastine alone. Studies in which 13-*cis*-retinoic acid was added to IFNα therapy give conflicting results (Aass *et al.* 2005). Another study compared the combination of IFNα and interleukin-2 (IL-2) with IL-2 continuous IV infusion or IFNα, both as single agent. The combination therapy showed a significantly higher response than both treatments as single agent. The disease-free survival was also higher in the combination arm; however the overall survival was not significantly different. Lastly, the efficacy of IFNα appears to be improved in patients with a prior tumour nephrectomy.

There is no rationale for administering IL-2 after failing on IFNα or vice versa, since response rates in second-line are less than 5%.

Although chemoimmunotherapy with IL-2, IFNα, and 5-fluorouracil has shown promising response rates in uncontrolled studies, its value has yet to be demonstrated in an ongoing EORTC/MRC study that compares this treatment with s.c. single-agent IFNα.

3.1.2 Melanoma

IFNα as a single agent has modest activity in advanced melanoma, with response rates of approximately 15% (Kirkwood 2000). Given its comparable efficacy but increased toxicity and more complicated administration compared with dacarbazine chemotherapy, it has no role in the treatment of advanced disease. Results of studies with combination chemo-immunotherapy have been disappointing. IFNα has been extensively studied as adjuvant treatment for high-risk melanoma. Although initial positive results were reported for its administration at high dose, currently there appears to be no role for IFNα in the standard adjuvant treatment of melanoma (Punt & Eggermont 2001). IFNα may prolong disease-free survival, but not overall survival. This result does not appear to be in balance with the toxicity and costs involved. The ongoing EORTC study in stage III melanoma with a pegylated formulation of IFNα versus observation has completed accrual but results are not yet available. For combination of IFNα with IL-2 see the following section on IL-2.

4 Interleukin-2

IL-2 is a cytokine produced by stimulated T cells, predominantly of T-helper 1 (Th1) cells. It has potent effects on the immune response against foreign antigens. Its main functions concern the clonal expansion of T cells, but also of non-specific effector cells such as natural killer (NK) cells and **lymphokine-activated killer (LAK) cells**. The availability of highly purified **recombinant** IL-2 has allowed the assessment of its *in vivo* biological activity. IL-2 has a serum half-life of less than 5 min after IV administration, but more prolonged serum levels have been observed after s.c. and i.p. administration. Pegylated IL-2 has a more prolonged half-life of several hours. Its primary route of elimination is through excretion by the kidneys. Recently IL-2 has been tested by inhalation in patients with lung metastases from renal cell cancer (Merimsky *et al.* 2004). Although the response rate was low, disease stabilisation was achieved in a significant percentage of patients.

In murine tumour models, IL-2 was consistently shown not only to prevent the outgrowth of tumour but also to eradicate established tumours. These effects were observed both by systemic and local IL-2 administration. Lymphocyte-depletion studies showed definite proof for immune cells as mediators of the effects of IL-2 (Mulé *et al.* 1987). IL-2 may be active against weakly- or non-immunogenic tumours through the activation of LAK cells, but also may stimulate specific anti-tumour responses against **tumour-associated antigens**.

The anti-tumour efficacy of IL-2 may be enhanced by its combination with other immunomodulating agents or strategies, but also with other treatment modalities such as chemotherapy and radiotherapy. In humans, an increase in the level of several cytokines such as tumour necrosis factor-α (TNFα), IL-4, IL-5, IL-6, IL-8, and IL-10 is detectable in serum after IL-2 administration.

4.1 Clinical results

The first pivotal clinical study in cancer patients involved the administration of high-dose IL-2 plus autologous LAK cells and was published in 1985 (Rosenberg *et al.* 1985). Comparable results were later achieved without the laborious and costly transfer of autologous cells. In this and subsequent studies, durable remissions were observed in patients with renal cell cancer and melanoma. However, toxicity was substantial and consisted primarily of constitutional symptoms such as fatigue, fever, and chills, and a vascular leakage syndrome with hypotension, oliguria, fluid retention, weight gain, peripheral oedema, and renal failure. Further possible toxic effects are cardiac arrhythmias and sometimes even myocardial infarction, interstitial pulmonary oedema, nausea and vomiting, diarrhoea, hyperbilirubinaemia, skin erythema, and pruritus followed by desquamation, thyroid dysfunction, infectious complications, and neurological symptoms such as somnolence, depression, disorientation, and even coma. The occurrence of auto-immune disorders such as thyroid dysfunction and vitiligo has been associated with a favourable outcome. The administration of low-dose s.c. IL-2 is associated with a much lower incidence of side-effects. With more experience gained over the years, the administration of IL-2 has become safe and feasible, although it should be stressed that its use should be restricted to experienced oncologists.

After more than 20 years of clinical research, the main anti-tumour effects of IL-2 are still limited to renal cell cancer and melanoma, with objective response rates of approximately 15–20%. In a small minority of responding patients, durable and ongoing remissions of several years have been observed, which in these tumour types is still quite uncommon with any other treatment. However it should be noted that, given the potential toxic effects, these studies were usually performed in a highly selected group of patients. Enormous efforts have been made to improve on these results by varying the dose, schedule, route of administration, and by combining IL-2 with other cytokines and/or chemotherapy. The large majority of these studies concerned uncontrolled phase I–II studies in small number of patients. In retrospect one may argue that the initial promising results in these treatment-resistant tumour types have led to overt optimism regarding this cytokine, resulting in a delay in the conduct of well-designed randomised clinical studies. To date, none of these studies have shown any benefit for IL-2 in combination therapies. The results of the most relevant studies will shortly be discussed.

4.1.1 Melanoma

In advanced melanoma, high-dose IV IL-2 resulted in a response rate of 16% in a highly selected group of 270 patients (Atkins *et al.* 1999). Median overall survival was 11.4 months. This result does not appear to be much different from treatment with less toxic and less costly chemotherapy with dacarbazine, with the results of this latter treatment usually being obtained in a less well-selected patient population. Of note, 59% of complete responders and 28% of all responders on IL-2 were durable, with no patient progressing after a response duration of 30 months. However this latter subgroup concerned only 5% of the total study population. A randomised study of high-dose IV IL-2 with or without IFNα was discontinued because of disappointing results (Sparano *et al.* 1993).

Three randomised phase III studies have investigated the addition of IL-2 plus IFNα to chemotherapy (Atkins *et al.* 2003; Del Vecchio *et al.* 2003), or

Table 9.2 Randomised studies with interleukin-2 in renal cell cancer and melanoma

Author	Tumour type	Treatment	n	Response rate	PFS (months)	OS (months)
Yang *et al.* 2003	RCC	HD IL-2 IV	156	21%[*]	ns	not significant
		LD IL-2 IV	150	13%		
		LD IL-2 s.c.	94	10%		
McDermott *et al.* 2005	RCC	HD IL-2 IV	95	23%[*]	3	17
		LD IL-2 s.c. + IFNα	91	10%	3	13
Rosenberg *et al.* 1999	melanoma	CDtam+IL-2+ IFNα	50	44%	ns	11
		CDtam	52	27%		16
Atkins *et al.* 2003	melanoma	CVD+IL-2+ IFNα	204	17%	5	8
		CVD	201	12%	3	9
Del Vecchio *et al.* 2003	melanoma	CVD+IL-2+ IFNα	76	33%	8	11
		CVD	75	22%	6	12
Keilholz *et al.* 2003	melanoma	CD+ IFNα	183	21%	ns	9
		CD+ IFNα+IL-2	180	23%		9

Abbreviations: RCC = renal cell carcinoma; PFS = progression-free survival; OS = overall survival; HD =high-dose; LD = low-dose; C = cisplatin; D = dacarbazine; tam = tamoxifen; V = vinblastine; ns = not stated.
[*] Statistically significant difference..

IL-2 to chemotherapy plus IFNα (Keilholz *et al.* 2005). No significant benefit for IL-2 was observed in any of these studies. In an earlier study the addition of IL-2 and IFNα to chemotherapy plus tamoxifen had a trend towards a worse outcome (Rosenberg *et al.* 1999) (Table 9.2).

4.1.2 Renal cell carcinoma

In advanced renal cell cancer, IL-2 continuous IV was compared with treatment with IFNα and with the combination of these two cytokines, with only a slight benefit in response rate and progression-free survival for the combination, as explained in the section on IFNα (Table 9.1) (De Mulder *et al.* 2004). Results of a study in which high-dose IL-2 IV was compared with low-dose s.c. IL-2 plus IFNα showed no difference for its primary endpoint of progression-free survival at 3 years (McDermott *et al.* 2005). However a significant benefit in response rate for high-dose IL-2 was observed, with durable complete remissions occurring in 7% and 0%, respectively. An increase in response duration (14 versus 7 months) and median overall survival (17 versus 13 months) was also noted but was not significant. Patients with bone or liver metastases or with the primary tumour *in situ* fared better with high-dose IV IL-2. In an earlier randomised study there was also a benefit for high-dose compared to low-dose IL-2, although this only reached statistical significance for the overall response rate, and the overall survival in the small subset of complete responders (Yang *et al.* 2003) (Table 9.2). Based on these results, the use of low-dose s.c. IL-2 should be discouraged, although its use as immunomodulator in combination with other immunotherapeutic strategies, such as vaccine therapy, may still be a valid option. Better selection criteria for treatment with high-dose IV IL-2 are badly needed.

5 Interleukin-12

IL-12 is mainly produced by phagocytic cells (macrophages and neutrophils), B cells, and dendritic cells (DCs) after encounter with infectious agents (Trinchieri 2003). IL-12 stimulates natural killer (NK) cells and T cells to produce interferon-γ (IFNγ), and also other cytokines such as GM-CSF and tumour necrosis factor (TNF). IL-12 is the key inducer of the T-helper 1 (Th1) response. The produced IFN acts on macrophages by increasing phagocytosis and killing of microbes and on B cells to stimulate production of IgG antibodies that opsonise microbes. Furthermore, Th1 cells stimulate differentiation of naïve CD8+ T cells into **cytotoxic T-lymphocytes** (CTLs). Next to its role in the modulation of the Th1 response, IL-12 induces the proliferation and activation of CTLs and NK cells. Lastly, IL-12 is a potent inhibitor of **angiogenesis** (Voest *et al.* 1995).

In experimental tumour models, treatment with IL-12 has been shown to have a marked anti-tumour effects (Colombo & Trinchieri 2002). In most experimental models, the IL-12 anti-tumour effect was shown to require the induction of IFNγ and a Th1 response. CD8+ T cells, NK cells, and NKT cells are often involved in the mechanism of action of IL-12. IFNγ and a cascade of induced cytokines have a direct toxic effect on the tumour cells and might activate potent anti-angiogenic mechanisms. In addition, IL-12 also augments the production of IgG2a antibodies that have been shown to have anti-tumour activity *in vivo*.

5.1 Clinical results

Several phase I studies have been performed with either intravenous (IV) or subcutaneous (s.c.) administration of IL-12, mainly in renal cell cancer and melanoma (Atkins *et al.* 1997; Bajetta *et al.* 1998; Gollob *et al.* 2000b; Motzer *et al.* 1998; Portielje *et al.* 1999; Rook *et al.* 1999). Toxicity was highly dependent on the schedule of administration (Leonard *et al.* 1997). The maximal tolerated dose of s.c. or IV administration of IL-12 varies between 500 and 1000 ng/kg, with varying frequencies of administration between the different studies. Toxicity mainly consisted of a flu-like syndrome. Dose-limiting toxicities consisted of elevated hepatic transaminases, cytopenias, hyperbilirubinaemia, triglyceridaemia, pulmonary toxicity, deterioration of performance status, fever, vomiting, and mental depression. IFNγ production was seen, which exhibited attenuation with subsequent administrations. Lymphopenia was observed, with recovery occurring within several days and without rebound lymphocytosis, as seen after IL-2 therapy. IL-12 may reverse defects in NK-cell and T-cell function (Robertson *et al.* 1999). Although not a primary endpoint, the number of responses in patients with advanced cancers in phase I studies was limited, i.e. five responders in 156 treated patients. It was shown that patients with tumour regression or prolonged disease-stabilisation were able to maintain IFNγ induction after repeated injections, while in patients with disease progression the IFNγ induction was attenuated (Gollob *et al.* 2000a). Lethal toxicity was observed in the first phase II study in patients with renal cell carcinoma. It appeared that the single priming dose of IL-12 two weeks before consecutive dosing, as was used in the phase I study but which was omitted in the phase II study, had a profound abrogating effect on IL-12-induced IFNγ production and toxicity (Leonard *et al.* 1997). Therefore careful attention to the schedule of administration of IL-12 is required. In three further phase II studies with systemic IL-12 in patients with advanced renal cell carcinoma (Motzer *et al.* 2001), ovarian cancer (Hurteau *et al.* 2001), and cervical cancer (Wadler *et al.* 2004) the response rate to rhIL-12 was between 3% and 7%. **Cell-mediated** immune responses to specific antigens after treatment were detected in cervical cancer.

Response rates of 21–43% were observed in phase II studies performed in patients with cutaneous T-cell lymphoma and non-Hodgkin's lymphoma (Rook *et al.* 2001;Younes *et al.* 2004). Biopsy of regressing lesions revealed an increase in numbers of CD8+ T lymphocytes, suggesting a role for these cells in the observed anti-tumour immunity.

Intra-tumoural IL-12 administration in patients with head and neck cancer resulted in significant biological effects on plasma concentrations of IFNg and IL-10, a decrease in T-bet mRNA (Th1 transcription factor), an increase of NK cells, and decrease of Th cells in lymph nodes and tumour, and an increase of IFNg-mRNA in lymph nodes. These changes were compatible with a switch from a **Th2** to a **Th1** profile (van Herpen *et al.* 2003, 2004).

Due to the low response rates in most phase II studies, there is currently no role for IL-12 as single agent in the treatment of cancer. However, since IL-12 appears to augment the cellular immune response, there is a rationale for its use as an adjuvant, i.e. together with T-cell directed vaccine strategies. Several phase I studies have been performed with low dose (30–100 ng/kg) IL-12 plus a peptide vaccine in melanoma patients. Preliminary results of combination therapy with other cytokines, such as IL-2, show immune activation and clinical efficacy. IL-12 has been administered together with s.c. IL-2 in an attempt to maintain IFN induction by rhIL-12 and to enhance its activity against melanoma and renal cell cancer IV (Gollob *et al.* 2003). This schedule was well-tolerated, restored and maintained immune activation by IL-12, and showed some clinical activity especially in melanoma patients. Based on synergistic effects in pre-clinical studies, the combination of s.c. IL-12 with IFN-α has been tested in patients with renal cell carcinoma or melanoma. This combination proved feasible, and immunological effects, i.e. induction of IP-10, MIG, and IFN mRNA expression, was observed (Alatrash *et al.* 2004). A phase I study in patients with B-cell non-Hodgkin lymphoma with the combination of s.c. IL-12 and rituximab, a **monoclonal antibody** that binds to CD20 on B lymphocytes, showed a response rate of 69% (Ansell *et al.* 2000). The efficacy of these combination regimens should be confirmed in further studies.

6 Summary

It would be reasonable to comment that despite a few 'successes' (e.g. IFN-α in renal cell cancer), single-agent cytokine use has failed to live up to its initial surrounding hype. As is the case with the evolution of most anticancer therapies, further translational research gives insight into more rational approaches, perhaps as an adjuvant to cell-based therapeutics or through identification and selection of those patients (and tumours) which have optimal response characteristics.

References

Aass, N., De Mulder, P. H. M., Mickish, G. H. J. *et al.* (2005) Interferon alpha-2a with and without 13-cis retinoic acid in patients with progressive metastatic renal cell carcinoma. A randomised phase II/III trial (EORTC 30951). *J Clin Oncol*, **23**, 4172–8.

Alatrash, G., Hutson, T. E., Molto, L., Richmond, A., Nemec, C., Mekhail, T. *et al.* (2004) Clinical and immunologic effects of subcutaneously administered interleukin-12 and interferon alfa-2b: Phase I trial of patients with metastatic renal cell carcinoma or malignant melanoma. *J Clin Oncol*, **22**, 14, 2891–900.

Ansell, S. M., Witzig, T. E., Kurtin, P. J., Jelinek, D. F., Howell, K. G., Markovic, S. N. *et al.* (2000) Phase I study of interleukin-12 in combination with rituximab in patients with B-cell non-Hodgkin's lymphoma (NHL). *Blood*, **96**, 11, 577A.

Atkins, M. B., Robertson, M. J., Gordon, M., Lotze, M. T., DeCoste, M., DuBois, J. S. *et al.* (1997) Phase I evaluation of intravenous recombinant human interleukin 12 in patients with advanced malignancies. *Clin Cancer Res*, **3**, 3, 409–17.

Atkins, M. B., Lotze, M. T., Dutcher, J. P., Fisher, R. I., Weiss, G., Margolin, K. *et al.* (1999) High-dose recombinant interleukin 2 therapy for patients with metastatic melanoma: Analysis of 270 patients treated between 1985 and 1993. *J Clin Oncol*, **17**, 7, 2105–2116.

Atkins, M. B., Lee, S., Flaherty, L. E. *et al.* (2003) A prospective randomised phase III trial of biochemotherapy with cisplatin, vinblastine, dacarbazine (CVD), IL-2 and interferon-alpha-2b versus CVD alone in patients with metastatic melanoma (E3695): an ECOG-coordinated intergroup trial. *Proc Am Soc Clin Oncol*, **22**, 708 (abstract 2847).

Bajetta, E., Del Vecchio, M., Mortarini, R., Nadeau, R., Rakhit, A., Rimassa, L. *et al.* (1998) Pilot study of subcutaneous recombinant human interleukin 12 in metastatic melanoma. *Clin Cancer Res*, **4**, 1, 75–85.

Caraglia, M., Marra, M., Pelaia, G., Maselli, R., Caputi, M., Marsico, S. A. *et al.* (2005) Alpha-interferon and its effects on signal transduction pathways. *J Cell Physiol*, **202**, 2, 323–35.

Colombo, M. P. & Trinchieri, G. (2002) Interleukin-12 in anti-tumour immunity and immunotherapy. *Cytokine Growth Factor Rev*, **13**, 2, 155–68.

Del Vecchio, M., Bajetta, E., Vitali, M. *et al.* (2003) Multicenter phase III randomized trial of cisplatin, vindesine, and dacarbazine (CVD) versus CVD plus subcutaneous interleukin-2 and interferon-alpha-2b in metastatic melanoma patients. *Proc Am Soc Clin Oncol*, **22**, 709 (abstract 2849).

De Mulder, P. H. M., van Herpen, C. M. L., & Mulders, P. A. F. (2004) Current treatment of renal cell carcinoma. *Ann Oncol*, **15**, 319–28.

Dranoff, G. (2002) GM-CSF-based cancer vaccines *Immunol Rev*, **188**, 147–54.

Fossa, S. D., Lehne, G., Gunderson, R., Hjelmaas, U., & Holdener, E. E. (1992) Recombinant interferon alpha-2a combined with prednisone in metastatic renal-cell carcinoma – treatment results, serum interferon levels and the development of antibodies. *Int J Cancer*, **50**, 6, 868–70.

Gollob, J. A., Mier, J. W., Veenstra, K., McDermott, D. F., Clancy, D., Clancy, M., *et al.* (2000a) Phase I trial of twice-weekly intravenous interleukin 12 in patients with metastatic renal cell cancer or malignant melanoma: ability to maintain IFN-gamma induction is associated with clinical response. *Clin Cancer Res*, **6**, 5, 1678–92.

Gollob, J. A., Mier, J. W., Veenstra, K., McDermott, D. F., Clancy, D., Clancy, M. *et al.* (2000b) Phase I trial of twice-weekly intravenous interleukin 12 in patients with metastatic renal cell cancer or malignant melanoma: ability to maintain IFN-gamma induction is associated with clinical response. *Clin Cancer Res*, **6**, 5, 1678–92.

Gollob, J. A., Veenstra, K. G., Parker, R. A., Mier, J. W., McDermott, D. F., Clancy, D. *et al.* (2003) Phase I trial of concurrent twice-weekly recombinant human interleukin-12 plus low-dose IL-2 in patients with melanoma or renal cell carcinoma. *J Clin Oncol*, **21**, 13, 2564–73.

Groopman, J. E., Molina, J. M., & Scadden, D. T. (1989) Hematopoietic growth-factors – biology and clinical-applications. *New England J Med*, **321**, 21, 1449–59.

Hurteau, J. A., Blessing, J. A., DeCesare, S. L., & Creasman, W. T. (2001) Evaluation of recombinant human interleukin-12 in patients with recurrent or refractory ovarian cancer: a gynecologic oncology group study. *Gynecol Oncol*, **82**, 1, 7–10.

Keilholz, U., Punt, C. J., Gore, M. *et al.* (2005) Dacarbazine, cisplatin and IFN-a2b with or without IL-2 in metastatic melanoma: a randomized phase III trial 18951 of the European organisation for Research and Treatment of Cancer Melanoma Group. *J Clin Oncol*, **23**, 6747–55.

Kikwood, J. M. (2000) Interferon-a and -b: clinical applications. Melanoma. In: *Principles and practice of the biologic therapy of cancer* (3rd edn) (S. A. Rosenberg, ed.), pp.224–51. Lippincott, Williams & Wilkins.

Leonard, J. P., Sherman, M. L., Fisher, G. L., Buchanan, L. J., Larsen, G., Atkins, M. B. *et al.* (1997) Effects of single-dose interleukin-12 exposure on interleukin-12-associated toxicity and interferon-gamma production. *Blood*, **90**, 7, 2541–8.

McDermott, D. F., Regan, M. M., Clark, J. I. *et al.* (2005) Randomised phase III trial of high-dose interleukin-2 versus subcutaneous interleukin-2 and interferon in patients with metastatic renal cell cancer. *J Clin Oncol*, **23**, 133–41.

Merimsky,O., Gez, E., Weitzen, R. *et al.* (2004) Targeting pulmonary metastases of renal cell carcinoma by inhalation of interleukin-2. *Ann Oncol*, **15**, 610–2.

Motzer, R. J., Rakhit, A., Schwartz, L. H., Olencki, T., Malone, T. M., Sandstrom, K. *et al.* (1998) Phase I trial of subcutaneous recombinant human interleukin-12 in patients with advanced renal cell carcinoma. *Clin Cancer Res*, **4**, 5, 1183–91.

Motzer, R. J., Rakhit, A., Thompson, J. A., Nemunaitis, J., Murphy, B. A., Ellerhorst, J. *et al.* (2001) Randomized multicenter phase ii trial of subcutaneous recombinant human interleukin-12 versus interferon-alpha2a for patients with advanced renal cell carcinoma. *J Interferon Cytokine Res*, **21**, 4, 257–63.

Mulé, J. J., Yang, J. C., Afreniere, R. L., Shu, S., & Rosenberg, S. A. (1987) Identification of cellular mechanisms operational invivo during the regression of established pulmonary metastases by the systemic administration of high-dose recombinant interleukin-2. *J Immunol*, **139**, 1, 285–94.

Ozer, H., Armitage, J. O., Bennett, C. L., Crawford, J., Demetri, G. D., Pizzo, P. A. *et al.* (2000) 2000 update of recommendations for the use of hematopoietic colony-stimulating factors: Evidence-based, clinical practice guidelines. *J Clin Oncol*, **18**, 20, 3558–85.

Portielje, J. E., Kruit, W. H., Schuler, M., Beck, J., Lamers, C. H., Stoter, G. *et al.* (1999) Phase I study of subcutaneously administered recombinant human interleukin 12 in patients with advanced renal cell cancer. *Clin Cancer Res*, **5**, 12, 3983–9.

Punt, C. J. A. & Eggermont, A. M. M. (2001) Adjuvant interferon-alpha for melanoma revisited: News from old and new studies. *Ann Oncol*, 12, 12, 1663–6.

Ribas, A., Butterfield, L. H., Glaspy, J. A., & Economou, J. S. (2003) Current developments in cancer vaccines and cellular immunotherapy. *J Clin Oncol*, 21, 12, 2415–32.

Robertson, M. J., Cameron, C., Atkins, M. B., Gordon, M. S., Lotze, M. T., Sherman, M. L. *et al.* (1999) Immunological effects of interleukin 12 administered by bolus intravenous injection to patients with cancer. *Clin Cancer Res*, 5, 1, 9–16.

Rook, A. H., Wood, G. S., Yoo, E. K., Elenitsas, R., Kao, D. M., Sherman, M. L. *et al.* (1999) Interleukin-12 therapy of cutaneous T-cell lymphoma induces lesion regression and cytotoxic T-cell responses. *Blood*, 94, 3, 902–8.

Rook, A. H., Zaki, M. H., Wysocka, M., Wood, G. S., Duvic, M., Showe, L. C. *et al.* (2001) The role for interleukin-12 therapy of cutaneous T cell lymphoma. *Cutaneous T Cell Lymphoma: Basic and Clinically Relevant Biology*, 941, 177–84.

Rosenberg, S. A., Lotze, M. T., Muul, L. M., Leitman, S., Chang, A. E., Ettinghausen, S. E. *et al.* (1985) Observations on the systemic administration of autologous lymphokine-activated killer cells and recombinant interleukin-2 to patients with metastatic cancer. *New Engl J Med*, 313, 23, 1485–92.

Rosenberg, S. A., Yang, J. C., Schwartzentruber, D. J., Hwu, P., Marincola, F. M., Topalian, S. L. *et al.* (1999) Prospective randomized trial of the treatment of patients with metastatic melanoma using chemotherapy with cisplatin, dacarbazine, and tamoxifen alone or in combination with interleukin-2 and interferon alfa-2b. *J Clin Oncol*, 17, 3, 968–75.

Sparano, J. A., Fisher, R. I., Sunderland, M., Margolin, K., Ernest, M. L., Sznol, M. *et al.* (1993) Randomized phase-III trial of treatment with high-dose interleukin-2 either alone or in combination with interferon alfa-2a in patients with advanced melanoma. *J Clin Oncol*, 11, 10, 1969–77.

Trinchieri, G. (2003) Interleukin-12 and the regulation of innate resistance and adaptive immunity. *Nat Rev Immunol*, 3, 2, 133–46.

Van Herpen, C. M. L., Huijbens, R., Looman, M. *et al.* (2003) Pharmacokinetics and immunological effects of a phase Ib study with intratumoural administration of recombinant human interleukin-12 in patients with head and neck squamous cell carcinoma: a decrease of T-bet in PBMCs. *Clin Cancer Res*, 9, 2950–6.

Van Herpen, C. M. L., Looman, M., Zonneveld, M. *et al.* (2004) Intratumoural administration of recombinant human interleukin-12 in head and neck squamous cell carcinoma patients elicits a T helper 1 profile in the locoregional lymphnodes. *Clin Cancer Res*, 10, 2626–35.

Voest, E. E., Kenyon, B. M., O'Reilly, M. S., Truitt, G., D'Amato, R. J., & Folkman, J. (1995) Inhibition of angiogenesis in vivo by interleukin 12. *J Natl Cancer Inst*, 87, 8, 581–6.

Wadler, S., Levy, D., Frederickson, H. L., Falkson, C. I., Wang, Y. X., Weller, E. *et al.* (2004) A phase II trial of interleukin-12 in patients with advanced cervical cancer: clinical and immunologic correlates Eastern Cooperative Oncology Group study E1E96. *Gynecol Oncol*, 92, 3, 957–64.

Williams, B. R. G. (2000) Interferon-a and -b: basic principles and Pre-clinical studies. In: *Principles and practice of the biologic therapy of cancer* (3rd edn) (S. A. Rosenberg, ed.), pp.194–209. Lippincott, Williams & Wilkins.

Wos, E., Olencki, T., Tuason, L. *et al.* (1996) Phase II trial of subcutaneously administered granulocyte-macrophage colony-stimulating factor in patients with metastatic renal cell carcinoma. *Cancer*, 77, 1149–53.

Yang, J. C., Sherry, R. M., Steinberg, S. M., Topalian, S. L., Schwartzentruber, D. J., Hwu, P. *et al.* (2003) Randomized study of high-dose and low-dose interleukin-2 in patients with metastatic renal cancer. *J Clin Oncol*, 21, 16, 3127–32.

Younes, A., Pro, B., Robertson, M. J., Flinn, I. W., Romaguera, J. E., Hagemeister, F. *et al.* (2004) Phase II clinical trial of interleukin-12 in patients with relapsed and refractory non-Hodgkin's lymphoma and Hodgkin's disease. *Clin Cancer Res*, 10, 16, 5432–8.

Chapter 10

Inhibitors of invasion and angiogenesis

Dirk Laurent

1 Introduction

The extracellular matrix (ECM) is an elaborate network of macromolecules that surrounds the cells of the body. Ultrastructurally, it consists of two identifiable domains, one that envelops cell sheets and the interstitial matrix, and a second, more condensed layer, termed the basement membrane, which is formed adjacent to the epithelial cells (Bosman & Stamenkovic 2003). The ECM is intricate and adaptable, serving both as structural support for tissues and as a complex microenvironment critical for modulating a wide variety of cell behaviours, from cell signalling, adhesion, and migration, to cellular proliferation, **differentiation**, and **apoptosis**. The architecture of the ECM is characterised by a three-dimensional collagen scaffold to which numerous specialised macromolecules adhere. It is a dynamic structure, subject to constant remodelling through the actions of different secreted and cell-associated proteolytic enzymes. This remodelling process allows tissues to respond to physiological changes such as development, pregnancy, growth, and wound repair.

The proteolytic enzymes that are involved in the remodelling of the ECM are known as **matrix metalloproteinases** (MMPs). They are a family of zinc-dependent endopeptidases uniquely capable of digesting the various structural components of the ECM (Nagase & Woessner 1999). Many of these MMPs are promiscuous, and are also able to cleave additional protein substrates, including other proteinases, proteinase inhibitors, secreted signalling molecules, latent growth factors, clotting factors, cell surface receptors, and adhesion molecules. MMPs are often overexpressed in human tumours, where they play key roles in facilitating tumour invasion and metastasis, neoplastic transformation, and **angiogenesis** stimulation (Egeblad & Werb 2002). As such, MMPs are seemingly attractive targets for novel cancer therapeutics, although clinical trials with MMP inhibitors (MMPIs) have in general failed to show a clear benefit for patients.

This chapter will briefly review the biology of the MMP family with specific emphasis on their roles in the development and progression of cancer, and discuss the results of important MMPI clinical trials and the direction of future research in this area.

2 MMPs: structure, function, roles, and cancer

2.1 The MMP family

MMPs are a large family of structurally and functionally related enzymes that are found ubiquitously from plants to humans (Bode 2003). They are synthesised as biologically inactive proteins that are either bound to the cell membrane or secreted into the extracellular space. There are 23 known human MMPs, many of which have overlapping functions, and they are produced by a wide range of cell types within the body, including epithelial cells, fibroblasts, chondrocytes, osteoclasts, endothelial cells, and leukocytes (Massova *et al.* 1998). They are, in general, characterised by several distinct and recognisable structural domains: an auto-inhibitory prodomain of approximately 80 amino acids that must be removed for the molecule to become active, a 175 amino acid catalytic domain, and a homopexin domain of almost 200 amino acids joined to the catalytic domain by hinge region (Fig. 10.1) (Visse & Nagase 2003). On the basis of substrate specificity, sequence similarity, and domain organisation, vertebrate MMPs can be further subdivided into six broad categories, which are briefly described below and summarised in Table 10.1 (Visse & Nagase 2003).

2.1.1 Collagenases

MMP-1, MMP-8, and MMP-13 are all members of the collagenase enzyme family. They are chiefly characterised by an ability to cleave interstitial collagens I, II, and III within a specific site near the C-terminus of the proteins. Collagenases are also capable of cleaving other ECM and non-ECM substrates.

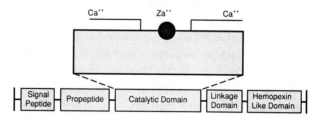

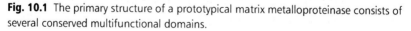

Fig. 10.1 The primary structure of a prototypical matrix metalloproteinase consists of several conserved multifunctional domains.

Table 10.1 Classification and key functions of human MMPs

Class/Family	Members	Key Substrates
Collagenases	MMP-1 MMP-8 MMP-13	Collagens, gelatin, aggrecan, L-selectin, IL-1β, decorin, laminin, proteoglycans, entactin, ovostatin, MMP-2, MMP-7, MMP-8, MMP-9, MMP-13
Gelatinases	MMP-2 MMP-9	Collagens, gelatin, aggrecan, entactin, elastin, fibronectin, osteonectin, plasminogen, MBP, IL-1β
Stromelysins	MMP-3 MMP-10 MMP-11	Collagens, gelatin, casein, aggrecan, elastin, MMP-1. MMP-8
Matrilysins	MMP-7 MMP-26	Collagens, gelatin, fibronectin, aggrecan, decorin, laminin, entactin, elastin, casein. transferrin, β4-integrin, MMP-1, MMMP-2, MMP-9, MMP-9/TIMP-1, α1-proteinase inhibitor, Fas-ligand, pro-TNF-2, E-cadherin, pro-α-defensin
Membrane-type MMPs Transmembrane	MMP-14 MMP-15 MMP-16 MMP-24	Collagens, gelatin, fibronectin, casein, laminin, vitreonectin, perlecan, entactin, proteoglycans, MMP-2, MMP-13, pro-gelatinase A
GPI Anchor	MMP-17 MMP-25	
Other MMPs	MMP-12 MMP-19 MMP-20 MMP-21 MMP-23 MMP-27 MMP-28	Collagens, gelatin, fibronectin, casein, amelogenin, cartilage oligomeric matrix protein, aggrecan, fibrin, plasminogen, perlecan, osteonectin, MMP-9

2.1.2 Gelatinases

MMP-2 and MMP-9, also referred to as gelatinase A and B, belong to the gelatinase family. Within their secondary structures, these enzymes possess type II fibronectin domains, which allow them to bind denatured collagens (gelatin), collagens, and laminin. Types I, II, and III collagen are specific substrates for MMP-2, which is thought to play an important role in bone development (Martigentti *et al.* 2001). MMP-2, the secreted inactive or proform of MMP-2, is bound and activated at the cell surface by MMP-14. Both MMP-2 and MMP-14 play important roles in angiogenesis.

2.1.3 Stromelysins

MMP-3 and MMP-10 are classified as stromelysins. MMP-3 is the more biologically active of the two enzymes. Among its many key functions, it is a specific activator of other MMPs, including MMP-1 (Suzuki *et al.* 1990).

2.1.4 Matrilysins

The matrilysins lack the characteristic homopexin domain found within most MMPs. MMP-7 and MMP-26 are members of this group, and both are capable of digesting numerous ECM components. MMP-7 also has activity processing cell surface molecules, including Fas-ligand, pro-TNF-3, E-cadherin, and pro-α-defensin (Visse & Nagase 2003).

2.1.5 Membrane-type MMPs

As the name suggests, the six membrane-type MMPs (MT-MMPs) are tethered to the cell membrane of a number of different cell types. Four of these enzymes (MMP-14, MMP-15, MMP-16, and MMP-24) are type I transmembrane proteins, and the remaining two (MMP-17 and MMP-25) are bound to the membrane via glycosylphosphatidylinositol (GPI) anchor domains (Visse & Nagase 2003). Aside from being able to digest components of the ECM, members of this enzyme family are also capable of cleaving and activating the latent form or pro-form of MMP-2, as previously discussed. MMP-14 is considered the cellular receptor for MMP-2. Endothelial cells produce both enzymes, and their synthesis is increased in response to signalling through the VEGF pathway (Pepper 2001). MMP-17 is a brain specific enzyme found predominantly within the cerebellum. MMP-25 is found on peripheral blood leukocytes and is expressed in astrocytomas and glioblastomas (Pei 1999; Velasco *et al.* 2000).

2.1.6 Other MMPs

The seven remaining MMPs tend to be specialised proteins, and are therefore not classified within these other groups. MMP-12, also called elastin, is produced by macrophages and is important for magrophage migration (Shipley *et al.* 1996). MMP-19 has been identified as a T-cell derived auto-antigen from patients with rheumatoid arthritis (Kolb *et al.* 1997). MMP-20 is found in newly formed tooth enamel and is commonly known as enamelysin (Li *et al.* 2001). MMP-22 has not yet been functionally characterised, though it is expressed in different human tissues including liver (Yang & Kurkinen 1998). MMP-23 is commonly expressed in reproductive tissue and lacks some of the structural features common to most MMPs, such as a homopexin domain and a specific activation sequence within the pro-domain (Pei *et al.* 2000). MMP-28, or epilysin, is made by keratinocytes and is thought to function in wound repair (Saarialho-Kere *et al.* 2002).

2.2 MMP structure and activation

To successfully develop novel therapeutics, an understanding of the structural features and mechanisms of action of the target molecules is required. In the case of MMPs, X-ray crystallographic and NMR studies of their three-dimensional structures, coupled with chemical analysis of these enzymes under laboratory conditions, have provided tremendous insight into the biology this class of molecules.

2.2.1 Common structural features of MMPs

The prodomain structures of MMP-2, MMP-3, and MMP-9 have been solved, revealing how this domain inhibits the catalytic activity of the molecule (Becker *et al.* 1995). Three N-terminal α-helices found within the prodomain serve to obstruct the active site and recruit enzymes that activate the proteinase. A protease-sensitive loop region between the first two helices is thought to be the 'bait region.' The third helix is the auto-inhibitory portion of the prodomain. It binds within the active site of the catalytic domain and contains a highly conserved amino acid motif termed the 'cysteine switch,' which inhibits the critical zinc ion in the catalytic site of the enzyme and is crucial for removal of the prodomain during the activation process. Cleavage and removal of the prodomain by chemical or biological means results in MMP activation, freeing it to bind and cleave its substrates.

The active site regions of MMPs are highly conserved and notably coordinate several consequential ions: one catalytic zinc ion, one structural zinc ion, and three calcium ions. The substrate-binding pocket (or S' pocket) within the active site varies in size and shape among MMPs and is thought to confer the substrate specificity to the individual molecule (Visse & Nagase 2003).

The homopexin domain is a versatile protein-binding region that functions differently depending on the MMP. It can facilitate MMP dimerisation, act as a substrate-binding region, as well as mediate the interaction between MMPs and their natural inhibitors known as TIMPs (tissue inhibitors of metalloproteinases) (Olson *et al.* 2000).

2.2.2 MMP activation

The mechanism of MMP activation has been extensively studied and is related to the aforementioned structural features of the molecule. Activation can occur either by chemical or biological means, with the key feature being the removal of the prodomain, resulting in the liberation of the catalytic region. Prodomain removal by biological means requires two basic steps (Nagase 1997). The first is its cleavage within the loop region between the first and the second α-helices by an exogenous proteinase. A specific sequence within the loop region determines the identity of the activating proteinase. Once the first cleavage is accomplished, the pro-MMP becomes partially active, as the inhibitory prodomain is destabilised. In turn, the partially active pro-MMP, via an intramolecular processing mechanism that is not altogether clear, activates itself, resulting in the complete removal of the prodomain.

Chemical activation of MMPs occurs differently, via the 'cysteine switch' region of the prodomain (Van Wart & Birkedal-Hansen 1990). Modification of the conserved cysteine residue by a number of different methods results in cleavage and partial activation of the pro-MMP. Once this is accomplished, full MMP activation is achieved as before, via an intramolecular mechanism. Although chemical activation of MMPs is most relevant to *in vitro* studies of these molecules, it has been observed *in vivo* in the activation of pro-MMP-9 by nitric oxide in instances of cerebral ischemia, and in response to the respiratory burst of neutrophils (Gu *et al.* 2002; Weiss *et al.* 1985).

Most MMPs are secreted into the extracellular space where they are subsequently activated by different proteinases or chemical agents, however, there are notable exceptions. MMP-11 undergoes intracellular activation by the enzyme furin convertase. Pro-MMP-11 contains a furin recognition sequence in its C-terminus and is cleaved and activated prior to secretion (Pei & Weiss 1995). This domain is also found on several other MMPs, suggesting that MMPs intracellular activation may be a more generalised phenomenon than previously thought. Clearly the myriad of mechanisms by which MMP activation occurs speaks to both the complexity of cell-matrix interactions and the biological diversity that exists within tissues. It is appears likely, then, that MMP activation is very much dependent on the physiological context within which these enzymes function.

2.3 Biological regulation of MMPs

Due to their vast degradative potential, MMPs are subject to numerous levels of regulation including transcriptional control, sequestration, complex formation, and catabolism. Overexpression of these enzymes is highly correlated with numerous pathological conditions (e.g. inflammation, tumour angiogenesis, tumour invasion), suggesting that in order to maintain tissue homeostasis, tight regulation of MMPs is essential. Each regulatory layer, therefore, ensures that the activities of these enzymes are controlled both spatially and temporally.

2.3.1 Transcriptional regulation

MMP gene expression within adult tissues is low and rapidly induced when remodelling of the ECM is required (Freije *et al.* 2003). Analyses of **promoter** sequences upstream of MMP genes have revealed that both AP-1 and phorbol-ester response elements are present, the former being a common downstream element common to numerous **cytokine** and growth factor signalling pathways. Other enhancer sequences, including TGF-β inhibitory elements, NFKB, SPRE (stromelysin-1 PDGF responsive element), RARE (retinoic acid response element), and NF-1 (nuclear factor-1), further underscore the point that MMP gene expression is influenced by a number of different cell stimuli (Freije *et al.* 2003). Moreover, pre-clinical studies of second messenger signalling pathways corroborate the gene analysis data, showing that MMP **transcription** is upregulated in response **protein kinase** C signalling. The MAP kinase pathway also increases transcription of certain MMPs, most likely through activation of the AP-1 complex. These studies are especially significant considering that these signalling cascades are mitogenic in nature and are often upregulated in cells that have undergone neoplastic transformation (Freije *et al.* 2003).

2.3.2 Sequestration

Spatial regulation is a concept central to the understanding of MMP function. In order to prevent the indiscriminate release of these enzymes, cells focus MMP activity by sequestering them to specific compartments within a tissue. This is accomplished by the association of MMPs with components of the cell membrane (Chakraborti *et al.* 2003). Numerous MMPs interact with cell surface macromolecules, such as **integrins**, CD44, and cell surface proteoglycans. Some MMPs, like MMP-2, require cell association for activation. Pro-MMP-2 forms a trimer at the cell surface with its natural inhibitor TIMP-2 and MMP-14, a cell anchored matrix metalloproteinase. This association is necessary because MMP-14 cleaves the prodomain from pro-MMP-2, resulting in its activation. Finally, interactions with the matrix provide a variety of cell types the necessary information to determine which MMP is required under a certain physiological circumstance. This information is relayed through surface receptors, such as integrins, to the cell **nucleus**, initiating transcription of the specific MMP (Chakraborti *et al.* 2003). Through all these mechanisms, MMP activity is both economised and channelled to prevent uncontrolled ECM degradation and ensure a measured and appropriate physiological response.

2.3.3 Complex formation

An important determinant in tissue homeostasis that is relevant to tumour invasion is the net balance that exists between biologically active MMPs and their endogenous protein inhibitors. Some of these inhibitors are specific to

MMPs, such as the membrane-bound RECK glycoprotein, while others, like α2 macroglobulin, are generalised enzymatic inhibitors. The most important and widely studied of all the MMP inhibitors, however, are the TIMPs. Often bound to the ECM, the four human TIMPs (TIMP-1 to -4) are secreted proteins that bind MMPs in tight non-covalent complexes in a 1:1 stoichiometry (Bode 2003; Freije *et al.* 2003). They are wedge-shaped, low-molecular-weight inhibitors that bind MMPs within the active site in a similar manner to the substrate. TIMPs inhibit all known MMPs with the exception of MMP-14, yet have a variety of biological functions apart form enzymatic inhibition. TIMPs have mitogenic activity, pro-apototic activity, erythroid-potentiating activity, as well as possible functions within the nucleus (Bode 2003; Chakraborti *et al.* 2003; Freije *et al.* 2003). While TIMPs are generally thought to be naturally occurring anti-invasive and anti-metastatic molecules, recent studies have suggested that they may also contribute to cancer spread as well. Immunohistochemical analysis of pathologically staged, resected, primary non-small cell lung cancers (NSCLCs) demonstrated that tissue overexpression of TIMP-1 is associated with adverse outcomes, and furthermore the abundance of TIMP-1 did not correlate to the presence of MMP-2 or MMP-9 in the same tissues (Aljada *et al.* 2004). These data suggest that TIMPs may have important non-inhibitory roles that in some instances are contributory factors to tumour progression, and may in fact be a relevant therapeutic target in the treatment of some NSCLCs.

2.4 MMPs: angiogenesis and cancer

The relationship between MMPs and cancer seems intuitively obvious. Tumours overproduce MMPs to degrade the basement membrane, invade the underlying connective tissue, and penetrate blood and lymphatic vessels resulting in metastasis. While there is evidence to support this model, recent research has demonstrated that MMPs also play a far more nuanced and complex role in tumourigenesis and metastasis than previously thought. Supporting the model are several key observations. MMPs are up-regulated in virtually all known human tumours and tumour cell lines, and several MMPs were in fact cloned as metastasis-specific tumour markers (Coussens *et al.* 2002). Moreover, overexpression or injection of TIMPs was found to halt tumour spread in mouse models of human cancer. These results, taken together, provide a strong rationale for targeting MMPs as a means for preventing tumour invasion and metastasis. Studies over the last few years, however, have muddied the waters with respect to an oversimplified notion of MMPs and cancer. It has been shown, for example, that it is not only tumours themselves, but also stromal cells within the neoplastic environment that are responsible for the majority of MMP production in cancers (Coussens *et al.*

2002). In other words, MMP production may represent a host response to tumourigenesis. Furthermore, while it is true that in cancer models, MMP leads to tumour invasion and metastasis, pre-clinical studies have shown that MMPs possess numerous other functions, including mediating cell proliferation, apoptosis, differentiation, and most significantly, angiogenesis (Fig. 10.2) (Coussens *et al.* 2002).

2.4.1 Tumour angiogenesis and MMPs

The critical contribution of angiogenesis to tumour growth is currently one of the most promising avenues of investigation in the study of tumour biology. Originally proposed by Judah Folkman in the 1970s, it is now accepted that for solid tumours to grow beyond microscopic dimensions, they require *de novo* blood vessel formation in order to access critical nutrients and oxygen from the peripheral blood supply (Folkman 1971). The complex process by which tumours recruit new blood vessels is called tumour angiogenesis. Tumour angiogenesis involves multiple signalling interactions among cancer cells, endothelial cells, pericytes, and smooth muscle cells. It requires degradation of the basement membrane surrounding an existing vessel, followed by migration, proliferation, and organisation of endothelial cells into a new luminal space (Pepper 2001). Tumour angiogenesis is thought to be initiated by tumour or inflammatory cell-secreted pro-angiogenic factors such as members of the VEGF family (vascular endothelial growth factors), bFGF (basic fibroblast growth factor), and TNFα, which activate endothelial cells and cause them to proliferate. These factors, once secreted by cells, are frequently sequestered to the ECM, forming micro-environments of local growth factor density. The contributions of MMPs to angiogenesis are not limited to their ability to degrade the vascular basement membrane, though certainly that is an important facet (Pepper 2001). MMPs also function by releasing ECM-bound pro-angiogenic factors that allow them to bind to endothelial cell surface receptors. Furthermore, MMP remodelling of the ECM reveals cryptic sites within the matrix that activate endothelial cell signalling through their integrin receptors (Rundhaug 2003). MMPs, however, also have anti-angiogenic functions, cleaving and activating angiogenesis inhibitors such as plasminogen to release angiostatin, activation of endostatin from collagen VIII, and autocatalytically generating homopexin domains. By and large, however, MMPs function as proangiogenic factors, and MMPIs have demonstrated **anti-angiogenic** activity in animal cancer models (Rundhaug 2003).

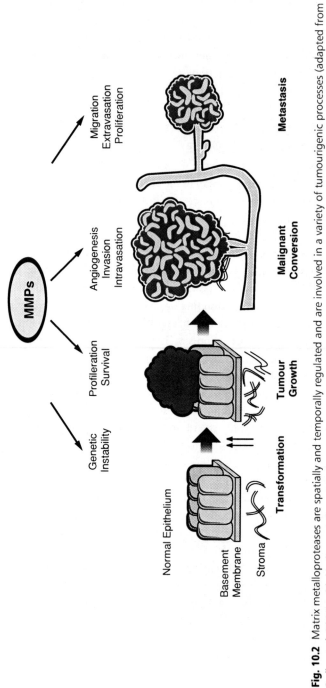

Fig. 10.2 Matrix metalloproteases are spatially and temporally regulated and are involved in a variety of tumourigenic processes (adapted from Freije et al. 2003, with kind permission of Springer Science and Business Media).

2.4.2   MMPs and cancer

As noted before, MMP expression is up-regulated in virtually every type of human cancer and correlates with an advanced disease stage, invasion and metastasis, and unfavourable outcomes. Tumour or stromal cell secreted MMPs remodel the ECM in early stages of cancer, creating a favourable environment for primary tumour growth. As tumour growth progresses, MMP-2 and MMP-9 are then responsible for facilitating the 'angiogenic switch' resulting in blood vessel recruitment. Subsequently, as the tumour enlarges, MMPs facilitate tumour invasion into the stroma and promote metastasis by degrading barriers between the tumour and the peripheral circulation and lymphatic system (Coussens *et al.* 2002; Freije *et al.* 2003). Once tumour cells have entered the circulation, MMPs also contribute to extravasation, or exit from the circulation, as well as establishment of tumour growth at a secondary metastatic site.

MMPs are clearly not functionally one-dimensional and many of their non-ECM roles are now thought to account for the significant contribution of MMPs to tumour growth and progression. One of the key observations from tumour models has been that MMP contributions to tumourigenesis are stage specific, and that effective application of anti-MMP therapy depends on the timing of its administration. Taken together, it is now apparent that MMPs are not simply targets for metastasis, but rather specific MMPs contribute to tumour progression at multiple stages.

3   MMPIs: strategies and clinical trials

Clinical approaches that have been developed to inhibit MMP function closely mirror the innate regulatory mechanisms discussed in the previous sections. There are three basic strategies for MMP inhibition: transcriptional inhibition, inhibition of MMP activation, and functional inhibition, which are the class MMPIs with the broadest clinical development. The results of trials thus far have been disappointing, with the majority of trials demonstrating either no effect, or in some cases deleterious effects of the drugs on cancer patients. This section will review the some interesting strategies for MMP inhibition in preclinical development, as well as the results of pivotal positive and negative trials with MMPIs over the last decade.

3.1   Strategies for MMP inhibition in pre-clinical development

3.1.1   Transcriptional inhibitors

As previously discussed, MMP genes are induced by a number different transcription factors that function downstream of key mitogenic signalling pathways. Compounds that influence these pathways are therefore very likely to have an effect on MMP transcription. Pre-clinical data with the MAPK inhibitor SB203580, for example, demonstrates significant transcriptional down-regulation of the MMP-1, MMP-9, and MMP-13 genes, coupled with decreased invasiveness in both keratinocyte and squamous cancer models (Freije *et al.* 2003). Furthermore, laboratory studies of the pan-RAR antagonist AGN193109 on tumour cell lines show a specific repression of NFKB-mediated transcription, with regulatory effects on MMP-9 and TIMP-1 gene expression (Andela & Rosier 2004). Compounds like the RAS farnesyl-transferase inhibitor manumycin A and the alkaloid halifunginone also have promising pre-clinical activity in cancer cell lines by modulating mitogenic signalling pathways (Freije *et al.* 2003). Finally, MMP-9 mRNA-targeted antisense and ribosyme approaches have also been developed and tested *in vitro* (Moore *et al.* 2003). It remains to be seen whether any of these compounds has potential value in the clinical setting.

3.1.2 Activation inhibitors

MMPIs that target specific MMP zymogen activation pathways are also being evaluated in pre-clinical studies. The selective furin convertase inhibitor alpha-1 PDX blocks the catalytic activation of a MMP-14 and MMP-2, and has shown potential in preventing invasion and tumourigenicity in different highly aggressive human cancer cell lines (Freije *et al.* 2003). Additionally, compounds that prevent the extracellular activation of pro-MMPs, such as thrombospondin, proteoglycans, and proteinase inhibitors are also being studied with respect to their roles in MMP. HIV proteinase inhibitors have demonstrated utility at inhibiting the conversion of the active form of MMP-2, and as a result, have recently been studied in a phase I clinical trial in nasopharyngeal carcinoma (Simonelli *et al.* 2004). Other molecules with potential in this class are inactivating **monoclonal antibodies** against membrane type MMPs, and green tea catechins, both of which have shown activity in preventing MMP activation (Freije *et al.* 2003).

3.2 Clinically evaluated synthetic MMPIs

By far the most widely studied of all the MMP inhibitors are synthetic MMPIs (Table 10.2). These compounds occur in three basic classes: peptide matrix, non-peptide matrix, and non-selective MMPIs. Peptide matrix molecules take advantage of the substrate specificity of MMPs and mimic the collagen cleavage site with an additional zinc-binding hydroxamate moiety necessary for chelating the active site zinc ion. All of these inhibitors are low molecular weight molecules with very tight binding kinetics, and exhibit powerful in vitro activity against MMPs.

Table 10.2 Key clinical trials with MMPIs

Compound	Cancer	Patients	Result	References
Marimastat				
Phase I	None (healthy volunteers)	31	Well tolerated; reversible increase in liver transa-minases noted, most significantly at 200 mg bid	Millat et al. (1998)
Phase II	Advanced cancers (pancre-atic, prostate, ovarian, and colorectal cancers)	415	Musculoskeletal side-effects; biological activity in patients with advanced cancer	Nemunaitis et al. (1998)
Phase III	Pancreatic (stages II, III, IV); unresectable	414	No significant difference in OS vs. gemcitabine	Bramhall et al. (2001)
	Pancreatic (stages II, III, IV); unresectable	239	No additional survival benefit with gemcitabine	Bramhall et al. (2002b)
	Pancreatic (stages I, II, III); respectable		Results pending	Coussens et al. (2002)
	Gastric	369	Modest OS benefit ($P = 0.07$); subset analysis, survival benefit for those with prior chemotherapy ($P = 0.045$)	Bramhall et al. (2002a)
	Glioblastoma (unresectable)	162	No survival benefit vs. placebo	Phuphaniah et al. (2001)
	SCLC (any; partial or com-plete response on first-line chemotherapy)	532	No survival benefit vs. placebo	Shepherd et al. (2002)
	NSCLC (stages IIIA or IIIB)	504	No survival benefit vs. placebo	Coussens et al. (2002)

(continued)

Table 10.2 (continued) Key clinical trials with MMPIs

Compound	Cancer	Patients	Result	References
	Ovarian (advanced)	300	Trial stopped due to lack of benefit	Coussens et al. (2002)
AG3340				
Phase I	Advanced cancers	75	Arthralgia and myalgia observed at doses >25 mg bid	Hande et al. (2004)
Phase III	NSCLC (stage IIIBT4 or IV)	686	No additional survival benefit with carboplatin + paclitaxel	Smylie et al. (2001)
	Prostate (metastatic, hormone refractory)	100	No difference in time to progression	Coussens et al. (2002)
BAY-12-9566				
Phase III	SCLC (extensive, partial or complete response on first-line chemotherapy)	474	Terminated prematurely due to poorer survival than placebo	Rigas et al. (2003)
	Pancreatic (metastatic, unresectable, no prior chemotherapy)	277	Terminated prematurely due to poorer survival than gemcitabine	Moore et al. (2003)
BMS-275291				
Phase II/III	NSCLC (stage IIB or IV)	774	No survival benefit	Leigh et al. (2005)
AE-941				
Phase II	RCC	22	Dose-dependent increase in median overall survival observed	Batistel et al. (2002)
Phase III	NSCLC	Currently accruing	Results pending	Lu et al. (2003)
	RCC (stage IV)	280	No survival benefit	Escudier et al. (2004)

bid: twice daily; OS: overall survival; NSCLC: non-small-cell lung cancer; SCLC: small-cell lung cancer; RCC: renal cell cancer.

3.2.1 Batimastat

The first synthetic MMPI to be evaluated clinically was batimastat. It was poorly soluble and had to be administered intrapleurally and intraperitoneally in the three clinical trials in which it was evaluated. While its pharmacokinetics were promising, none of the 50 patients treated exhibited any form of response. As a result of this, clinical development of this compound was halted (Beattie & Smyth 1998).

3.2.2 Marimastat

Marimastat, an orally bioavailable hydroxamate, has shown promise in clinical studies. In phase I studies in patients with advanced solid tumours, marimastat showed good tolerability at single doses up to 800 mg (Millat *et al.* 1998). The dose-limiting toxicity was an inflammatory polyarthritis that persisted after discontinuation of treatment. Subsequent phase II studies of marimastat were conducted in patients with advanced ovarian, prostate, colorectal, and pancreatic cancers. A dose-dependent decrease in serum tumour markers, the clinical endpoint of the study, was observed. While an increase in overall survival was not observed, patients exhibiting a biological response did live longer in the trial (Nemunaitis *et al.* 1998). In addition, a phase II trial in patients with advanced pancreatic cancer showed similar one-year survival in both the marimastat and gemcitabine arms, although the combination arm did not display any synergism between the two drugs (Bramhall *et al.* 2001).

Phase III evaluation of marimastat was done in several different treatment settings with ostensibly the same result. First, it was evaluated in a study of untreated or stable patients with advanced gastric cancer. The trial of 369 patients, was disappointing overall, showing only a modest increase in disease-free survival and overall survival with no statistical significance ($P = 0.07$). A subset analysis of the data from these patients, however, did demonstrate a significant two-year survival benefit (from 5% to 18%) for patients who had received prior chemotherapy. While this was an exciting observation, it still requires prospective validation. As previously reported, severe musculoskeletal side-effects were observed in this trial and 10% of the marimastat treated patients had to withdraw due to pain (Bramhall *et al.* 2002a). Phase III trials of this drug has also been reported for patients with unresected pancreatic cancer, glioblastoma, non-small-cell lung cancer, and small-cell lung cancer (Bramhal *et al.* 2002b; Phuphanich *et al.* 2001; Shepherd *et al.* 2002; Coussens *et al.* 2002). In all of these studies, no convincing therapeutic effect was observed. Phase III results of this drug in patients with resectable pancreatic cancer in combination with gemcitabine are still pending.

3.2.3 BAY12–9566

This compound is an orally bioavailable, selective non-peptide matrix MMPI that is a potent inhibitor of MMP-2, MMP-3, and MMP-9. Its clinical development was suspended due to a prematurely terminated phase III study in patients with pancreatic cancer when those who received the compound demonstrated shortened survival times compared to gemcitabine (Moore *et al.* 2003). A similar result was also observed in a randomised study of small-cell lung cancer patients (Rigas *et al.* 2003).

3.2.4 SS-3304

This drug is a D-tryptophan derivative currently in phase II development. It binds the S' pocket of MMP2 and MMP-9 and hence is referred to as a 'deep pocket' MMPI. Phase I studies have shown that the drug is well tolerated without serious side-effects (Creaven *et al.* 2002). MMP inhibitory effects were also reported in the study by in situ zymography.

3.2.5 Col-3 (metastat)

Col-3 is a chemically altered tetracycline that inhibits MMP2 and MMP-9 in pre-clinical prostate cancer models. This drug has shown promise in the treatment of **AIDS**-related Kaposi's sarcoma, where a phase I study reported one complete response and seven partial responses. Also, in the same study, serum concentrations of MMP-2 were found to be significantly lower in patients who responded to COL-3 (Cianfrocca *et al.* 2002). This drug is currently in phase II evaluation.

3.2.6 Other clinically promising MMPIs

A number of other MMPIs have been tested or are currently under investigation. BMS-275291, an MMP-2 and MMP-9 inhibitor, is currently in phase II testing for prostate cancer, as is CGS-27023A, a similar compound. BMS-275291 failed to show a survival benefit in patients with NSCLC (Leigh *et al.* 2005). The shark cartilage extract AE-941 (Neovastat), a potent *in vitro* anti-angiogenic and MMPI, was evaluated in a phase II study in patients with advanced solid tumours (Baptist *et al.* 2002). While an overall benefit was not reported, a subset analysis of the data did reveal a statistically significant survival advantage for renal cell patients. A phase III study of AE-941in patients with metastatic renal cell cancer carcinoma who failed **immunother-apy**, however, failed to show any additional survival benefit (Escudier *et al.* 2004). A phase III study in non-small cell lung cancer is currently underway (Lu *et al.* 2003).

4 Conclusion

The metabolic pathways that regulate the ECM are important components of a variety of physiological and pathological processes. Studies of cell-matrix interactions have demonstrated both the complexities of these pathways and their extraordinary adaptability. MMPs, in particular, play critical roles in ECM biology, and are emerging therapeutic targets in the treatment of cancer. MMPs are overexpressed in the vast majority of human tumours and play multiple important roles in different stages of cancer development and progression. While clinical trials with MMPIs have experienced some setbacks in recent years, several compounds have shown promise and there is certainly reason for optimism. As the biological roles of MMPs in cancer progression are elucidated, new therapies that are both specifically targeted and administered at specific disease stages will undoubtedly emerge.

References

Aljada I, Ramnath N, Donohue K, Harvey S, Brooks JJ, Wiseman SM *et al.* (2004) Upregulation of the tissue inhibitor metalloproteinase-1 protein is associated with progression of human non-small-cell lung cancer. *J Clin Oncol*; 22: 3218–29.

Andela VB, Rosier RN (2004) The proteosome inhibitor MG132 attenuates retinoic acid receptor trans-activation and enhances trans-repression of nuclear factor kappaB. Potential relevance to chemo-preventive interventions with retinoids. *Mol Cancer*; 3(1): 8.

Batist G, Patenaude F, Champagne P, Croteau D, Levinton C, Hariton C *et al.* (2002) Neovastat (AE-941) in refractory renal cell carcinoma patients: report of a phase II trial with two dose levels. *Ann Oncol*; 13(8): 1259–63.

Beattie GJ, Smyth JF (1998) Phase I study of intraperitoneal metalloproteinase inhibitor BB-94 in patients with malignant ascites. *Clin Can Res*; 4: 1899–902.

Becker JW, Marcy AI, Rokosz LL, Axel MG, Burbaum JJ, Fitzgerald PM *et al.* (1995) Stromelysin-1: three-dimensional structure of the inhibited catalytic domain and of the C-truncated proenzyme. *Protein Sci*; 4(10): 1966–76.

Bode W (2003) Structural basis of matrix metalloproteinase function. *Biochem Soc Symp*; 70: 1–14.

Bosman FT and Stamenkovic I (2003) Functional structure and composition of the extracellular matrix. *J Pathol*; 200: 423–8.

Bramhall SR, Rosemurgy A, Brown PD, Bowry C, Buckels JA (2001) Marimastat Pancreatic Cancer Study Group. Marimastat as first-line therapy for patients with unresectable pancreatic cancer: a randomized trial. *J Clin Oncol*; 19(15): 3447–55.

Bramhall SR, Hallissey MT, Whiting J, Scholefield J, Tierney G, Stuart RC *et al.* (2002a) Marimastat as maintenance therapy for patients with advanced gastric cancer: a randomised trial. *Br J Cancer*; 86(12): 1864–70.

Bramhall SR, Schulz J, Nemunaitis J, Brown PD, Baillet M, Buckels JA (2002b) A double-blind placebo-controlled, randomised study comparing gemcitabine and marimastat with gemcitabine and placebo as first line therapy in patients with advanced pancreatic cancer. *Br J Cancer*; 87(2): 161–7

Chakraborti S, Mandal M, Das S, Mandal A, Chakraborti T (2003) Regulation of matrix metalloproteinases: an overview. *Mol Cell Biochem*; 253: 269–85.

Cianfrocca M, Cooley TP, Lee JY, Rudek MA, Scadden DT, Ratner L *et al.* (2002) Matrix metalloproteinase inhibitor COL-3 in the treatment of AIDS-related Kaposi's sarcoma: a phase I AIDS malignancy consortium study. *J Clin Oncol*; 20(1): 153–9.

Coussens LM, Fingleton B, Matrisian LM (2002) Matrix metalloproteinase inhibitors and cancer: trials and tribulations. *Science*; 295: 2387–92.

Creaven PJ, Sullivan DM, Eckhardt G, Bukowski KM, Bonomi P, Rao S *et al.* (2002) A phase I study of S-3304 a matrix metalloproteinase inhibitor in patients with solid tumours. *Eur J Cancer*; 38: S77.

Egeblad M and Werb Z (2002) New functions for the matrix metalloproteinases in cancer progression. *Nature Rev Cancer*; 2: 161–74.

Escudier B, Venner P, Stern L, Donovan M, Croteau D, Champagne P *et al.* (2004) Prognostic factors in metastatic renal cell carcinoma after failure of immunotherapy: lessons from a large phase III study. *Proc ASCO*; 22(14S): 4547.

Folkman J (1971) Tumour angiogenesis: therapeutic implications. *N Engl J Med*; 285(21): 1182–6.

Freije JM, Balbin M, Pendas AM, Sanchez LM, Puente XS, Lopez-Otin C (2003) Matrix metalloproteinases and tumour progression. *Adv Exp Med Biol*; 532: 91–107.

Gu Z, Kaul M, Yan B, Kridel SJ, Cui J, Strongin A *et al.* (2002) S-nitrosylation of matrix metalloproteinases: signaling pathway to neuronal cell death. *Science*; 297(5584): 1186–90.

Hande KR, Collier M, Paradiso L, Stuart-Smith J, Dixon M, Clendeninn N *et al.* (2004) Phase I and pharmacokinetic study of prinomastat, a matrix metalloprotease inhibitor. *Clin Cancer Res*; 10(3): 909–15.

Kolb C, Mauch S, Peter HH, Krawinkel U, Sedlacek R (1997) The matrix metalloproteinase RASI-1 is expressed in synovial vessels of a rheumatoid arthritis patient. *Immunol Lett*; 57: 83–8.

Leigh NB, Paz-Ares L, Douillard JI, Peschel C, Arnold A, Depierre A *et al.* (2005) Randomized phase III study of matrix metalloproteinase inhibitor BMS-275291 in combination with paclitaxel and carboplatin in advanced non-small-cell lung cancer: National Cancer Institute of Canada–clinical trials group study br.18. *J Clin Oncol*; 23(12): 2831–9.

Li W, Gibson CW, Abrams WR, Andrews DW, DenBesten PK (2001) Reduced hydrolysis of amelogenin may result in X-linked amelogenesis imperfecta. *Matrix Biol*; 19: 755–60.

Lu C, Komaki R, Herbst RS, Evans WK, Smith TL, Moore CA *et al.* (2003) A phase III study of Æ-941 with induction chemotherapy (IC) and concomitant chemoradiotherapy (CRT) for stage III non-small cell lung cancer (NSCLC) (NCI T99–0046, RTOG 02–70, MDA 99–303): an interim overall toxicity report. *Proc Am Soc Clin Oncol*; 22: 663 (abstr 2665).

Martigenetti JA, Aqeel AA, Sewairi WA, Bournah CE, Kambouris M, Maouf SA *et al.* (2001) Mutation of the matrix metalloproteinase 2 gene (MMP2) causes a multicentric osteolysis and arthritis syndrome. *Nat Genet*; 28: 261–5.

Massova I, Kotra LP, Fridman R, Mobashery S (1998) Matrix metalloproteinases: structure, evolution and diversification. *FASEB J*; 12: 1075–95.

Millar AW, Brown PD, Moore J, Galloway WA, Cornish AG, Lenehan TJ *et al.* (1998) Results of single and repeat dose studies of the oral matrix metalloproteinase inhibitor marimastat in healthy male volunteers. *Br J Clin Pharmacol*; 45: 21–6.

Moore MJ, Hamm J, Dancey J, Eisenberg PD, Dagenais M, Fields A *et al.* (2003) National Cancer Institute of Canada Clinical Trials Group. Comparison of gemcitabine versus the matrix metalloproteinase inhibitor BAY 12–9566 in patients with advanced or metastatic adenocarcinoma of the pancreas: a phase III trial of the National Cancer Institute of Canada Clinical Trials Group. *J Clin Oncol*; 21(17): 3296–302.

Nagase H (1997) Activation mechanisms of matrix metalloproteinases. *Biol Chem*; 378: 151–60.

Nagase H, Woessner JF Jr (1999) Matrix metalloproteinases. *J Biol Chem*; 274: 21491–4.

Nemunaitis J, Poole C, Primrose J, Rosemurgy A, Malfetano J, Brown P *et al.* (1998) Combined analysis of studies of the effects of the matrix metalloproteinase inhibitor marimastat on serum tumour markers in advanced cancer: selection of a biologically active and tolerable dose for longer-term studies *Clin Cancer Res*; 4(5): 1101–9.

Olson MW, Bernardo MM, Pietila M, Gervasi DC, Toth M, Kotra LP *et al.* (2000) Characterisation of the monomeric and dimeric forms of latent and active matrix metalloproteinase-9. Differential rates for activation by stromelysin 1. *J Biol Chem*; 275(4): 2661–8.

Pei D (1999) Leukolysin/MMP25/MT6-MMP: a novel matrix metalloproteinase specifically expressed in the leukocyte lineage. *Cell Res*; 9: 291–303.

Pei D, Weiss SJ (1995) Furin-dependent intracellular activation of the stromelysin 3 zymogen. *Nature*; 375: 244–47.

Pei D, Kang T, Qi H (2000) Cysteine array matrix metalloproteinase (CA-MMP)/MMP-23 is a type II transmembrane matrix metalloproteinase regulated by a single cleavage for both secretion and activation. *J Biol Chem*; 275: 33988–97.

Pepper MS (2001) Extracellular proteolysis and angiogenesis. *Thromb Haemost*; 86: 346–55.

Phuphanich S, Levin V, Yung W, Forsyth P, Maestro R, Perry J, The Marimastat Glioblastoma Study Group, Elliott M, Baillet M (2001) A multicenter, randomized, double-blind, placebo (PB) controlled trial of marimastat (MT) in patients with glioblastoma multiforme (GBM) or gliosarcoma (GS) following completion of conventional, first-line treatment. *Proc ASCO*; (abstr 205).

Rigas JR, Denham CA, Rinaldi DA, Moore TD, Smith JW, Winston RD *et al.* (2003) Randomized placebo-controlled trials of the matrix metalloproteinase inhibitor (MMPI), BAY12–9566 as adjuvant therapy for patients with small cell and non-small cell lung cancer. *Proc Am Soc Clin Oncol*; 22 (abstr 2525).

Rundhaug JE (2003) Matrix metalloproteinases, angiogenesis, and cancer. *Clin Cancer Res*; 9: 551–4.

Saarialho-Kere U, Kerkela E, Johkola T, Suomela S, Keski-Oja J, Lohi J (2002) Epilysin (MMP-28) expression is associated with cell proliferation during epithelial repair. *J Invest Dermatol*; 119: 14–21.

Shepherd FA, Giaccone G, Seymour L, Debruyne C, Bezjak A, Hirsh V *et al.* (2002) Prospective, randomized, double-blind, placebo-controlled trial of marimastat after response to first-line chemotherapy in patients with small-cell lung cancer: a trial of the National Cancer Institute of Canada-Clinical Trials Group and the European Organisation for Research and Treatment of Cancer. *J Clin Oncol*; 20(22): 4434–9.

Shipley JM, Wesselschmidt RL, Kobayashi DK, Ley TJ, Shapiro SD (1996) Metalloelastase is required for macrophage-mediated proteolysis and matrix invasion in mice. *Proc Natl Acad Sci USA*; 93: 3942–6.

Simonelli C, Vaccher E, Martellotta F, Tedeschi R, Salvi E, Scadari C *et al.* (2004) Assessment of safety and feasibility of HIV protease inhibitors (PI) as anti-angiogenic agents in the treatment of advanced nasopharangeal carcinoma (NPC) [abstract]. *Proc ASCO*; 23: 255.

Smylie M, Mercier R, Aboulafia D (2001) Phase III study of the matrix metalloprotease (MMP) inhibitor prinomastat in patients having advanced non-small cell lung cancer (NSCLC). *Proc ASCO*; 20: 1226

Suzuki K, Enghild JJ, Morodomi T, Salvesen G, Nagase H (1990) Mechanisms of activation of tissue procollagenase by matrix metalloproteinase 3 (stromolysin). *Biochemistry*; 29: 10261–10270.

Van Wart HE, Birkedal-Hansen H (1990) The cysteine switch: a principle of regulation of metalloproteinase activity with potential applicability to the entire matrix metalloproteinase gene family. *Proc Natl Acad Sci USA*; 87(14): 5578–82.

Velasco G, Cal S, Merlos-Suarez A, Ferrando AA, Alvarez S, Nakano A *et al.* (2000) Human MT6-matrix metalloproteinase: identification, progelatinase A activation, and expression in brain tumours. *Cancer Res*; 60: 877–82.

Visse R and Nagase H (2003) Matrix metalloproteinases and tissue inhibitors of metalloproteinases; structure, function and biochemistry. *Circ Res*; 92: 827–39.

Weiss SJ, Peppin G, Ortiz X, Ragsdale C, Test S (1985) Oxidative autoactivation of latent collagenase by human neutrophils. *Science*; 227: 727–49.

Yang M, Kurkinen M (1998) Cloning and characterisation of a novel matrix metalloproteinase (MMP) CMMP, from chicken embryo fibroblasts, *Xenopus* XMMP, and human MMP19 have a conserved unique cysteine in the catalytic domain. *J Biol Chem*; 273: 17893–900.

Chapter 11

Proteins, peptides, and DNA vaccines for cancer

Aniruddha Choudhury and Håkan Mellstedt

1 Introduction

The concept of vaccinating patients against their cancers has advanced over time (as outlined in Chapter 2). What started out as hypotheses, was succeeded with empirical studies and observations in the laboratory and clinic, and currently represents an established scientific discipline with constantly expanding frontiers. Approaches to cancer **vaccination** can be broadly grouped into two categories:

(1) approaches that rely on the whole tumour cell or fractions derived from it as the source of **immunogen**; and

(2) approaches that utilise a synthetic immunogen that immunologically mimics a molecule associated with the tumour cell. Such a molecule is called a **tumour-associated antigen**(s) (TAA).

This chapter discusses the most common modes of using defined TAA as antigens for cancer **immunotherapy** namely peptide, protein and DNA vaccines.

2 Tumour-associated antigens: the ideal and the reality

Harnessing immune responses for the therapy of cancer necessitates that the evoked immune responses have the capability to kill tumour cells, maintain a protracted effect over a substantial period of time, and cause little or no collateral damage to normal, non-malignant tissue. The characteristics of the TAA that are used as cancer vaccines is therefore of critical importance. The ideal TAA should have the following characteristics:

it should elicit strong responses in the various immune compartments including **helper T cells**, **cytotoxic** T cells, and humoral immune responses;

it should be uniquely expressed on the malignant cells and ideally be completely absent on normal tissues;

it should be essential to the survival and growth of the tumour cells, since immune response against a redundant tumour molecule may result in the generation of escape variants of the tumour;

the immune response should not be restricted to a single **HLA allele**.

In reality, TAA with all these attributes are very few, if any. Oncogenic proteins of **viruses** such as Epstein–Barr virus or human papilloma virus, associated with human tumours normally are better suited as TAA than 'self' proteins associated with the vast majority of human cancers. Typically, emphasis is placed on certain characteristics over others when making a choice of an antigen, depending on the nature of the disease and the clinical settings in which vaccination therapy is to be employed. The majority of TAA belong to one of the classes of molecules listed in Table 11.1.

3 Vaccination with whole proteins

The idea of immunising individuals with a protein is not novel. Indeed, all modes of vaccine therapy that use whole tumour cells or cell fractions rely on the ability of proteins derived from tumour cells to stimulate the appropriate antigenic response. Moreover, a large number of animal studies have conclusively demonstrated that **immunisation** with a whole TAA protein is an effective approach to bring about regression of established tumours or to prevent the development of tumours following challenge with live tumour cells. With the advent of **recombinant** technology, it is now feasible to produce a specific protein in sufficiently large quantities and with the high purity required for clinical therapy. The disadvantage of protein vaccination is that the administered protein has to be processed by **antigen-presenting cells** for the induction of immune responses. The logistics and expense of producing recombinant proteins under conditions stipulated for generating a clinical product are also greater than some alternate approaches, e.g. synthetic peptides or DNA-based vaccines. Vaccination with whole protein however has its distinct advantages. Most proteins contain several immunodominant **epitopes** within their primary structure that can potentially induce polyvalent immune responses that normally are more efficacious in controlling tumours. Additionally, whole protein vaccinations are not restricted to a subpopulation of patients with a particular HLA type, unlike synthetic peptides, which are

Table 11.1 Some of the main categories of tumour-associated antigens (TAA) and their description

Type of antigen	Example	Description	Malignancy
Overexpressed normal, non mutated protein.	Her-2/neu, EGFR	Member of the EGF-receptor family.	Breast, ovarian, colorectal cancers.
	Telomerase	Enzyme responsible for maintaining telomere length.	Pancreatic, colorectal, breast cancers.
	EpCAM	Cell surface glycoprotein.	Breast, colorectal, ovarian cancers.
Abnormal protein produced due to genetic or chromosomal aberration associated with the malignancy.	Bcr-Abl fusion protein	Abnormal protein resulting from the t(9;22) chromosomal translocation.	Chronic myelogeneous leukaemia.
Differentiation antigen.	Idiotype	Portion of the immunoglobulin produced by malignant clone of B cells.	Lymphoma, myeloma.
Mutated oncogene.	Ras	Single amino acid substitutions in the Ras oncogene (H, K and N-ras).	Lung, pancreatic cancers.
Oncofetal antigen.	Carcinoembryonic antigen	CEA is a protein found at high levels in the foetal colon, in a variety of cancers and at very low levels in the normal adult colon.	Colorectal, pancreatic, bladder cancers.
Cancer testis antigen.	MAGE-1, NY-ESO-1	Cancer testis antigens are a group of antigen expressed on a variety of malignancies and normal testis.	Melanoma, lung cancers.

restricted to a single HLA allele. Through a process called cross-presentation, peptides derived from proteins can be presented on both **MHC class I** and **class II** molecules of antigen-presenting cells and thereby induce a **CD4**, as well as **CD8** T-cell response critical for effective anti-tumour immunity.

As mentioned in Table 11.1, carcinoembryonic antigen (CEA) is a member of the **immunoglobulin** superfamily and its level is greatly increased in several different cancers including gastrointestinal and breast cancer. In one study, colorectal cancer patients were vaccinated with recombinant CEA protein produced in a baculovirus sytem (Ullenhag *et al.* 2004). The immune-enhancing **cytokine**, granulocyte macrophage-colony stimulating factor (GM-CSF) was co-administered as an immune **adjuvant** to some of the patients. The vaccinated patients were followed for a median of 6 years after start of therapy. Some of the observations made in this study are pivotal to the general theme of vaccine therapy. First, all of the patients who received the protein along with GM-CSF developed **humoral** and **cell-mediated** immune response, whereas only a fraction of the patients who received the protein alone developed such responses. This finding clearly reveals that whole proteins can be suitably processed by antigen-presenting cells *in vivo* to stimulate both humoral and T-cell immunity. It also emphasises the requirement of immune adjuvants to optimally elicit immune responses. The second observation of importance was that the survival of the patients correlated in a statistically significant manner to the levels of anti-CEA antibodies elicited by the vaccine. This observation implies that vaccination with a whole protein can not only reverse **tolerance** to a 'self antigen' like CEA resulting in immune responses, but that these immune responses may be clinically beneficial in terms of improving patient survival. The third observation is that over the relatively long follow-up period of 6 years, none of the patients developed any immunopathologic disease resulting from an immune response to a self antigen. Therefore, at least in the context of colorectal cancer and CEA, vaccination with a whole protein was not associated with **auto-immunity**.

MUC-1 is a deglycosylated mucin abundantly expressed by several epithelial tumours (e.g. lung, ovarian, breast, and gastrointestinal carcinomas), as well as haematological malignancies (e.g. myeloma). Patients have been vaccinated with this protein enveloped in lipid-A containing **liposomes**. Lipid A is a bacterial cell wall derived adjuvant and incorporation of lipid A into liposomes containing the immunogen is known to increase uptake of the complex by antigen-presenting cells and preferential processing through the MHC class I pathway. Vaccination of non-small cell lung cancer patients, stage IIIB, in remission or stable disease using this approach improved overall as well as progression-free survival compared to patients who did not receive vaccine therapy. T-cell responses to MUC-1 were also noted in these patients.

Another prototype protein vaccination approach that has yielded good clinical success is **idiotype** vaccination in **B-cell** malignancies. The idiotype is the region of the immunoglobulin molecule, arranged by the combination of the heavy and light chains that determine the antigen-biding characteristics of the antibody (Fig. 11.1). Each immunoglobulin has a specific idiotype that is made of a unique sequence of peptides. Since the majority of B-cell malignancies are clonal in origin, i.e. the progeny of a single B cell causes the disease; the idiotype represents a unique and specific TAA. The drawback of this strategy, however, is that idiotype vaccines are patient-specific, since no two patients express exactly identical idiotypes on their malignant clones. The necessity for purifying the idiotype of each individual patient and formulating a vaccine restricts the large-scale application of this approach for cancer therapy. Nevertheless, clinical trials have demonstrated that this vaccine approach produces potent immune responses and significant clinical benefit for the patients. Clinical trials with lymphoma patients, where the tumour immunoglobulin was used as the vaccine together with immunological adjuvants, have demonstrated statistically significant improvement in survival and freedom from progression (Hsu *et al.* 1997). Idiotype vaccination was also tested in myeloma patients who demonstrated strong immune responses in several patients and minor clinical responses (Osterborg *et al.* 2000).

The idiotypic network theory of Niels Jerne (Jerne 1973) postulates that immune homeostasis is maintained by a cascade of humoral and cellular immune responses against idiotypic determinants of the B- and T-cell receptors. Figure 11.2 depicts a schematic representation of the concept for humoral responses. The idiotype of an antibody and its potential as an antigen is discussed in the preceding paragraph. An antibody generated against the idiotype of

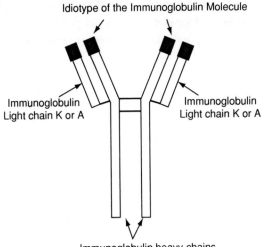

Idiotype of the Immunoglobulin Molecule

Immunoglobulin Light chain K or A

Immunoglobulin Light chain K or A

Immunoglobulin heavy chains

Fig. 11.1 Structure of an immunoglobulin molecule. Two heavy and two light chains make up the basic immunoglobulin molecule. The idiotype represents the antigen binding region formed by the combination of heavy and light chains.

another antibody molecule (Ab_1) is called an **anti-idiotypic** antibody (Ab_2). A third induction of antibodies in the cascade against Ab_2 results in the generation of anti-anti-idiotypic antibodies (Ab_3). As is apparent, Ab_3 has the same reactivity against the antigen as Ab_1 (hence Ab_3 is often referred to as Ab_1')

Ab_2 or anti-idiotypic antibodies can serve as a surrogate for the original tumour antigen for the purposes of vaccine development. Ab_2 may have similarities in its 3D structure or the amino acid sequence of the CDR3 region with the original antigen. Ab_2 have been produced by immunising animals with Ab_1 or from patients who generate a humoral response against **monoclonal antibodies** (Ab_1) used in therapy. There are some advantages of using Ab_2 compared with the original tumour antigen. With anti-idiotype antibodies the structure of the original antigen need not be chemically characterised but merely defined through serological reactivity to an antibody (Ab_1). Large quantities of the immunising entity can be readily and cheaply produced. Additionally the antigenic structures are presented in a setting and context that is different from the original tumour antigen, which may be more effective in generating an immune response.

Anti-idiotype antibodies mimicking antigens like CEA, EpCAM, CD55, and gangliosides have been utilised for vaccination. Humoral and cellular immune responses against the tumour antigens have been induced post-vaccination. The clinical effects of this approach, however, have been limited with the exception of CEA anti-idiotype, which when used to vaccinate colorectal cancer patients in adjuvant settings appeared to improve progression free as well as overall survival. However, at present, protein, peptide, and DNA vaccines are favoured for cancer immunotherapy compared to anti-idiotype antibodies.

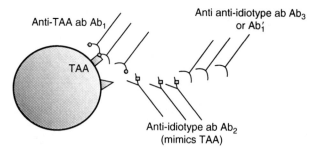

Fig. 11.2 Jerne's idiotypic network. A TAA can elicit an antibody (**Ab**)$_1$ with its own unique idiotype. A second antibody **Ab**$_2$ against the idiotype of **Ab**$_1$, may serve as a surrogate immunogen eliciting the same immune response as the original TAA. Thus the reactivity of **Ab**$_3$ may be similar to **Ab**$_1$.

4 Peptide vaccines: the nominal, defined antigen for anti-tumour immunity

The pathways for uptake, processing, and presentation of intracellular or extracellular antigens by antigen-presenting cells have been described in Chapter 2. The result of intracellular processing of protein antigens is the generation of peptides that are presented on the cell surface in conjunction with MHC class I or class II molecules. Generally peptides bound to class I molecules are 8–9 amino acids (aa) long whereas those binding class II molecules can vary from 11 to 20 amino acids. An immune response is initiated when a T cell carrying the cognate receptor recognises the MHC-peptide complex. These minimal units of immune recognition or 'epitopes' can effectively serve as substitutes for whole proteins for the purpose of stimulating anti-tumour effector cells. The advantages of using peptides rather than whole proteins are that they can be chemically synthesised with high consistency between batches, are less expensive to produce than recombinant proteins, and represent defined immunological moieties against which immune responses can be specifically and sensitively measured. Disadvantages of short peptide (8–10 aa) vaccination are that they are restricted to a single HLA allele, which limits their use to patients who carry that HLA gene. Moreover, tumour cell variants that have lost or modified the expression of the target epitope are unaffected by the immune response to the peptide vaccine. Both of these disadvantages can be partially mitigated by the identification and use of multiple peptide epitopes for vaccination.

5 The mechanics of defining T-cell epitopes

The first T-cell epitopes were defined by Boon and his colleagues using T cells isolated from melanoma patients. T cells were stimulated *in vitro* with tumour cells and used to screen for reactivity against a library of genes expressed by the tumour. The process led to the identification of three gene families called MAGE, GAGE and BAGE (van den Bruggen *et al.* 1991). MHC class I restricted epitopes were subsequently delineated and used for clinical therapy of melanoma patients with varying clinical success. The use of **cytotoxic T lymphocytes (CTL)** for identifying novel epitopes that correspond to TAA is now extensively used and has been successfully utilised to discover epitopes that can potentially be used for a wide variety of cancers.

A second approach to discovering novel epitopes for cancer vaccination is through the use of a technology called SEREX. Michael Pfreundschuh and his colleagues developed this technique, which was called 'serological identification of antigens by recombinant expression cloning' and abbreviated to SEREX (Tureci *et al.* 1997). In contrast to using CTL for screening antigens, the SEREX method employs **autologous** serum from the patients to screen a library of potential antigens. It is established that patients with tumours have circulating antibodies against a variety of antigens presented by the tumour cells. These antibodies can react specifically against antigens produced by an expression library generated from autologous tumour cells. The putative TAA can then be further characterised using modern molecular biology techniques and can be evaluated for their ability to induce tumour-specific immune responses. SEREX technology has produced a large number of potential vaccine candidates which are at various stages of pre-clinical and clinical testing.

A direct approach to detecting peptide epitopes involves the extraction and analysis of peptides from MHC molecules. MHC class I molecules bind peptides endogenously produced within intracellular compartments and present them on the cell surface. Immunoproteomics involves the chemical extraction of these peptides from surface MHC, their high-definition separation by reverse phase-high performance liquid chromatography (RP-HPLC) and sequence analysis by Edman's chemistry and mass spectrometry. Peptide epitopes corresponding to the derived sequences can then be chemically synthesised and screened for their ability to stimulate anti-tumour T cells. The drawback of this approach compared with the previous approaches is that a large number of peptides bound to the MHC complexes may not be relevant to tumour rejection or be **immunogenic** enough to stimulate effective immune responses.

In contrast to the above methods of epitope identification that utilises biological or chemical reagents as a starting point, recent advances in computer technology, as well as insight into peptide-MHC interactions, now permits the delineation of potential epitopes *in silico*. Such predictive or 'reverse immunology' begins with the selection of a potential TAA whose amino acid sequence has been previously established. Sophisticated computer algorithms then scan the entire length of TAA for small peptide sequence that can bind to a designated MHC class I or II molecule. Based on the nature of the 'anchor residues', which are amino acids in positions critical to bind the MHC molecules, as well as general considerations for all the amino acids in a selected peptide sequence, a list of all potential peptide epitopes and their predictive binding scores to the designated MHC molecule is generated. The peptides with the highest binding affinities are then chemically synthesised and used to stimulate T-cell responses, which in turn are studied for their tumouricidal properties. With this approach, it is essential to conclusively demonstrate that the T cells elicited to the synthetic peptide possess the ability to react with the naturally processed epitope of the TAA presented on the tumour cell.

6 Improving immune responses to peptide vaccines

Irrespective of the methodology used to identify peptides for cancer vaccination, the cumulative results of numerous studies *in vitro*, in animal models, and in human trials strongly indicate that mere vaccination with a single peptide epitope is inadequate in the vast majority of instances for generating a robust, therapeutic immune response. It is therefore essential to explore methods to increase the magnitude of the immune response induced by peptide vaccination. Low immunogenic potential of most peptides derived from TAA is principally due to the fact that these TAA generally represent 'self' antigens to which the immune system is anergic. Generation of immune responses to peptide vaccines therefore depend on reversing the immune tolerance to the antigens. One approach to increasing the **immunogenicity** of peptides is switching some of the amino acids in their sequence. These substitutions generally fall into two categories:

1. Amino acid substitutions that cause the peptide to bind to the MHC molecule with greater affinity. The substitutions typically are made at the anchor residues and various studies have demonstrated that the immunogenicity of a peptide correlates to its MHC binding capacity.
2. Amino acid substitutions that result in greater recognition of the MHC-peptide complex by T-cell receptors. These 'heteroclitic' peptides as they are termed can potentially be used to augment the immunogenicity of a weakly antigenic peptide. However, caution must be exerted to ensure that the immune response elicited by the heteroclitic analogue maintains its cross reactivity to the native epitope presented by the tumour cell.

Another means of increasing the immune response to peptide vaccines is by administering them together with adjuvants. The simplest adjuvant involved the emulsification of an aqueous solution of the peptide with oil, which prevented the rapid clearance of the delivered peptide and facilitated protracted release, as well as inflammatory responses at the site of the injection. Subsequently, **Bacillus Calmette-Guérin (BCG)** or *Corynebacterium parvum* was added to these preparations. Currently, bacterial DNA, which is rich in unmethylated cytosine guanine (CpG) motifs or immunostimulatory cytokines such as IL-2, IL-12, GM-CSF, and interferons are used to provide activation signals to antigen presenting for improving immune responses.

Peptides are also administered with **dendritic cells** as 'cellular adjuvants'. Dendritic cells are described in greater detail in Chapter 12.

7 Optimising the use of peptide vaccines for cancer therapy

Natural immune responses involve a complex interplay between antigen-presenting cells, helper and cytotoxic T cells, as well components of humoral immunity. A plethora of studies *in vitro* and *in vivo* have established that immune responses to a single peptide epitope are normally not sustained and are inadequate in their efficacy to control tumours. It is becoming increasingly clear that effective vaccine strategies using peptides would involve the use of multiple peptides directed at stimulating both helper and cytotoxic T cells. Vaccination with several peptides simultaneously poses certain logistic challenges. Manufacturing the peptides for vaccination independently with appropriate quality control and testing makes it more expensive and labour intensive. Making a longer peptide with appropriate junction sequences, which can be cleaved *in vivo* to generate the individual epitopes, is a possible alternative. However, the correct cleavage of the linker region is critical for the generation of functional and relevant epitopes. Besides these issues, one has to consider the immunodominance of the peptides, i.e. the nature of the immune system to bias the response more towards one epitope than the other, as well as the tendency of peptides to compete for binding with a given HLA allele. A greater understanding of the immune system and the development of more versatile algorithms to predict the nature of the response to competing epitopes would allow these issues to be resolved in the future.

8 Clinical experiences with peptide-based vaccine therapy

MHC class I restricted, monoepitopic peptides derived from $MAGE_1$, tyrosinase, and survivin have been used to vaccinate melanoma patients with varying but generally limited clinical effects. A mixture of short (8-aa) ras-derived peptides and a long (16-aa) **telomerase**-derived peptide that is capable of being presented in conjunction with multiple alleles of MHC class I and class II, have been used to immunise advanced pancreatic carcinoma patients. In a non-randomised trial, prolonged progression free and overall survival was noted in those patients who responded immunologically to the vaccine, compared to patients who were immune non-responders.

9 DNA vaccination: transcribing and translating a vaccine *in vivo*

In 1990, the remarkable observation was made by Felgner and his colleagues that injection of a circular segment of DNA under the control of a **promoter** active in mammalian cells resulted in the expression of the gene coded by the DNA in muscle cells at the site of injection (Wolff *et al.* 1990). This was the first unequivocal evidence that such DNA plasmids were capable of expressing encoded gene products, not only in bacteria but also could be directly taken up by the mammalian cells, transcribed, and translated into proteins. Vaccination with plasmids offers some distinct advantages. The plasmids are constructed, scaled-up, and purified with relative ease. They are easily manipulated to modify the encoded gene product and once taken up by the cell, achieve sustained expression of the antigen over a period of time. The disadvantage of plasmid vaccination is that injection of naked plasmids results in very low frequency of uptake by the cells. Unmodified plasmids are also very prone to degradation by nucleases and, finally, uptake of plasmids and expression of the encoded 'transgene' following vaccination typically occurs in muscle cells that are not involved in immune response to antigens. Nevertheless, Margaret Liu and her colleagues demonstrated for the first time that immunisation with plasmid DNA resulted in the generation of antigen-specific T-cell responses (for an excellent review on DNA vaccines refer to: Liu 2003). It was subsequently established that while the initial uptake and expression of the transgene occurred in muscle cells following plasmid vaccination, the stimulation of immune responses to the encoded protein occurred as a result of cross priming of antigen presenting cells. Many of the initial studies on plasmid vaccination focused on antiviral immunity; however, generation of anti-tumour responses by vaccinating with plasmids encoding TAA epitopes have also been shown by several independent investigators.

10 Modifying plasmids to increase the safety and efficacy

As described above, the elementary component for plasmid vaccination consists of a mammalian promoter driving the **transcription** of the gene coding for the tumour antigen. A basic feature of most plasmid backbones composed of bacterial DNA is that they contain unmethylated CpG **nucleotides** that inherently serve as immune adjuvants. Several modifications have been suggested to this basic unit to increase the safety and efficacy of plasmid vaccination for cancer therapy (Table 11.2 and Fig. 11.3). TAA with oncogenic

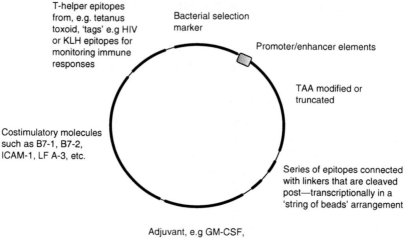

Fig. 11.3 A schematic representation of the elements commonly incorporated in genetic vaccine against cancer. The immunising TAA or epitopes are used independently as a vaccine or together with one or two other immune enhancing elements like adjuvants and/or co-stimulatory molecules.

Table 11.2 Modifications to plasmid DNA vaccines

Modification	Description
Truncations, deletions or mutations of the TAA	Ensures that a plasmid coding for a TAA with oncogenic potential (such as mutated ras or Her-2/neu) does not cause transformation when taken up by cells.
Codon substitution	Changes anchor residues resulting in heteroclitic epitope presentation.
Multiple epitopes	'String of beads' constructs such that multiple epitopes capable of stimulating cytolytic and helper T cells are joined with linkers (see text).
Costimulatory molecules	Molecules such as CD80, CD86 (B7-1, B7-2) facilitate T-cell stimulation when present on the surface of cells presenting TAA epitopes.
Cytokines genes	Genes encoding cytokines like GM-CSF, CD40 ligand, IL-2 or IL-12 serve as chemoattractants for antigen presenting cells, facilitate cross-priming and stimulate T-cell responses.

potential are truncated or have regions deleted to prevent expression of the functional protein in the cells that have taken up the plasmid, thereby abrogating the possibility of causing neocarcinogenesis. Various modifications to the primary sequence of the antigenic epitope aimed at increasing their immunogenicity have also been evaluated. Multiple epitopes can be delivered as plasmid DNA vaccines using the 'string of beads' approach. This method involves connecting multiple epitopes capable of stimulating helper and cytotoxic T cells with linkers that can be potentially cleaved within the cells following transcription and **translation**. Strong antigenic epitopes derived from viral proteins can also be included in these string-of-bead constructs that serve as surrogate markers for evaluating the efficacy of vaccination and resulting immune responses. In addition to the immunising epitopes, incorporation of genes encoding for co-stimulatory molecules or immunostimulatory cytokines into plasmid vaccines have been tested and demonstrated to enhance the immune response.

11 Modes of delivery of plasmid DNA vaccines

The conventional method for immunising with plasmid DNA is by injecting them intramuscularly, subcutaneously, or intradermally. However, new strategies for plasmid delivery have shown promise with regard to their ability to enhance the resultant immune response. The 'gene gun' strategy involves coating the plasmid DNA on submicron gold particles and propelling them directly into the epidermis. This method has been demonstrated to result in increased uptake of the plasmid DNA and animals or patients who do not respond immunologically to conventional immunisation produce antibodies and/or T cells after immunisation via gene gun. Cationic lipids and liposomes have also been successfully tested as vehicles for plasmid delivery. Electroporation has been demonstrated to be an effective mode for delivering plasmid vaccines in animal model. The mild electric current may also cause minor local inflammatory responses facilitating an immune response. However, safety and ethical concerns have to be addressed before this method finds application in clinical settings.

12 Viral delivery of cancer vaccines

Viruses have traditionally been recognised for their ability to introduce their genetic material into host cells where they undergo replication. The life cycle of typical viruses can therefore be broadly divided into an infective phase, which involves the mechanisms of entering the cell, and a replicative phase, when the cell's protein synthesis machinery is usurped by the viral pathogen to produce its own proteins. The use of viruses as vectors to deliver vaccines involves the engineering of the viral **genome** such that then modified virus has identical infectivity to the **wild type** virus but has other genes critical for its replication and pathogenesis replaced with genes encoding for tumour antigens. Infection of a host cell with such an engineered virus results in an abortive or dead-end infectious cycle but in the process facilitates the expression of its recombinant payload within the host cell.

Viral vectors offer certain distinct advantages. The accompanying viral proteins serve as potent immune adjuvants enhancing the immunogenicity of the antigen payload. This system of antigen delivery can be harnessed to directly deliver antigen to critical components of the immune system, such as antigen-presenting cells and infection of cells results in high expression levels of endogeneously produced antigens. Disadvantages of viral vectors include issues of safety and also the observation that use of most viral vectors result in humoral immunity to viral structural components. These antibodies preclude the repeated use of viral vector vaccines for boosting immunity to the antigens they carry.

Viral vectors expressing a combination of tumour antigens with co-stimulatory molecules or cytokines have been previously demonstrated in animal studies to be potent stimulators of anti-tumour immunity. Several immunotherapy trials in humans based on antigen delivery using viral vectors is currently ongoing. Some of the common viruses used to deliver antigenic genes are described briefly below.

12.1 Retroviruses

Retroviruses are double-stranded **RNA** viruses that utilise a DNA intermediate for replication. The loading capacity into retrovirus vectors is relatively small up to 8 kb of DNA. The use of retroviruses is limited due to their requirement of dividing cells as targets of infection and also because they have a DNA intermediate which poses the risk of mutagenesis. Vectors based on lentiviruses are however being developed that can overcome the first problem by infecting non-dividing cells.

12.2 Herpesvirus

Herpes simplex 1 (HSV-1) is a double-stranded DNA virus that replicates in the **nucleus** of infected cells. A recently developed HSV-based vector named DISC-HSV (disabled infectious single cycle) has shown high efficacy and safety in animal models of colorectal cancer. Although HSV vectors have a large loading capacity (30 kb) they carry the potential risk of integration into the host genome due to the characteristics of their replication.

12.3 Adenovirus

Adenovirus is a double-stranded DNA virus that does not integrate the host chromosome. Replication-incompetent adenoviruses have been overwhelmingly used for cancer immunotherapy, both for *ex vivo* transfection of dendritic cells, as well as for direct administration. Clinical trials using adenovirus vectors encoding antigens like gp100 or Mart-1 have been performed with melanoma patients. New adenovirus vectors in which all the viral genes are deleted and only the viral-inverted terminal repeats are retained have been produced that can package as much as 32 kb payload. The capsids of these viruses are known to induce the secretion of pro-inflammatory cytokines, which provide an added benefit to the use of these vectors for cancer immunotherapy

12.4 Poxvirus

Poxvirus is a double-stranded DNA virus that replicates in the **cytoplasm** of the cell. They probably represent the most advanced and widely tested viral vectors with a massive amount of human and animal testing data. The most frequently used pox virus vectors are highly attenuated vaccinia virus strains such as modified virus ankara (MVA), generated after hundreds of passages in chick embryo fibroblasts. Other pox virus vectors include strains of fowl pox virus and canary pox virus (ALVAC).

12.4 Alphaviruses

The development of alphaviruses for immunotherapy is still in its infancy compared to other vectors like poxviruses and adenoviruses. Alphaviruses are enveloped positive-stranded RNA viruses. Once the virus enters the cell, the viral genome serves as a mRNA molecule. Expression systems based on Sindbis virus and Semliki Forest viruses have been developed. Such vectors have been proven to be effective delivery systems of heterologous genes for vaccination and gene therapy in animal models.

12.5 Virus-like particles (VLP)

Virus-like particles (VLP) are a highly effective mode of delivering antigens for vaccine therapy and consist of the assembled structural components of the virus that are completely devoid of viral genetic material. VLPs can be used to delivery proteins, peptides or **plasmids** as antigens. By removing all viral genetic materials, the concerns of recombination, re-assortment, and reversion are completely abrogated. These particles are based on the fact that in many instances a combination of viral structural proteins can spontaneously assemble into functional capsids that resemble the wild-type virus. The process can be modified to include proteins, peptides, or plasmids that can be then introduced into cells through a process of 'pseudo-infection'. Administrations of VLP have been demonstrated to induce not only humoral immunity but also helper and cytotoxic T-cell responses to the payload antigen.

TAA packaged in viruses have been successfully used in clinical trials for generating anti-tumour immune responses in patients. Jeffrey Schlom and his colleagues (Marshall *et al.* 2005) have generated vaccinia and replication-defective avipox virus encoding the tumour antigen CEA and three co-stimulatory molecules, B7–1 (CD80), ICAM-1, and LFA-3. The combination of the three co-stimulatory molecules have been designated TRICOM. In a recent phase I clinical trial, patients with CEA-positive cancers were initially vaccinated with vaccinia or avipox TRICOM-CEA and then sequentially boosted with the alternate vector construct. GM-CSF was used as an adjuvant in a group of patients. Significant clinical effects were noted in some of the patients including decrease in circulating CEA, prolongation of progression free survival and a complete response in one patient. The responses were noted in the absence of significant toxicity and strongly support the further development of viral vector-based vaccination strategies for cancer.

13   Mixed modality vaccines: the 'prime-boost' concept

Each of the vaccine strategies discussed have their potential advantages and disadvantages. Viral delivery systems are known to have potent immunoadjuvant properties, but antibodies to structural proteins of the virus can limit their repeated administration to boost immunity. Vaccination strategies involving administration of the same TAA through different delivery vehicles can be carried out such that the benevolent effects of the individual strategies are exploited and the disadvantages are minimised at the same time. Such 'prime-boost' approaches involve initial vaccination with one modality, such as synthetic peptides or whole proteins, followed by booster immunisations of the same antigen as plasmid DNA or viral vectors. The hope is that development of better vaccination strategies with advances in identification of potent TAA and an improved understanding of therapeutic immune responses can bring cancer vaccination from the realms of experimental therapy to the front lines of cancer therapy.

References

Hsu FJ, Caspar CB, Czerwinski D, Kwak LW, Liles TM, Syrengelas A *et al.* (1997). Tumour-specific idiotype vaccines in the treatment of patients with B-cell lymphoma–long-term results of a clinical trial. *Blood*, 89, 3129–35.

Jerne NK (1973). Towards a network theory of the immune system. *Annals of Immunology*, 125C, 373–89.

Liu MA (2003). DNA vaccines: a review. *Journal of Internal Medicine*, 253, 402–10.

Marshall JL, Gulley JL, Arlen PM, Beetham PK, Tsang KY, Slack R *et al.* (2005). Phase I study of sequential vaccinations with fowlpox-CEA(6D)-TRICOM alone and sequentially with vaccinia-CEA(6D)-TRICOM, with and without granulocyte-macrophage colony-stimulating factor, in patients with carcinoembryonic antigen-expressing carcinomas. *Journal of Clinical Oncology*, 23, 720–31

Osterborg A, Henriksson L, Mellstedt H (2000). Idiotype immunity (natural and vaccine-induced) in early stage multiple myeloma. *Acta Oncologogica*, 39, 797–800.

Tureci O, Sahin U, Pfreundschuh M (1997). Serological analysis of human tumour antigens: molecular definition and implications. *Molecular Medicine Today*, 3, 342–9.

Ullenhag GJ, Frodin JE, Jeddi-Tehrani M, Strigard K, Eriksson E, Samanci A *et al.* (2004). Durable carcinoembryonic antigen (CEA)-specific humoral and cellular immune responses in colorectal carcinoma patients vaccinated with recombinant CEA and granulocyte/macrophage colony-stimulating factor. *Clinical Cancer Research*, 10, 3273–81.

van der Bruggen P, Traversari C, Chomez P, Lurquin C, De Plaen E, Van den Eynde B *et al.* (1991). A gene encoding an antigen recognized by cytolytic T lymphocytes on a human melanoma. *Science*, 254, 1643–7.

Wolff JA, Malone RW, Williams P, Chong W, Acsadi G, Jani A *et al.* (1990). Direct gene transfer into mouse muscle *in vivo*. *Science*, 247, 1465–8.

Chapter 12

Cell-based immunotherapy

Neil Steven

1 Introduction

T lymphocytes and other immune effectors offer potentially attractive agents with which to treat cancer. They can mediate selective killing of malignant cells that express a molecular repertoire differing from that within normal cells. **Immunotherapy** for malignancy is more difficult than vaccination against infections and remains largely an experimental modality.

The basic concepts underlying cellular immunotherapy have been outlined in Chapter 2 and are summarised below. There are four key steps:

(1) the abnormal molecules (i.e. the antigens) from malignant cells must be taken up, processed and presented to the immune system;

(2) antigen-specific effectors must be activated;

(3) the effectors must migrate to the tumour site; and

(4) they recognise and selectively kill malignant cells.

Tumour cells have been injected so as to challenge the immune system with their entire macromolecular contents (Fig. 12.1B). A different approach is to harvest components of the cellular immune cascade for analysis and modulation *ex vivo* before re-injection, allowing a better understanding about the factors that might lead to or limit an effective immune response against cancer cells. Specialised antigen-presenting cells termed **dendritic cells** (DC) can be activated and loaded with antigen *ex vivo*. These are potentially powerful vehicles for vaccination to generate a T-cell response *in vivo* (Fig. 12.1C). T cells activated and selected *ex vivo* can be infused as a ready-made antigen-specific immune response (Fig. 12.1D). Genes might be transfected into cells before injection to modify immune processes (Larin *et al.* 2004). The host might be treated systemically so as to create a better environment for an effective immune response. Events *in vivo*, i.e. the recruitment, activation, and migration of immune effectors, are known only indirectly using imperfect markers of immune and tumour response and the correlation with clinical benefit is uncertain.

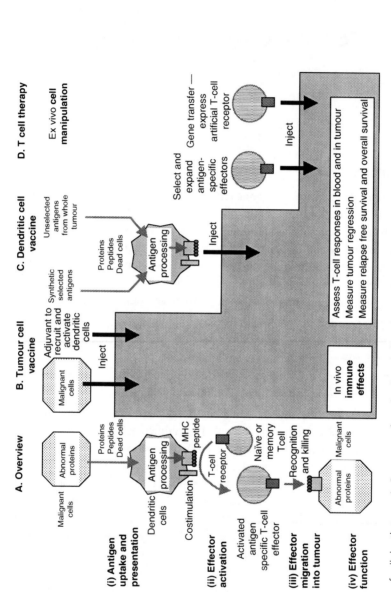
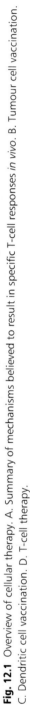

Fig. 12.1 Overview of cellular therapy. A. Summary of mechanisms believed to result in specific T-cell responses *in vivo*. B. Tumour cell vaccination. C. Dendritic cell vaccination. D. T-cell therapy.

2 The key components of cellular immunotherapy

2.1 Malignant cells

Malignant cells express a range of proteins that might be the basis of selective immune killing, summarised in Fig. 12.2. In considering **tumour-associated antigens (TAA)**, there are two main concepts:

(1) unique versus shared antigens; and
(2) strong versus weak antigens.

Genetic instability is a characteristic of many malignancies and results in expression of many self-derived proteins containing mutations unique to the individual. In contrast, aberrant expression of particular proteins is highly conserved between malignancies of the same type and even between different types of malignancy. Unique antigens might be the basis of highly selective immune responses using vaccines derived from autologous tumour, whereas shared antigens are more readily standardised into widely-used immunother-apy approaches.

Many shared antigens that have been described are expressed in limited cell lineages that include both the malignancy and the normal tissue of origin. These include proteins such as melan A, gp100 and tyrosinase expressed in melanoma and melanocytes. Physiological mechanisms that limit **auto-immunity** are likely to permit only weak immune responses to such antigens. By contrast, there may be a higher likelihood of generating strong immune responses against proteins new to the mature immune system. Such TAA include mutated self proteins, viral

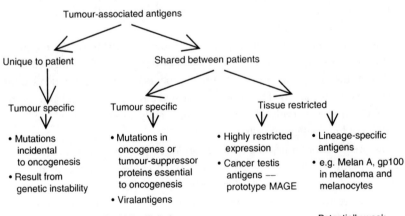

Fig. 12.2 Tumour-associated antigens (TAA).

antigens in **virus**-induced malignancy, and proteins normally expressed only in the foetus or in sites protected from **immune surveillance** such as the testis.

Malignant tumours are clearly sites of immune interactions involving macrophages, DC, neutrophils, eosinophils, lymphocytes, and endothelial cells. **Cytokines** and chemo-attractant cytokines (**chemokines**) released both by the malignant cells and by immune components create a complex network of signals. In this dysregulated immune micro-environment, the malignant cells are poorly **immunogenic**.

2.2 Dendritic cells

Dendritic cells are components of **innate immunity** that act as a link to the highly specific **adaptive immune** responses. Central functions of DC are to take up exogenous antigen in peripheral tissue sites and migrate to secondary lymphoid tissue to present antigen to T cells.

DC share with most cell types the ability to target endogenously synthesised proteins to a proteolytic complex, the **proteosome**. This digests them to short peptides. These are transported to the **endoplasmic reticulum** where they stabilise the folding of **major histocompatibility complex (MHC) class I**. The MHC–peptide complex moves via the **Golgi apparatus** to the cell surface. Peptide **epitopes** presented by MHC class I are typically recognised by CD8+ **cytotoxic T lymphocytes (CTL)**.

Exogenous antigens are degraded in endosomes/**lysosomes** to peptides that are loaded onto **MHC class II**. This is also exported to the surface. Epitopes presented on MHC class II are typically recognised by **CD4+** T cells, including **helper T cells (Th)**. T-helper cells can, in turn, switch on the ability of dendritic cells to stimulate CTL as well as carrying out other functions that enhance cellular immunity.

Unlike other cell types, DC express a number of antigen uptake receptors that enable exogenous antigens in the form of dead cells, virus-infected cells, and immune complexes to be acquired, processed, and presented on both MHC class I and class II. This process is termed cross-presentation and means that DC can activate both CTL and Th against antigens expressed within other cells, including malignant cells.

The presentation of peptide epitopes on MHC provides what is regarded as 'signal 1' for T-cell responses. It selects T-cell clones from the total T-cell repertoire. These express a **T-cell receptor (TCR)** that specifically recognises the MHC–epitope complex. The strength of signal 1 is made up of the affinity with which the T-cell receptor can bind to the MHC–peptide and the number of MHC peptide complexes on the DC surface (i.e. epitope density). The additional co-stimulation provided by DC is termed collectively 'signal 2'. This includes expression of cell surface molecules such as CD80 and CD86 (**ligands** for CD28 on T cells), 41BB ligand, CD70 (ligand for CD27), and the release of cytokines such as **interleukin**-12 (IL-12).

Maturation is a key concept in understanding the role of DC in cellular immunotherapy for cancer. In the maturation process, DC integrate signals from the inflammatory micro-environment, including cytokines, pathogen-associated molecules, and interactions with other immune cells such as Th. This influences their ability to present antigen (signal 1) and to provide co-stimulation (signal 2) to T cells. T cells are stimulated to differentiate differently depending on the strength and nature of signal 1 and 2. DC are very effective in activating T-cell responses and can influence the functional properties of the effectors. However, they can also render antigen-specific cells inert, i.e. they can induce immune **tolerance.**

DC do not only present protein antigens. Lipid and glycolipids derived from cells and pathogens can be presented on CD1 molecules that are structurally similar to MHC. A wide range of lymphocytes carry receptors for CD1 including CD3+ **natural killer** (NK) T cells.

2.3 T lymphocytes

The T-cell population is heterogeneous. Of particular relevance are those components of adaptive immunity bearing the αβ TCR that can specifically recognise MHC-bound peptide epitopes. During thymic **differentiation**, re-combination of gene segments, plus the random insertion and deletion of **nucleotides**, results in the generation of a diverse population of clonotypes each expressing unique TCRαβ variants. This population undergoes positive and negative selection by thymic epithelial and bone marrow-derived cells expressing MHC and peptides derived from normal self proteins. T cells that recognise self peptides with high avidity are deleted. Additional mechanisms operate in and outside the thymus to shape a naïve circulating T-cell population fitted to the recognition of self MHC, but with reduced recognition of peptides derived from normal self proteins. This reduces the potential for auto-immunity but limits the potential recognition of shared TAA that are expressed in both malignant and normal cells.

T lymphocytes exhibit diverse **phenotypes** and function that reflect thymic programming and subsequent events on exposure to antigen. **CD8+** CTL can potentially recognise any cell type, including malignant cells, which presents endogenous antigen as MHC class I-bound epitopes. Activated CTL express interferon gamma (IFNγ) and tumour necrosis factor alpha (TNFα). They also can selectively kill target cells through the release of **perforin** and granzymes that initiate **apoptosis.** Cells expressing CD4 interact with MHC class II expressed on specialised **antigen-presenting cells.** CD4+ T-helper cells type I (**Th1**) release IL-2, IFNγ, and TNFα and interact to support CTL responses. Th2 cells release IL-4 and typically support germinal centre reactions enhancing **humoral** responses. Regulatory T cells (T_RC) resulting from thymic programming express the nuclear **transcription** factor foxP3 and the IL-2 receptor CD25. They mediate suppression of antigen-specific T cells by unclear mechanisms.

3 Tumour cell vaccination

Whole cell vaccines, usually killed by irradiation to prevent *in vivo* growth, deliver a wide array of antigens as targets for potential immune responses. In contrast to non-cellular highly synthetic vaccination methods (e.g. peptide vaccines, **DNA** vaccines), the tumour cells may include both the known well-characterised TAA and many others not yet identified. One approach has been to create a dissociated cell suspension from harvested **autologous** tumour. Such cells potentially express a wide array of unique TAA. The dissociation to a cell suspension may reduce interactions within the intact tumour that had prevented immune recognition *in vivo*. Alternatively, vaccination using tumour cell lines, that express shared TAA, is more easily standardised for large trials compared to preparation from autologous tumour.

Tumour cell vaccines have been given with **adjuvant**—material known to increase vaccine **immunogenicity.** One of the most commonly used is **Bacillus Calmette-Guérin (BCG).** Such adjuvants contain many pathogen-associated molecules that are potentially recognised by receptors expressed on immune cells. Such interactions play key immune regulatory roles, including the activation of DC to stimulate Th1 and CTL responses.

Early phase clinical trials using whole cell tumour vaccines have been undertaken for patients with prostate, renal, and breast cancer. Three phase III trials (723 patients) have been reported of vaccination using autologous cancer with BCG following resection of stage II and III colon cancer. These showed improved recurrence-free survival and demonstrated the importance of centralised quality controlled vaccine preparation (Hanna Jr *et al.* 2001). A phase III trial is ongoing of an **allogeneic** whole-cell vaccine containing three cell lines expressing shared TAA, given with BCG, to treat melanoma. In a report on 54 patients with skin or soft tissue recurrence of melanoma, nine had an objective clinical response to this vaccine (Hsueh *et al.* 1999).

Both autologous tumour cell suspensions and allogeneic cell lines have been genetically modified to enhance their efficacy as cancer vaccines. Using diverse vectors, three classes of proteins have been expressed: **cytokines**, co-stimulatory ligands, and MHC class II, as summarised in Fig. 12.3. Conceptually, there are two strategies incorporating genetically modified tumour cells. Firstly, the tumour cells are vehicles for delivering their complement of TAA to DC *in vivo*. Cross-presentation enables the antigen load from allogeneic cell lines and from MHC-negative cells to be efficiently processed and presented to initiate an immune cascade that results in both Th and CTL effectors. Expression by the tumour cells of the cytokine, granulocyte macrophage colony stimulating factor (GMCSF), has been shown to be very effective in recruiting DC. The co-stimulatory ligand CD154 expressed on the tumour cells can ligate CD40 on DC, mimicking the signal given by Th that licenses DC to activate CTL responses.

The second strategy is aimed at re-programming the tumour cell to act as a specialised antigen-presenting cell, directly activating T-cell responses against its TAA. MHC class II has been expressed in tumour cells, in theory to permit presentation of TAA to Th. The most widely used co-stimulatory molecule has been CD80 that ligates CD28 on T cells during effective antigen priming. However, although the strategy is intended to mimic DC function, there is evidence that the dominant immunostimulatory pathway of CD80-transduced tumour cells is through cross-presentation on DC rather than by direct T-cell

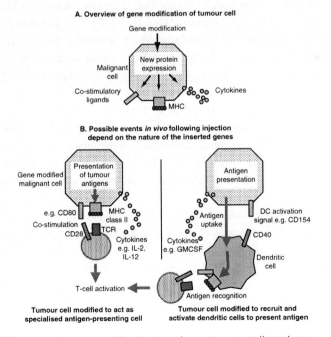

Fig. 12.3 Concepts in gene modification to enhance tumour cell vaccines.

activation. In a phase I trial, 30 women with metastatic breast cancer received an allogeneic breast cancer cell line, modified to express CD80. Tumour-specific immune responses were detected in a minority of patients but no objective tumour regressions were observed (Dols *et al.* 2003).

In theory, the selective exposure of patients to cytokines such as IL-12 and IL-2 at the site of tumour cell injection might enhance T-cell priming yet limit toxicities associated with systemic cytokine administration. Genes have been inserted within tumour cells to create cellular vaccines that express cytokine. Alternatively, malignant cells have been mixed with fibroblasts that are easier to manipulate *in vitro* and that have been gene-modified to provide sustained cytokine release (Sobol *et al.* 1999).

4 Dendritic cell vaccination

4.1 Types of dendritic cells used in clinical trials

DC constitute multiple populations of cells *in vivo* with overlapping but not identical functions and occupying different anatomical niches (O' Neill *et al.* 2004). In human blood, DC are typically negative for the cell surface markers of B cells, T cells, and natural killer cells, but express MHC class II, i.e. they are HLA DR+. This population has been divided according to the appearance under light microscopy and the expression of surface markers CD11c and CD123 into populations termed myeloid (MDC) and plasmacytoid DC (PDC). PDC and MDC differ greatly in their functional properties and tissue distribution. PDC have hardly been used in clinical immunotherapy trials because of their scarcity. In the first DC trials for malignancy, MDC were isolated from peripheral blood by a series of differential centrifugation steps. The limiting step has been to isolate large numbers of MDC (Figdor *et al.* 2004). This can be enhanced by treating the patient with Flt3-ligand, which enhances DC differentiation from bone marrow precursors, and by harvesting a large number of peripheral blood mononuclear cells using **leukapharesis** (Fong *et al.* 2001). MDC have instead been generated *in vitro* from other, more abundant, precursors in blood, such as proliferating CD34+ cells (Banchereau *et al.* 2001). The most widely reported source of MDC has been peripheral blood mononuclear preparations enriched for CD14+ monocytes either by immunomagnetic selection or by harvesting cells adherent to plastic after overnight culture (Fig. 12.4). Differentiation to immature DC is induced by culture for up to a week in IL-4 and GMCSF. Different approaches have then been used to load antigen and to induce DC maturation (Schuler *et al.* 2003).

Generation of dendritic cells from blood precursors for vaccination

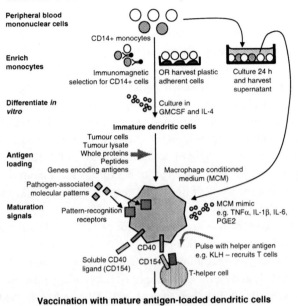

Fig. 12.4 Generation of dendritic cells from blood precursors for vaccination.

4.2 Maturation of dendritic cells in clinical trials

Different strategies for maturing DC (Reis e Sousa 2004) are summarised in Fig. 12.4. A widely used approach was to generate a cytokine mix from peripheral blood mononuclear cells, cultured for 24 h in an **immunoglobulin coated** Petri dish in complete medium including 1% human serum. The supernatant, termed macrophage conditioned medium (MCM), contained several cytokines and other biologically active molecules and was used to supplement the growth medium of differentiated DC. In many more recent clinical trials, a combination of synthetic cytokines and prostaglandins (PG) including IL-1b, IL-6, TNFα and PGE$_2$ has been used as a substitute that can be more readily standardised between patients (Schuler-Thurner *et al.* 2002).

In many trials, DC have been pulsed not only with target antigen but with proteins known to induce Th responses, such as tetanus toxoid or keyhole limpet haemocyanin. These enable measurement of predictable immune responses *in vivo* and might recruit Th *in vivo*. Activated Th express CD154 that ligates CD40 on DC and delivers a potent maturation stimulus. Alternatively, soluble CD154 has been used to mature DC *in vitro*.

Natural killer T cells are a lymphocyte population that express CD3 and a particular T-cell receptor Va14Vb8. This interacts with a non-polymorphic MHC termed CD1d on the surface of DC that presents the lipid a-galactosyl ceramide. NKT can stimulate DC maturation.

DC express a repertoire of pattern-recognition receptors that can interact with pathogen-associated molecular patterns (PAMP) directing the pathway of maturation. The best characterised family of such receptors are the Toll-like receptors (TLR). *In vitro* differentiated DC have been reported as expressing, among others, TLR 2 (that recognises bacterial lipoteichoic acid and lipoproteins), TLR 4 (bacterial lipopolysccharide), and TLR3 (double-stranded RNA). Detailed evidence of the effect of PAMP on DC maturation and on the differentiation pathways of the T cells responding to DC stimulation will inform future clinical trials

DC maturity is regarded as a critical issue for vaccination. Healthy volunteers vaccinated with matured peptide-coated DC resulted in detectable specific immune responses, whereas immature DC vaccination caused a decline in T cells releasing IFNγ and an increase in specific cells releasing the immunosuppressive cytokine, IL-10 (Banchereau *et al.* 2001; Dhodapkar *et al.* 2001).

4.3 Loading antigen on dendritic cells in clinical trials

An approach that has been used to pilot the development of DC vaccination has been to incubate DC with synthetic short peptides using the sequences of known MHC class I-restricted epitopes from TAA (Nestle *et al.* 1998). Many strategies are in development to load more complex antigens on DC for vaccination resulting in more diverse responses that include Th and CTL and that are not limited to the epitopes that have already been identified. These can be usefully split according to two criteria:

(1) single known synthetic antigens versus the whole antigen repertoire from malignant cells; and

(2) delivery of exogenous antigen versus endogenous gene expression within the DC.

The delivery of single synthetic antigens is a very useful experimental approach that might result in highly focused immune responses that can be monitored. The delivery of the content of whole malignant cells markedly increases the number of potentially antigenic molecules available to the DC. These might include unique antigens if the source of antigens is the autologous tumour rather than a cell line. However, in principle, TAA may have to compete for antigen presentation with normal sequence proteins. Furthermore, effective DC vaccination might result in auto-immunity against normal proteins.

DC uniquely express a number of receptors mediating uptake of exogenous antigen, either in the form of long peptides, proteins, or whole cells, that target antigens for endogenous processing and cross-presentation on MHC class I and II. The immunoglobulin receptors, FcgRI and FcgRII, mediate uptake of proteins complexed with antibody and also of opsonised whole cells. The receptors aVb5 and CD36 both mediate uptake of apoptotic cells. LOX-1 and CD91 are receptors for heat-shock proteins that are chaperone molecules binding to other proteins. It is likely that these are important mechanisms for the uptake of the complex molecular mix within disrupted autologous tumour cells or allogeneic cell lines. Such cell lysates have been widely used as a ready source of TAA in DC vaccination trials, and a few clinical and immune responses have been described (Nestle *et al.* 1998; Stift *et al.* 2003).

DC have been loaded with a **chimeric** protein in the context of vaccination against prostate cancer. The construct included prostatic acid phosphatase fused to GMCSF. A small number of patients showed reduction in the tumour marker, prostate-specific antigen, in response to vaccination (Small *et al.* 2000). An interesting model for DC vaccination has exploited the unique B-cell receptor, termed the **idiotype**, expressed by B cell-derived malignancies such as myeloma and lymphoma. Full-length idiotype or just the unique variant sequences, alone or coupled to the Th antigen KLH, have been used in several trials. In the most extensive series of 35 patients, clinical responses have been reported (Timmerman *et al.* 2002).

DC vaccines have been created using gene therapy to express TAA within DC. Both total RNA from malignant cells and synthetic RNA encoding single antigens have been effectively delivered to DC by electroporation and used in clinical vaccination (Heiser *et al.* 2002). DNA **plasmids** complexed with a cationic peptide are efficiently taken up by DC (Irvine *et al.* 2000). A promising strategy for future clinical trials is electrofusion of an irradiated tumour cell line with mature MDC resulting in DC hybrids that can cross-present antigens on both MHC class I and II (Parkhurst *et al.* 2003).

5 Infusion of effectors

A summary of approaches to the infusion of specific T lymphocytes to treat malignancy is shown in Fig. 12.5. Key issues are to consider:

(1) the source of the cells, whether from an allogeneic lymphocyte donor versus autologous cells from the patient;

(2) whether the cells have undergone specific stimulation and selection during culture to enrich effectors that recognise TAA;

(3) whether the T cells have been pre-activated *in vivo* before harvest; and

(4) how modification of the host might improve the survival and function of T cells following infusion.

5.1 Unselected donor lymphocyte infusion

Allogeneic haematopoietic stem cell transplantation (allo-HSCT) has been used for more than two decades to treat patients with leukaemia refractory to maximum tolerated doses of conventional cytotoxic treatment (Slavin *et al.* 2003). This approach has more recently been used for a wider range of malignancies, particularly non-Hodgkins lymphoma, Hodgkins disease, and some solid cancers.

It is now recognised that the key elements of allo-HSCT are:

(1) a conditioning regimen that suppresses host immunity and enables engraftment; and

(2) supplying allogeneic immunocompetent effectors capable of recognising and killing malignant cells, where the cancer had evaded the patient's native immune responses.

This understanding has led to two important developments. First, there is now widespread use of selective lymphoablative (or non-myeloablative) conditioning. This is better tolerated than using very intense cytotoxic regimens with intent to ablate the recipient haematopoietic cells and maximise cancer cell kill ahead of transplantation. Following conditioning, patients receive HLA-matched donated bone marrow or, more recently, peripheral blood stem cells mobilised by GMCSF treatment *in vivo* and harvested by leukapharesis. The second key development has been the subsequent administration of donor lymphocyte infusions (DLI) to treat various indications, including malignant relapse (Fig. 12.5A).

Allo-HSCT has profound effects on the patients' immunity (Riddell *et al.* 2003). Individuals are susceptible to opportunistic infection but also suffer from immune responses against their tissues, termed **graft versus host disease** (GVHD). Additional immune modulation is required to reduce the risk and severity of GVHD including depletion of T cells from transplanted stem cells, treating the recipient with immunosuppressive medication and carefully titrating the cell numbers given in DLI.

These sequelae of immune dysfunction are a major cause of treatment related morbidity and mortality. However, there is also evidence for a graft versus leukaemia (GVL) effect that is related to immunological interactions between donor-derived and host cells. The risk of relapse of leukaemia is less for recipients of grafts from HLA-matched siblings compared to identical twins. T-cell depletion of donor graft increases the risk of recurrent cancer.

Malignancy can regress following cessation of immune suppression. DLI is directly effective against malignancy: it has been reported as bringing about complete response in about 70% of cases of chronic myelogenous leukaemia (CML) and about 20–30% of cases of acute leukaemia relapsing following allo-HSCT.

It appears that some of the antigens that contribute GVL are shared with normal tissues because evidence of GVL is more common in patients with GVHD. Stem cell transplants are matched as far as possible for major histocompatibility antigens, i.e. for the polymorphic human leukocyte antigens (HLA) that present peptides to T cells. However, polymorphisms in other components of the **genome** (termed minor histocompatibility antigens— mHAg) result in donor and recipient differing in the complement of peptides that are actually presented by their shared HLA **alleles**. Transplantation of female HSC into a male recipient results in greater GVHD and a lower risk of leukaemia relapse (i.e. a greater GVL effect) than other gender combinations, indicating that mHAg encoded by the Y **chromosome** are targets for allogeneic immune recognition. Several immunogenic polymorphic peptide sequences from autosomal genes restricted through a number of different MHC class I alleles have also been described.

In some patients, GVL (and graft versus tumour, GVT) has been reported as dissociated from GVHD, suggesting that donor cells may recognise antigens with selective expression within malignant cells. Candidate leukaemia-associated antigens include transformation-associated proteins, such as mutated *ras* and the bcr-abl chimaeric protein characteristic of CML, and normal proteins overexpressed in leukaemic cells, such as proteinase-3, myeloperoxidase, Wilms tumour protein (WT-1), and survivin.

5.2 Selection and expansion of antigen-specific effectors

Following allo-HSCT, particularly using T-cell depleted grafts, patients are susceptible to secondary lymphoma termed post-transplant lymphoproliferative disease (PTLD). These comprise B cells transformed by the human γ-herpes virus, Epstein–Barr virus (EBV) that is resident in the malignant cells as an extra-chromosomal plasmid. The viral antigens expressed within EBV-transformed cells are targets for CTL and Th responses that are abundant within the blood of healthy individuals but barely detectable soon after allo-HSCT at the time of greatest susceptibility to PTLD. DLI results in a 10–50-fold increase in the frequency of EBV-specific effectors detectable in blood. In a further development, the EBV-specific component has been selectively expanded by successive rounds of *in vitro* stimulation using whole irradiated EBV-transformed cells (Fig. 12.5B). Infusion of such effectors following

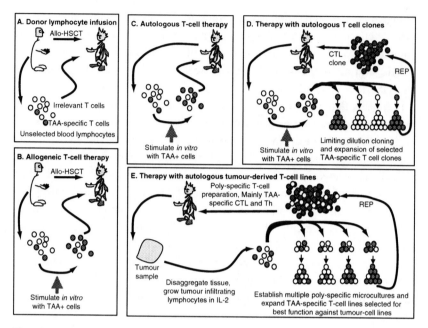

Fig. 12.5 Concepts in T-cell therapy. Tumour antigen-specific T cells are shown as filled circles, those specific for irrelevant antigens shown as open circles. A. Donor lymphocyte infusion. This takes place following allogeneic haematopoietic stem cell transplantation, and involves the transfer of blood-derived lymphocytes without a step selecting for antigen-specific effectors. This is widely used for treating relapse of CML, acute leukaemia, lymphoma, Hodgkins disease, and other malignancies following allo-HSCT. B. Allogeneic T-cell therapy. This has a particular indication for the treatment of EBV+ secondary lymphoma following allo-HSCT. The blood-derived T cells are enriched for EBV-specific effectors by stimulations with an EBV-transformed cell line before infusion. The approach has also been used for leukaemia using irradiated malignant cells to stimulate the T-cell preparation. C. Autologous T-cell therapy. This is an extension of (B). Autologous blood-derived EBV-specific T-cell preparations are used to treat EBV+ Hodgkins disease. D. Therapy with autologous T-cell clones. Autologous blood-derived lymphocytes are first enriched for TAA-specific effectors by bulk stimulation *in vitro* and then cloned by limiting dilution to generate homogeneous cultures. Only cultures showing TAA specificity are expanded by a rapid expansion protocol (REP) to very high numbers before infusion. This has been used as experimental treatment for advanced melanoma. E. Therapy with autologous tumour-derived T-cell lines. Autologous tumour infiltrating lymphocytes are first expanded in high dose IL-2 then established as multiple microcultures. TIL may be enriched for tumour-specific T cells compared to blood. Only cultures showing TAA specificity are grown by a rapid expansion protocol (REP) to very high numbers before infusion. These are not clonal and contain both Th and CTL, although are enriched for tumour-specific T cells. This has been used as experimental treatment for advanced melanoma.

allo-HSCT resulted in reduction of EBV genome levels in peripheral blood, prevention of PTLD and regression of established PTLD (Rooney *et al.* 1998).

EBV+ tumours offer a human model for extending the use of *in vitro* selected antigen-specific T cells outside the allo-HSCT setting (Fig. 12.5C). In about 40% of cases of Hodgkins disease, EBV is present within the malignant Hodgkin Reed Sternberg (HRS) cells and a viral antigen, LMP2, is expressed in HRS cells. Circulating LMP2-specific responses are suppressed in patients with Hodgkins disease compared to healthy controls but can be expanded *in vitro* by stimulating peripheral blood lymphocytes with EBV-transformed cells. The resulting T-cell lines were predominantly CD8+ CTL but all contained at least a small CD4+ T-cell component that might act as Th. Of 14 patients receiving infused T cells, four had sustained complete remissions. Circulating infused T cells expanded by 100-fold after infusion and were detectable 3–12 months after treatment. The effectors were functional *in vivo* and could accumulate selectively in disease sites (Bollard *et al.* 2004).

The specificity of the T-cell lines used for infusion can be selected with more precision by establishing microcultures from T-cell lines already enriched for antigen-specific effectors by several rounds of *in vitro* stimulation. These are set up to achieve limiting dilution cloning, i.e. such that each microculture is likely to have grown from just one T cell. Growing microcultures are screened in assays of antigen-specific T-cell function and selected cultures are expanded to very high numbers by a rapid expansion protocol, that typically includes irradiated allogeneic lymphocytes and a culture medium containing IL-2 and anti-CD3 stimulating **monoclonal antibody** (Fig. 12.5D). Using such an approach, 10 patients with metastatic melanoma received very large numbers (greater than one billion) of highly specific autologous T cells. No major clinical responses occurred but there was evidence of clinical effect for 8 patients in the form of stabilisation of previously progressive disease or minor or mixed responses. T cells accumulated in tumour sites (Yee *et al.* 2002).

5.3 Use of T cells pre-activated *in vivo*

A further refinement in T-cell therapy is to harvest and to expand to large numbers of T cells that have already been activated by exposure to antigen *in vivo*. This concept can be seen in several different immunotherapy strategies. First, patients have been immunised ahead of lymphocyte harvest. Second, lymphocytes can be harvested from tissue sites other than blood. Several trials have re-infused **tumour-infiltrating lymphocytes** (TIL), on the grounds that these are likely to include tumour-specific T cells that have proven ability to migrate to the site of malignancy. For example, 13 patients with melanoma who had previously received gp100 peptide vaccination subsequently received autologous T-cell therapy. The effectors were derived by limiting dilution cloning from gp100 peptide-stimulated blood lymphocytes or from bulk TIL cultures grown up in high dose IL-2. Two patients experienced clinical benefit with minor or mixed responses (Dudley *et al.* 2001).

5.4 The fate of T cells following infusion

Infused *in vitro*-activated TAA-specific T cells or CTL clones localise rapidly initially to the lungs and are then found at 24 h in the liver and spleen. In two trials, TAA-specific CTL clones detectable in blood were at their most abundant one day after infusion and showed a 100-fold decline in frequency over the next two weeks. Interestingly, the use of low-dose IL-2 given systemically following T-cell infusion extended the median duration of persistence of the circulating TAA-specific T cells by one week (Yee *et al.* 2002). This is supporting evidence for the widely held impression that IL-2 may have beneficial effects following specific immunotherapy.

There is evidence that transferred CTL only persist as functional memory cells if delivered with antigen-specific CD4+ Th. This might limit the efficacy of infused homogenous T-cell preparations, such as a cloned CTL specific for a single MHC class I restricted epitope.

5.5 The use of conditioning before infusion

As discussed above, DLI and specific T-cell therapy clearly show clinical benefit in the context of allo-HSCT in which the recipient has also undergone lymphoablative conditioning to enable acceptance of the graft. Lymphocyte depletion might stimulate homeostatic cytokines that promote lymphocyte growth *in vivo* and may diminish regulatory T-cell populations that suppress tumour-specific responses. Thus effectors are infused into an environment that supports their survival, expansion, and function. The use of lymphoablative conditioning with fludarabine and cyclophosphamide before autologous T-cell therapy was piloted in a trial including 15 patients with advanced melanoma. They received homogenous cloned epitope-specific CTL derived from blood or from TIL and subsequent high dose systemic IL-2. Five patients experienced a tumour reduction that fell short of a major response (Dudley *et al.* 2002b).

In subsequent clinical reports from the same group, the approach was modified such that infused lymphocytes were derived from poly-specific TIL cultures selected for their ability to recognise melanoma cell lines, i.e. the selected cultures were not clones and contained CTL and Th. In the initial report 7/13 patients had a major tumour response (Dudley *et al.* 2002a). Subsequent reports indicate that this 50% response rate continues (Rosenberg and Dudley 2004). Five patients experienced auto-immunity against non-malignant pigmented cells. For some patients, the circulating CD8+ T-cell compartment regenerating after conditioning was repopulated almost completely with a single melanoma-specific clone.

6 Summary

Cellular therapy for malignancy remains an experimental modality. There is clear evidence of promise with sporadic tumour responses seen in many vaccination trials. The manipulation of T cells *ex vivo* and their delivery to a prepared lymphoid compartment *in vivo* can generate an overwhelming immune response and regression of malignancy. These approaches are labour intensive and demanding on investment. *In vitro* experiments continue to develop novel ways of manipulating antigen presenting cells and effectors. However, the clinical challenge is more mundane: the techniques for generating cellular materials for immunotherapy must be standardised and reproduced in multiple centres to support larger scale trials.

References

Banchereau, J., Palucka, A., Dhodapkar, M. *et al.* (2001) Immune and clinical responses in patients with metastatic melanoma to CD34(+) progenitor-derived dendritic cell vaccine. *Cancer Research,* **61,** 6451–8.

Bollard, C. M., Aguilar, L., Straathof, K. C. *et al.* (2004) Cytotoxic T lymphocyte therapy for Epstein-Barr virus+ Hodgkin's disease. *Journal of Experimental Medicine,* **200,** 1623–33.

Dhodapkar, M. V., Steinman, R. M., Krasovsky, J., Munz, C., and Bhardwaj, N. (2001) Antigen-specific inhibition of effector T cell function in humans after injection of immature dendritic cells. *Journal of Experimental Medicine,* **193,** 233–8.

Dols, A., Smith, J. W., 2nd, Meijer, S. L. *et al.* (2003) Vaccination of women with metastatic breast cancer, using a costimulatory gene (CD80)-modified, HLA-A2-matched, allogeneic, breast cancer cell line: clinical and immunological results. *Human Gene Therapy,* **14,** 1117–23.

Dudley, M. E., Wunderlich, J., Nishimura, M. I. *et al.* (2001) Adoptive transfer of cloned melanoma-reactive T lymphocytes for the treatment of patients with metastatic melanoma. *Journal of Immunotherapy,* **24,** 363–73.

Dudley, M. E., Wunderlich, J. R., Robbins, P. F. *et al.* (2002a) Cancer regression and auto-immunity in patients after clonal repopulation with antitumor lymphocytes. *Science,* **298,** 850–4.

Dudley, M. E., Wunderlich, J. R., Yang, J. C. *et al.* (2002b) A phase I study of nonmyeloablative chemotherapy and adoptive transfer of autologous tumor antigen-specific T lymphocytes in patients with metastatic melanoma. *Journal of Immunotherapy,* **25,** 243–51.

Figdor, C. G., de Vries, J. M., Joost Lesterhuis, W., and Melief, C. J. M. (2004) Dendritic cell immunotherapy: mapping the way. *Nature Medicine*, 10, 475–480.

Fong, L., Hou, Y., Rivas, A. *et al.* (2001) Altered peptide ligand vaccination with Flt3 ligand expanded dendritic cells for tumor immunotherapy. *Proceedings of the National Acadamy of Science U S A*, 98, 8809–14.

Hanna Jr, M., Hoover, H., Vermoken, J., Harris, J., and Pinedo, H. (2001) Adjuvant active specific immunotherapy of stage II and stage III colon cancer with an autologous tumor cell vaccine: first randomized phase III trials show promise. *Vaccine*, 19, 2576–2582.

Heiser, A., Coleman, D., Dannull, J. *et al.* (2002) Autologous dendritic cells transfected with prostate-specific antigen RNA stimulate CTL responses against metastatic prostate tumors. *Journal of Clinical Investigation*, 109, 409–17.

Hsueh, E. C., Nathanson, L., Foshag, L. J. *et al.* (1999) Active specific immunotherapy with polyvalent melanoma cell vaccine for patients with in-transit melanoma metastases. *Cancer*, 85, 2160–9.

Irvine, A. S., Trinder, P. K., Laughton, D. L. *et al.* (2000) Efficient nonviral transfection of dendritic cells and their use for in vivo immunization. *Nat Biotechnol*, 18, 1273–8.

Larin, S. S., Georgiev, G. P., and Kiselev, S. L. (2004) Gene transfer approaches in cancer immunotherapy. *Gene Therapy*, 11, S18-S25.

Nestle, F. O., Alijagic, S., Gilliet, M. *et al.* (1998) Vaccination of melanoma patients with peptide- or tumor lysate-pulsed dendritic cells. *Nature Medicine*, 4, 328–32.

O'Neill, D. W., Adams, S., and Bhardwaj, N. (2004) Manipulating dendritic cell biology for the active immunotherapy of cancer. *Blood*, 104, 2235–46.

Parkhurst, M., DePan, C., Riley, J., Rosenberg, S., and S, S. (2003) Hybrids of dendritic cells and tumor cells generated by electrofusion simultaneously present immunodominant epitopes from multiple human tumor-associated antigens in the context of MHC class I and class II molecules. *The Journal of Immunology*, 170, 5317–25.

Reis e Sousa, C. (2004) Activation of dendritic cells: translating innate into adaptive immunity. *Current Opinion in Immunology*, 16, 21–5.

Riddell, S. R., Berger, C., Murata, M., Randolph, S., and Warren, E. H. (2003) The graft versus leukaemia response after allogeneic hematopoietic stem cell transplantation. *Blood Reviews* 17, 153–62.

Rooney, C. M., Smith, C. A., Ng, C. Y. *et al.* (1998) Infusion of cytotoxic T cells for the prevention and treatment of Epstein-Barr virus-induced lymphoma in allogeneic transplant recipients. *Blood*, 92, 1549–55.

Rosenberg, S. A. and Dudley, M. E. (2004) Cancer regression in patients with metastatic melanoma after the transfer of autologous antitumor lymphocytes. *Proceedings of the National Acadamy of Science U S A*, 101(Suppl 2), 14639–45.

Rosenberg, S. A., Yang, J. C., and Restifo, N. P. (2004) Cancer immunotherapy: moving beyond current vaccines. *Nature Medicine*, 10, 909–15.

Schuler, G., Schuler-Thurner, B., and Steinman, R. M. (2003) The use of dendritic cells in cancer immunotherapy. *Current Opinion in Immunology*, 15,138–47.

Schuler-Thurner, B., Schultz, E. S., Berger, T. G. *et al.* (2002) Rapid induction of tumor-specific type 1 T helper cells in metastatic melanoma patients by vaccination with mature, cryopreserved, peptide-loaded monocyte-derived dendritic cells. *Journal of Experimental Medicine*, 195, 1279–88.

Slavin, S., Morecki, S., Weiss, L., and Or, R. (2003) Immunotherapy of hematologic malignancies and metastatic solid tumors in experimental animals and man. *Critical Reviews in Oncology / Hematology*, 46, 139–43.

Small, E. J., Fratesi, P., Reese, D. M. *et al.* (2000) Immunotherapy of hormone-refractory prostate cancer with antigen-loaded dendritic cells. *Journal of Clinical Oncology,* 18, 3894–903.

Sobol, R. E., Shawler, D. L., Carson, C. *et al.* (1999) Interleukin 2 gene therapy of colorectal carcinoma with autologous irradiated tumor cells and genetically engineered fibroblasts: a Phase I study. *Clinical Cancer Research,* 5, 2359–65.

Stift, A., Friedl, J., Dubsky, P. *et al.* (2003) Dendritic cell-based vaccination in solid cancer. *Journal of Clinical Oncology,* 21, 135–42.

Timmerman, J. M., Czerwinski, D. K., Davis, T. A. *et al.* (2002) Idiotype-pulsed dendritic cell vaccination for B-cell lymphoma: clinical and immune responses in 35 patients. *Blood,* 99, 1517–26.

Yee, C., Thompson, J. A., Byrd, D. *et al.* (2002) Adoptive T cell therapy using antigen-specific CD8+ T cell clones for the treatment of patients with metastatic melanoma: in vivo persistence, migration, and antitumor effect of transferred T cells. *Proceedings of the National Acadamy of Science U S A,* 99, 16168–73.

Chapter 13

Gene therapy for cancer— approaches and ethical considerations

Deborah Beirne and Leonard Seymour

1 Introduction

The development of gene therapy as a potential therapeutic modality for both inherited and acquired disease has continued to gain momentum and sustained interest among the scientific and medical community. The number of gene therapy clinical trials conducted in the UK and elsewhere has risen year on year since its infancy in the early 1990s. In the UK, the Gene Therapy Advisory Committee (GTAC) has approved 96 trials in its 11-year history, 11 in 2004 compared with 3 in 1993 (GTAC 2005; Nevin 1998).

Whilst significant interest continues in **monogenic** diseases, like cystic fibrosis and haemophilia, and recent success achieved in the treatment of children with X-linked Severe Combined Immunodeficiency (X-SCID), around 70% (7 of 11 GTAC approved trials in 2004) of the gene therapy strategies and clinical trials to date have been directed towards the treatment of cancer (GTAC 2005).

Advancement in our knowledge of molecular cell biology, vector virology, and the role genes play in the development of cancer, including the sequencing of the human **genome**, is providing researchers with the necessary tools to develop novel gene therapy approaches to cancer. Such treatment modalities may have potential utility in a wide range of neoplastic diseases for which standard therapies have limited efficacy, significant treatment-limiting toxicity, or where no standard therapy currently exists.

One of the major goals of any new therapy for cancer is to develop agents with a high degree of toxicity to target cancer cells but with minimal pathogenicity to normal tissue. The benefit obtained by a particular treatment in terms of specific cell killing with minimal toxicity to other cells is frequently referred to as the 'therapeutic index'. Gene therapy strategies harness the infective ability of bacteria and **viruses** to enter and deliver gene products to the **nucleus** of target cells. The concept of specific viruses that might contain the necessary discriminatory power to treat human cancers will be addressed later in this chapter.

Current cancer gene therapy strategies include suicide gene therapy, **tumour suppressor gene** replacement and immunotherapeutic approaches. Whilst there are undoubtedly many hurdles to overcome before gene therapy becomes a viable and effective treatment for neoplastic disease, in particular adequate delivery of the therapeutic gene to the target cell, there is increasing pre-clinical evidence that gene therapy can be successful in targeting and killing tumour specific cells (Zeh and Bartlett 2002).

Furthermore, a large number of clinical trials in human subjects have revealed that the treatments have low morbidity and mortality and are continually being refined as we learn more about virology, molecular biology, and the pathogenesis of cancer. Theoretically, gene therapy may also prove to be useful as an adjunct to existing therapeutic modalities. Whilst there have been disappointments and concerns about the potential of gene therapy to deliver on its early promise, generally the debate has shifted away from questioning whether gene therapy approaches can selectively kill cancer cells, to one of which method will be most successful (McCormick 2001).

Gene therapy is a complex field of medical research. Public interest requires that specialist ethical review be undertaken in examining proposals involving human subjects. The role and considerations of the UK Gene Therapy Advisory Committee and the wider ethical debate around 'genetic engineering' in general and gene therapy in particular are important aspects of current gene therapy research. Transparency, shared knowledge and a willingness to engage with the general public are crucial if the field is to deliver on its early promise.

2 Ethical considerations

2.1 The role of the UK Gene Therapy Advisory Committee (GTAC)

Newly emerging fields of medicine frequently evoke concerns about the ethical acceptability, safety, and monitoring of novel therapeutic strategies in human subjects. Following the Clothier Report (Department of Health 1992), The Gene Therapy Advisory Committee was established by the British Government in 1993, to oversee the field of gene therapy research conducted in human subjects in the UK.

The committee consists of the chair, secretariat (responsible for the day to day functioning of the committee), and a panel drawn from expert and lay members. Their remit is to consider and advise on the acceptability of proposals for gene therapy research on human subjects on ethical grounds, taking into account the scientific merit, potential benefits and risks of each proposal. The primary aim of the decisions taken by the committee is that of the safety and welfare of patients. The committee also provides advice to UK Health Ministers on developments in gene therapy research and their implications.

GTAC works closely with other agencies that have statutory responsibilities such as the Medicines and Healthcare Products Regulatory Agency (MHRA), the Health and Safety Executive (HSE), and the Department for Environment, Food and Rural Affairs (DEFRA). In doing so a cohesive approach is achieved between all those with an interest in seeing the safe, but speedy translation of gene therapy research from the laboratory to the bedside.

Its advisory role extends to applicants/researchers in the regulatory aspects of gene -therapy research, expert feedback, and advice on the scientific aspects of the proposal, information, and counselling for patients, and the long-term surveillance of research subjects in a bid to try and monitor long-term consequences of gene therapy interventions.

More recently, in recognition of GTACs role as a specialist Multi-centre Research Ethics Committee (MREC), the government has specifically named it in the new Clinical Trials Regulations as the sole MREC to review gene therapy proposals in the UK (enacted into UK law in May 2004).

3 Cancer therapeutic strategies

Cancer gene therapy differs from most other diseases in that the central aim is to use the genetic material to kill target cells, not restore their normal function. There are several different molecular strategies to achieve this, and the main ones are outlined here:

3.1 Gene-supplementation therapy for cancer

Gene-supplementation therapy is the main technology used for treating genetic disorders, notably monogenic diseases, where supplementation of a cell with a **wild type** copy of a diseased gene can lead to restoration of normal function. The most obvious example of this is in the field of cystic fibrosis therapy, where supplementation of a wild type copy of the gene encoding the 'Cystic Fibrosis Membrane Transport Conductance Regulator' (CFTR) protein can overcome the deficiency (Griesenbach *et al.* 2004). Cancer is a more complex disease, however, and clinical tumours usually contain several genetic mutations. Accordingly, gene supplementation strategies for cancer do not aim to restore all mutated genes, rather they aim to kill tumour cells by restoring the cell's ability to undergo **apoptosis** or programmed cell death. Programmed cell death is a central feature of multicellular organisms, and mutations in genes controlling it (often referred to as 'tumour-suppressor genes') can produce tumour cells that fail to die in response to the correct signals. Many tumours have mutations in the **p53** gene, and this is a key cellular effector molecule in mediating apoptosis. Accordingly there has been a range of gene therapy studies evaluating the ability of wild-type copies of the p53 gene to cause cell death in tumours. Following encouraging pre-clinical studies (Horowitz 1999; Morrissey *et al.* 2002), the early clinical trials were generally disappointing, although recent studies in China are reported to have shown good efficacy for this approach, particularly in combination with chemotherapy. Full data have not yet been released, although preliminary related studies have already been reported (Guan *et al.* 2005), and a product licence has recently been issued in China for **adenovirus** expressing wild-type p53 for **adjuvant** treatment of head and neck cancer. This is the first gene therapy to receive a product licence anywhere in the world.

3.2 Gene-directed enzyme prodrug therapy (GDEPT or suicide gene therapy)

Gene-directed enzyme **prodrug** therapy involves the delivery of a novel gene encoding an enzyme that metabolises a relatively non-toxic drug into a substance toxic to the host or cancer cell (Brown and Lemoine 2004; Denny 2002; Fillat *et al.* 2003; McCarthy *et al.* 2003). This approach is essentially gene-delivered chemotherapy, and has the advantage over normal chemotherapy in that the effect of the therapeutic agent is amplified *in situ*, since each gene copy produces many copies of mRNA, each of which produces many copies of the enzyme, which in turn metabolises many prodrugs. This amplification can be combined with great selectivity, since targeting of the delivery vector (so called '**transductional** targeting') may be combined with selective **transcription**, by placing the **transgene** under the control of a tumour-associated **promoter** to restrict expression to tumour cells (Barnett *et al.* 2002). Coupled with the intrinsic selectivity of most chemotherapy agents for cancer cells, these attributes combine to promise an extremely powerful and yet highly selective approach that should show improved anticancer action without unwanted side-effects (Denny 2002). Several enzyme–prodrug combinations are currently being evaluated in early phase I clinical trials. The herpes simplex virus thymidine kinase (HSV-tk) converts the non-toxic pro-drug ganciclovir into the toxic anti-metabolite ganciclovir triphosphate,

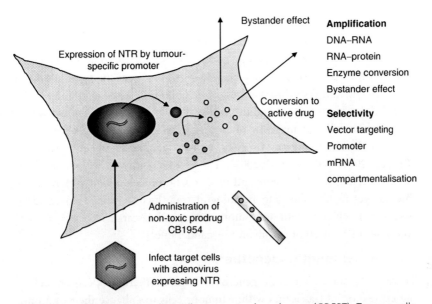

Bystander effect

Amplification

DNA–RNA

RNA–protein

Enzyme conversion

Bystander effect

Expression of NTR by tumour-specific promoter

Conversion to active drug

Selectivity

Vector targeting

Promoter

mRNA

compartmentalisation

Administration of non-toxic prodrug CB1954

Infect target cells with adenovirus expressing NTR

Fig. 13.1 An example of gene-directed enzyme prodrug therapy (GDEPT). Tumour cells are infected with a replication-deficient adenoviral vector encoding the *Escherichia coli* enzyme nitroimidazole reductase (NTR). Expressed NTR converts the administered prodrug CB1954 from a relatively weak, mono-functional alkylating agent into a potent bifunctional alkylating species that binds DNA and induces cell death. Tumour targeting and amplification of the anti-tumour effects are achieved by a variety of mechanisms.

which becomes incorporated into **DNA**, and has been shown to easily diffuse across cell membranes and have **cytotoxic** effects by the inhibition of DNA synthesis on surrounding tumour cells. Delivery of the *Escherichia coli* bacterial enzyme nitroimidazole reductase (NTR) by means of a replication-deficient adenoviral vector, converts the prodrug CB1954 from a relatively weak, mono-functional alkylating agent into a potent bifunctional alkylating species that binds DNA and induces cell death (see Fig. 13.1).

3.3 The bystander effect

GDEPT approaches are attractive for several reasons. First, only cells expressing the therapeutic gene product should be directly susceptible to cell killing by the relevant prodrug, thereby enhancing tumour 'selectivity'. Second, in most cases both the transgene and the prodrug are relatively non-toxic when given separately, and in combination have thus far demonstrated only modest and transient toxic side-effects. However, the real strength of the approach is that it provides a possible means to overcome limitations on delivery of transgene to every tumour cell. Efficient gene delivery is always an issue, and normally only a fraction of the target tumour cell population can be transduced to express the therapeutic gene. However, with some GDEPT approaches the activated drug may be able to diffuse from the transduced cell into adjacent, non-transduced, tumour cells and exert a toxic effect. This is the so-called 'bystander effect' and in practice a powerful bystander effect would be useful to kill the majority of non-expressing tumour cells with drug produced by the minority, which have taken up the therapeutic transgene (Chester 2004; Wilson *et al.* 2004). The phenomenon of 'bystander effect' has been demonstrated *in vitro* and *in vivo* (Chung-Faye *et al.* 2001), however this has yet to translate into meaningful transduction within surrounding tissues and subsequent tumour suppression, and research into this concept continues in an attempt to enhance bystander effects.

3.4 Cancer immunogenetherapy

There are several strategies for gene-based immunotherapy of cancer, including expression of transgenes within tumour cells to enhance their immunogenicity, genetic modification of immune effector cells to strengthen their response to the cancer, or use of cellular vaccines. This is a very popular field and many variations have already been proposed and several taken forward into clinical trial. Enhancing the immunogenicity of tumour cells directly could be achieved, for example, by engineering them to secrete immune-stimulating cytokines or by expressing B cell co-presentation antigens to enable the tumour cells to present their surface antigens directly to T cells, potentially leading to induction of an immune response against the tumour cells (Searle and Young 1996; Souberbielle *et al.* 1998; von Mehren *et al.* 2000). An alternative approach is aimed directly at immune effector cells, such as dendritic cells, and involves expressing cytokines or tumour-associated antigens within them to improve antigen presentation (see also Chapter 12). A development of this is the heterolgous prime-boost system, where two different genetic vectors are employed sequentially, to focus the response on the encoded tumour antigen (and away from the components of the vector). This approach is now undergoing clinical assessment (Bonnet *et al.* 2000; Irvine *et al.* 1997; Kaufman *et al.* 2004). A third promising strategy is cellular vaccination; again a large field with many possible strategies. Several vaccines have been constructed by *ex vivo* transduction of tumour cells that are then irradiated and re-introduced to the patient (Nemunaitis *et al.* 2004; Salgia *et al.* 2003), but probably the most promising at present are the GVAX vaccines, entering phase III trial for prostate cancer, which are non-patient-specific and include two irradiated prostate cancer cell lines transduced to express GM-CSF.

3.5 Virotherapy for cancer

An intriguing new approach to cancer gene therapy exploits the similarities between the cellular changes that occur when a cell becomes a cancer cell, and the changes that a virus induces during infection of normal cells. One of the most fundamental changes is manifest in the interferon response pathways, intrinsic to cellular resistance against virus infection (and therefore suppressed by successfully infecting viruses) and also very frequently deficient in cancers (Russell 2002). This can make cancers very sensitive to virus infection. In the case of lytic viruses (viruses that replicate within the cell and then lyse it in order to spread to adjacent cells) the net effect is that viruses may show selectivity towards killing cancer cells (Rainov and Ren 2003). There have been several reports where cancers have responded when patients have had exposure to viruses, for example, in vaccination programmes, although it is difficult to assess how much of this effect is due to stimulation of the immune response and how much is due to a direct effect of the virus on the tumour.

These observations have spawned a new approach to cancer therapy, based on using the cell killing activity of **lytic** viruses to kill tumours. In early clinical trials, injecting wild-type adenovirus into cervical cancers produced a high response rate, and the approach seems worthy of further exploration using a range of wild-type viruses. Great tumour selectivity and safety can be introduced by including mutations within the viruses, designed to complement the mutations that are already present in the tumours. For example, the Onyx-015 virus was deleted in the protein known as E1B 55K, which is normally responsible for inactivating cellular p53 and thereby preventing programmed cell death in response to virus infection (which would be undesirable for the virus, as its replication would be prevented). Deleting E1B 55K is intended to prevent the virus replicating in normal cells (which have normal p53 function) but enable it to replicate in tumour cells that already have inactive p53 (Heise *et al.* 1997). In this way, it should be possible to produce a virus that spreads throughout a solid p53-mutant tumour, lysing all the tumour cells, and then stop when it reaches normal tissue. In fact the mechanism of action of the virus is still under intensive discussion (McCormick 2000; O'Shea *et al.* 2004), but the results of clinical trials were promising, with the virus showing good therapeutic activity when combined with chemotherapy (Ganly *et al.* 2000; Kirn 2001; Nemunaitis *et al.* 2001; Reid *et al.* 2002).

The studies with Onyx-015 have stimulated substantial interest in this field, with groups trying to develop safe lytic viruses that will spread throughout a solid tumour and destroy it (Kirn 2003; Liu *et al.* 2005; Thorne and Kirn 2004; Varghese and Rabkin 2002; Vile *et al.* 2002). Interestingly one of the factors that impedes this approach is the patient's immune system, which often appears to destroy the virus before the virus has completely eradicated the tumour. Nevertheless, this field promises an immensely powerful way to destroy solid tumours and is likely to grow in significance and popularity rapidly in the next few years.

4 Vectors for cancer gene therapy

There are a range of gene-delivery vectors that can be applied to cancer, although nearly all of these have been based on viruses. Historically **retroviruses** have seen most usage, mainly because their selectivity for infection of proliferating cells was expected to give them an edge towards infecting tumours with high growth fraction. They have encountered problems of bloodstream stability (Shimizu *et al.* 1995; Takeuchi *et al.* 1994) and poor efficiency of infection, although the use of non-lytic replicating retrovirus to enable spread of GDEPT enzymes through solid tumours is an extremely attractive approach (Logg and Kasahara 2004; Wang *et al.* 2003). In fact, treatment of cancer is probably the main application of retrovirus where the risk of insertional mutagenesis would generally be tolerated. Nevertheless, adenovirus is now more widely used as a vector for gene delivery to cancer (Searle and Mautner 1998). Adenovirus has several advantages—it has a reasonable packaging capacity, it can be produced to high titre, it infects cells efficiently and independently of the cell cycle, and it does not integrate into the genome (see Fig. 13.2). In its simplest form adenovirus is also highly **immunogenic**, and this limits its usefulness for most diseases but may actually be useful in promoting a response against the tumour in cancer patients.

Adenovirus is also being developed further for cancer virotherapy—either by placing key virus genes (such as the E1A gene) under transcriptional control of tumour-associated promoters to restrict replication to tumours, or using the concept of complementary deletions described above. Other viruses are also being assessed for virotherapy—most notably including Newcastle Disease Virus, herpes simplex virus, measles virus, vaccinia, vesicular stomatitis virus, myximitosis virus, and cardiovirus, either in wild-type forms or following genetic modification.

Many gene-therapy clinical trials to date have involved direct injection of the therapeutic agent into solid tumours, mainly because of the challenges faced in remote targeting of vectors to disseminated cancer. However, to achieve useful therapy of metastatic disease it is necessary to develop strategies enabling intravenous delivery of vectors that can target selectively to cancer cells that

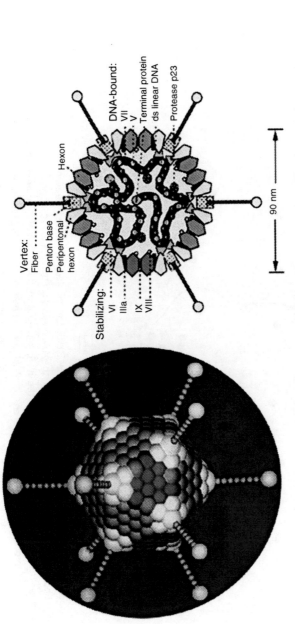

Fig. 13.2 Adenovirus type 2. Increasingly used as a vector for cancer gene therapy, the icosahedral adenovirus particle is approximately 90 nm in diameter, and is composed of an outer capsid and an inner DNA-associated core with a 36-kbp linear dsDNA, two terminal proteins, and the DNA-condensing proteins V and VII. The chromosome also contains about ten copies of the cysteine protease p23. The capsid itself consists mainly of hexon proteins and stabilising proteins IIIa, VIII, and IX. The vertices of the capsid are made up of pentameric penton base and protruding trimeric fibres. The fibres are composed of a linear shaft and a carboxy-terminal globular head domain of about 200 amino acids containing the receptor binding component. © Urs Greber; reproduced with permission.

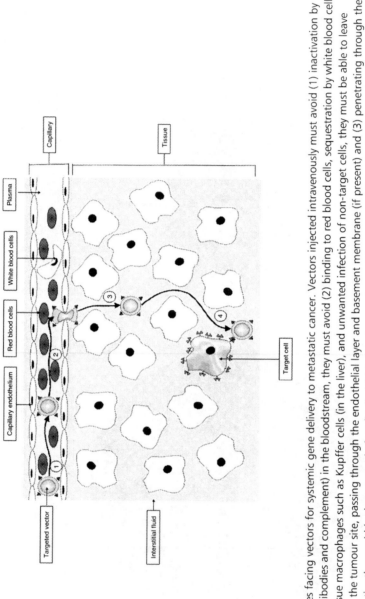

Fig. 13.3 Challenges facing vectors for systemic gene delivery to metastatic cancer. Vectors injected intravenously must avoid (1) inactivation by factors (notably antibodies and complement) in the bloodstream, they must avoid (2) binding to red blood cells, sequestration by white blood cells, phagocytosis by tissue macrophages such as Kupffer cells (in the liver), and unwanted infection of non-target cells, they must be able to leave the bloodstream at the tumour site, passing through the endothelial layer and basement membrane (if present) and (3) penetrating through the extracellular connective tissue within the tumour before finally (4) binding to receptor-positive tumour cells and selectively transducing them. © Simon Briggs 2005; reproduced with permission.

are spread throughout the body. Some of the challenges are shown in Fig. 13.3; they include potential neutralisation by protein or antibodies in the plasma, possible non-specific capture by the liver, infection of irrelevant cells, possible restrictions on leaving the bloodstream to gain access into solid tumours, and finally effective penetration through the tumour extracellular milieu and receptor-mediated entry into the target tumour cells. This is a difficult goal to achieve, although several attempts are underway to develop vectors capable of systemic targeting using genetic modification (Akiyama *et al.* 2004; Bauerschmitz *et al.* 2004) or physical 'cloaking' of the vectors using polymeric coats (Fisher *et al.* 2001; Green *et al.* 2004).

5 The future of cancer gene therapy

Every chapter in this book demonstrates how molecular biology continues to inform our understanding of the mechanisms that influence genetic mutations, and how this translates to malignant transformation. These insights provide new opportunities for therapeutic intervention with ever greater selectivity, aiming to maximise efficacy and minimise toxicity. The field of gene therapy is the most subtle of therapeutic approaches, since it seeks to express the therapeutic agent actually within the cancer cell itself, thereby maximising action and preventing exposure of non-target cells to the active agent.

Nevertheless, despite the promise, the reality of gene therapy is hard to bring about. Current exploration of ways to influence or correct cellular function, regulate immunogenicity, overcome the barriers to effective gene delivery, quantify and predict the risk of insertional mutagenesis, reduce the risk of generalised viral toxicity or early viral degradation, all remain a challenge. However, we must not forget that the field of gene therapy has steadily progressed in its first 15 years, and elegant strategies are in development that aim to learn from and improve upon the results of earlier laboratory work and phase I/II clinical trials in human subjects. It is important to recognise that as with all other therapeutic treatment modalities, some treatment-related toxicity is almost inevitable, despite attempts to reduce this as far as possible, and so the safety of gene therapy as well as efficacy will always be paramount.

As well as the scientific challenges, **somatic** cell gene therapy research has generated a great deal of ethical debate. This has ranged from questions regarding the appropriate application of gene therapy approaches (currently, genetic disorders and acquired life-threatening disease), concerns about the immediate safety or unknown long-term consequences of genetic manipulation, and accusations of creating unusually positive 'hype' about the therapeutic possibility of such strategies. In addition, there has been extensive debate and warnings around the notion of a 'slippery slope' from purportedly therapeutic intentions towards the possibility for, and attraction towards, *eugenic enhancement* for non-therapeutic aims; or to extend gene therapy approaches towards permanent alterations to the human genome by means of intentional germ line genetic manipulation (Rabino 2003).

Novel approaches to the treatment of human cancers necessitate stringent evaluation within the context of clinical trials. Such therapies are often first introduced in patient groups who have failed all conventional treatment options and have far advanced metastatic disease. In such patients and their families, expectation of, and faith in, the medical profession and science in general runs high. Partly, the level of expectation can be explained by the publicity that 'medical breakthroughs' and 'promising scientific discoveries' generates within the media.

Several ethical issues, therefore, are pertinent to the current application of gene therapy research. Patients who have exhausted conventional treatment options, have limited life-expectancy, and few or no existent treatment options, are a vulnerable group for whom any opportunity to try something, however experimental, can be very appealing (Dettweiler *et al.* 2001).

Decisions by the patient to participate in gene-therapy clinical trials may be said to reflect both an expectation (or hope), however remote, to derive personal benefit (perhaps through desperation), and an altruistic beneficence towards future persons similarly afflicted. Patients frequently give consent to participate in clinical research because they trust the doctor, the cancer centre, and believe in the research process overall (Kass *et al.* 1996). Similarly the way in which people assess 'risk' when in good health differs greatly when faced with terminal disease.

Gene-therapy approaches themselves are complex but must be clearly explained in terms that the general population can readily understand. Clinical trials generally require a great deal from the subjects who agree to participate both in terms of time, willingness to undergo additional safety procedures and tests, and to long-term follow-up. Furthermore the physician–patient relationship can become more complex when the physician is also the researcher (Dettweiler *et al.* 2001). Conflicting interests may arise between the exclusive care of the patient and the research objectives of a study, particularly when applied to current gene-therapy trials, where no direct benefit to the patient is expected.

Respect for personal autonomy in clinical trials is incorporated into the guidelines and frameworks governing clinical trial conduct (ICH Harmonised Tripartite Guideline for Good Clinical Practice 1996; Declaration of Helsinki World Medical Association 2002). The Helsinki Declaration makes clear that the responsibility for the patient's well-being remains with the medically qualified person and never rests on the subject of the research, despite the subject having given consent. Adoption of independent counselling of patients prior to gene-therapy trial entry may be one way of facilitating an informed and voluntary decision, independent of the researcher. This may also help to redress questions regarding potential vested interests between academia and commercial organisations, for example, or the dependent relationship of patients to their doctors/researchers (Kong 2004). Researchers have a duty towards current and future gene therapy recipients to ensure that the science is robust, that trials are carried out to the highest standards, and that transparency and vested interests are declared.

It has been suggested that the words 'treatment' or 'therapy' should be avoided altogether when mentioning current gene-therapy clinical trials as they can be misleading, indicating a degree of efficacy that cannot be substantiated (Kong 2004). Thus far, the majority of all gene-therapy trials are phase I/II safety, feasibility, proof of principle, or dose-finding studies, where efficacy is not the primary objective. Caution is therefore required when talking with patients and preparing patient information sheets, so that the proposed study does not create over-optimism about possible benefits or induce false hope (Sikora 1996). Patients require clear, unambiguous, and realistic information upon which to base their decision to participate in gene therapy research.

Moreover, there is the issue of unforeseen risks, especially pertinent in gene-therapy trials. Pre-clinical research, no matter how extensive, cannot exactly replicate the situation in human subjects. Whilst it is crucial to obtain as much information as possible before introducing a new approach in humans, early clinical trials in human subjects are the only way in which to assess safety and quantify as yet unknown risk. Two recently reported events, that of the death of 18-year-old Jesse Gelsinger following the use of an experimental gene-therapy approach for a rare metabolic disorder in 1999, and the recent cases of a 'leukaemia like' illness, secondary to un-intentional insertional mutagenesis, in children who received gene therapy for the immunodeficiency disorder X-SCID in 2002, highlighted concerns about the viability of gene therapy as an approach to treating illness (Thomas *et al.* 2003). However, as with any other modality, gene therapy is not without risk. Whilst every effort should be made to quantify, minimise, and learn from such events, and inform patients adequately about known or potential risks, **iatrogenic** effects remain a possibility.

It has been suggested that gene-therapy approaches should start earlier in the disease process, when it might have a better chance of preventing deterioration in the patient's condition (Rabino 2003). Presently, gene-therapy trial participation is offered where no effective alternative exists or where patients have exhausted known therapeutic options for their particular disease. Risk of potential harm is weighed in situations where no personal benefit is expected. Placing gene therapy amongst the early armament of treatment options is some distance away, and ethically is likely to occur only when the efficacy of gene therapy approaches have been more clearly and consistently demonstrated. Efficacy of gene delivery has yet to translate into therapeutic benefit in large numbers of patients with cancer. Nevertheless, it remains a viable and logical modality to explore and develop much needed strategies to target cancer.

Lastly, as the field develops further, the question of how far genetic manipulation technology can be developed and the justification for its application in a particular disease site—perhaps 'prevention' rather than 'treatment'—will require careful, thorough and widespread ethical debate.

References

Akiyama, M., Thorne, S., Kirn, D., Roelvink, P. W., Einfeld, D. A., King, C. R. *et al.* (2004). Ablating CAR and integrin binding in adenovirus vectors reduces nontarget organ transduction and permits sustained bloodstream persistence following intraperitoneal administration. *Mol Ther* 9, 218–30.

Barnett, B. G., Tillman, B. W., Curiel, D. T., and Douglas, J. T. (2002). Dual targeting of adenoviral vectors at the levels of transduction and transcription enhances the specificity of gene expression in cancer cells. *Mol Ther* 6, 377–85.

Bauerschmitz, G. J., Kanerva, A., Wang, M., Herrmann, I., Shaw, D. R., Strong, T. V. *et al.* (2004). Evaluation of a selectively oncolytic adenovirus for local and systemic treatment of cervical cancer. *Int J Cancer* 111, 303–9.

Bonnet, M. C., Tartaglia, J., Verdier, F., Kourilsky, P., Lindberg, A., Klein, M. *et al.* (2000). Recombinant viruses as a tool for therapeutic vaccination against human cancers. *Immunol Lett* 74, 11–25.

Brown, N. L. and Lemoine, N. R. (2004). Clinical trials with GDEPT: cytosine deaminase and 5-fluorocytosine. *Methods Mol Med* 90, 451–7.

Chester, J. (2004). Cancer gene therapy. In: *Cellular and molecular biology of cancer* (4th edn) (ed., Selby, P. L.). Oxford University Press, Oxford pp. 458–79.

Chung-Faye, G., Palmer, D., Anderson, D., Clark, J., Downes, M., Baddeley, J. *et al.* (2001). Virus-directed, enzyme prodrug therapy with nitroimidazole reductase: a phase I and pharmacokinetic study of its prodrug, CB1954. *Clin Cancer Res* 7, 2662.

Declaration of Helsinki (1964; last updated 2002). Ethical principles for medical research involving human subjects (policy document 17.c). World Medical Association. Available online at http://www.wma.net/e/policy/pdf/17c.pdf.

Denny, W. A. (2002). Nitroreductase-based GDEPT. *Curr Pharm Des* 8, 1349–61.

Dettweiler, U. and Simon, P. (2001). Points to consider for ethics committees in human gene therapy trials. *Bioethics* 15, 491.

Department of Health (1992) *Report of the Committee on the Ethics of Gene Therapy.* London HMSO; Cm 1788.

Fillat, C., Carrio, M., Cascante, A., and Sangro, B. (2003). Suicide gene therapy mediated by the Herpes Simplex virus thymidine kinase gene/Ganciclovir system: fifteen years of application. *Curr Gene Ther* 3, 13–26.

Fisher, K. D., Stallwood, Y., Green, N. K., Ulbrich, K., Mautner, V., and Seymour, L. W. (2001). Polymer-coated adenovirus permits efficient retargeting and evades neutralising antibodies. *Gene Ther* 8, 341–8.

Ganly, I., Kirn, D., Eckhardt, G., Rodriguez, G. I., Soutar, D. S., Otto, R. *et al.* (2000). A phase I study of Onyx-015, an E1B attenuated adenovirus, administered intratumorally to patients with recurrent head and neck cancer. *Clin Cancer Res* 6, 798–806.

Green, N. K., Herbert, C. W., Hale, S. J., Hale, A. B., Mautner, V., Harkins, R. *et al.* (2004). Extended plasma circulation time and decreased toxicity of polymer-coated adenovirus. *Gene Ther* 11, 1256–63.

Griesenbach, U., Geddes, D. M., and Alton, E. W. (2004). Advances in cystic fibrosis gene therapy. *Curr Opin Pulm Med* 10, 542–6.

GTAC (2001). *Eighth Annual Report.* Department of Health: London.

GTAC (2005). *Eleventh Annual Report of the Gene Therapy Advisory Committee.* Department of Health: London.

Guan, Y., Liu, Y., Zhou, X., Li, X., He, Q., and Sun, L. (2005). p53 gene (Gendicine) and embolisation overcame recurrent hepatocellular carcinoma. *Gut.* 54(9), 1318–19.

Heise, C., Sampson-Johannes, A., Williams, A., McCormick, F., Von Hoff, D. D., and Kirn, D. H. (1997). ONYX-015, an E1B gene-attenuated adenovirus, causes tumor-specific cytolysis and antitumoral efficacy that can be augmented by standard chemotherapeutic agents. *Nat Med* 3, 639–45.

Horowitz, J. (1999). Adenovirus-mediated p53 gene therapy: overview of preclinical studies and potential clinical applications. *Curr Opin Mol Ther* 1, 500–9.

International Conference on Harmonisation of Technical Requirements for Registration of Pharmaceuticals for Human Use (1996). *ICH Harmonised Tripartite Guideline for Good Clinical Practice.* Available online at: *http://www.ich.org/MediaServer.jser?@_ID =482&@_MODE=GLB* (last accessed 20 June 2005).

Irvine, K. R., Chamberlain, R. S., Shulman, E. P., Surman, D. R., Rosenberg, S. A., and Restifo, N. P. (1997). Enhancing efficacy of recombinant anticancer vaccines with prime/ boost regimens that use two different vectors. *J Natl Cancer Inst* 89, 1595–601.

Kaufman, H. L., Wang, W., Manola, J., DiPaola, R. S., Ko, Y. J., Sweeney, C. *et al.* (2004). Phase II randomized study of vaccine treatment of advanced prostate cancer (E7897): a trial of the Eastern Cooperative Oncology Group. *J Clin Oncol* 22, 2122–32.

Kass, N. E. S., J. Faden, R., and Schoch-Spana, M. (1996). Trust, the fragile foundation of contemporary biomedical research. *Hastings Centre Report* 25.

Kirn, D. (2001). Oncolytic virotherapy for cancer with the adenovirus dl1520 (Onyx-015): results of phase I and II trials. *Expert Opin Biol Ther* 1, 525–38.

Kirn, D. (2003). Oncolytic virotherapy as a novel treatment platform for cancer. *Ernst Schering Res Found Workshop,* 43, 89–105.

Kong, W. M. (2004). The Regulation of Gene Therapy Reserach In Competent Adult Patients, Today and Tomorrow: Implications of EU Directive 2001/20/EC. *Medical Law Review,* 12, 164.

Liu, X. Y., Qiu, S. B., Zou, W. G., Pei, Z. F., Gu, J. F., Luo, C. X. *et al.* (2005). Effective gene-virotherapy for complete eradication of tumor mediated by the combination of hTRAIL (TNFSF10) and plasminogen k5. *Mol Ther* 11, 531–41.

Logg, C. R. and Kasahara, N. (2004). Retrovirus-mediated gene transfer to tumors: utilizing the replicative power of viruses to achieve highly efficient tumor transduction *in vivo*. *Methods Mol Biol* **246**, 499–525.

McCarthy, H. O., Yakkundi, A., McErlane, V., Hughes, C. M., Keilty, G., Murray, M. *et al.* (2003). Bioreductive GDEPT using cytochrome P450 3A4 in combination with AQ4N. *Cancer Gene Ther* **10**, 40–8.

McCormick, F. (2000). ONYX-015 selectivity and the p14ARF pathway. *Oncogene* **19**, 6670–2.

McCormick, F. (2001). Cancer gene therapy: fringe or cutting edge? *Nat Rev Cancer* **1**, 130.

Morrissey, R. E., Horvath, C., Snyder, E. A., Patrick, J., Collins, N., Evans, E. *et al.* (2002). Porcine toxicology studies of SCH 58500, an adenoviral vector for the p53 gene. *Toxicol Sci* **65**, 256–65.

Nemunaitis, J., Khuri, F., Ganly, I., Arseneau, J., Posner, M., Vokes, E. *et al.* (2001). Phase II trial of intratumoral administration of ONYX-015, a replication-selective adenovirus, in patients with refractory head and neck cancer. *J Clin Oncol* **19**, 289–98.

Nemunaitis, J., Sterman, D., Jablons, D., Smith, J. W., 2nd, Fox, B., Maples, P. *et al.* (2004). Granulocyte-macrophage colony-stimulating factor gene-modified autologous tumor vaccines in non-small-cell lung cancer. *J Natl Cancer Inst* **96**, 326–31.

Nevin, N. C. (1998). Experience of gene therapy in the United Kingdom. *Ann N Y Acad Sci* **862**, 184–7.

O'Shea, C. C., Johnson, L., Bagus, B., Choi, S., Nicholas, C., Shen, A. *et al.* (2004). Late viral RNA export, rather than p53 inactivation, determines ONYX-015 tumor selectivity. *Cancer Cell* **6**, 611–23.

Rabino, I. (2003)Gene therapy: ethical issues. *Theor Med Bioeth* **24**, 31.

Rainov, N. G. and Ren, H. (2003). Oncolytic viruses for treatment of malignant brain tumours. *Acta Neurochir* **88**, 113–23.

Reid, T., Galanis, E., Abbruzzese, J., Sze, D., Wein, L. M., Andrews, J. *et al.* (2002). Hepatic arterial infusion of a replication-selective oncolytic adenovirus (d11520): phase II viral, immunologic, and clinical endpoints. *Cancer Res* **62**, 6070–9.

Russell, S. J. (2002). RNA viruses as virotherapy agents. *Cancer Gene Ther* **9**, 961–6.

Salgia, R., Lynch, T., Skarin, A., Lucca, J., Lynch, C., Jung, K. *et al.* (2003). Vaccination with irradiated autologous tumor cells engineered to secrete granulocyte-macrophage colony-stimulating factor augments antitumor immunity in some patients with metastatic non-small-cell lung carcinoma. *J Clin Oncol* **21**, 624–30.

Searle, P. F. and Mautner, V. (1998). Adenoviral vectors: not to be sneezed at. *Gene Ther* **5**, 725–7.

Searle, P. F. and Young, L. S. (1996). Immunotherapy II: antigens, receptors and costimulation. *Cancer Metastasis Rev* **15**, 329–49.

Shimizu, K., Miyao, Y., Tamura, M., Kishima, H., Ohkawa, M., Mabuchi, E. *et al.* (1995). Infectious retrovirus is inactivated by serum but not by cerebrospinal fluid or fluid from tumor bed in patients with malignant glioma. *Jpn J Cancer Res* **86**, 1010–3.

Sikora, K. (1996) Scope and limitations of gene therapy. In: *Gene therapy* (ed., Lemoine, N. R. Cooper, D.N). BIOS Scientific Publishers Ltd, Oxford pp. 9–27.

Souberbielle, B. E., Westby, M., Ganz, S., Kayaga, J., Mendes, R., Morrow, W. J. *et al.* (1998). Comparison of four strategies for tumour vaccination in the B16-F10 melanoma model. *Gene Ther* **5**, 1447–54.

Takeuchi, Y., Cosset, F. L., Lachmann, P. J., Okada, H., Weiss, R. A., and Collins, M. K. (1994). Type C retrovirus inactivation by human complement is determined by both the viral genome and the producer cell. *J Virol* **68**, 8001–7.

Thomas, C. E., Ehrhardt, A., and Kay, M. A. (2003) Progress and problems with the use of viral vectors for gene therapy. *Nat Rev Genet* **4**, 346.

Thorne, S. H. and Kirn, D. H. (2004). Future directions for the field of oncolytic virotherapy: a perspective on the use of vaccinia virus. *Expert Opin Biol Ther* **4**, 1307–21.

Varghese, S. and Rabkin, S. D. (2002). Oncolytic herpes simplex virus vectors for cancer virotherapy. *Cancer Gene Ther* **9**, 967–78.

Vile, R., Ando, D., and Kirn, D. (2002). The oncolytic virotherapy treatment platform for cancer: unique biological and biosafety points to consider. *Cancer Gene Ther* **9**, 1062–7.

von Mehren, M., Arlen, P., Tsang, K. Y., Rogatko, A., Meropol, N., Cooper, H. S. *et al.* (2000). Pilot study of a dual gene recombinant avipox vaccine containing both carcinoembryonic antigen (CEA) and B7.1 transgenes in patients with recurrent CEA-expressing adenocarcinomas. *Clin Cancer Res* **6**, 2219–28.

Wang, W. J., Tai, C. K., Kasahara, N., and Chen, T. C. (2003). Highly efficient and tumor-restricted gene transfer to malignant gliomas by replication-competent retroviral vectors. *Hum Gene Ther* **14**, 117–27.

Wilson, W. R., Pullen, S. M., Hogg, A., Hobbs, S. M., Pruijn, F. B., and Hicks, K. O. (2004). *In vitro* and *in vivo* models for evaluation of GDEPT: quantifying bystander killing in cell cultures and tumors. *Methods Mol Med* **90**, 403–31.

Zeh, H. J. and Bartlett, D. L. (2002). Development of a replication-selective, oncolytic poxvirus for the treatment of human cancers. *Cancer Gene Ther* **9**, 1001–12.

Chapter 14

Individualising cancer therapy

Wan-Teck Lim and Howard L. McLeod

1 Introduction

1.1 The scope of the problem

Cancer is a complex disease with variable **phenotypes** determined by different genes. Aside from curative surgery in the early stages of cancer, treatment of advanced cancer includes cytotoxics, biologics, or radiation. These modalities affect both tumour and normal tissue, leaving in its wake significant toxicity. The benefits of **cytotoxic** drugs are determined to different extents by patient biology, absorption, distribution, metabolism, excretion, and by tumour biology. In patients with advanced disease, where the goal is palliative and not curative, the best modern therapies still only benefit the minority in terms of improving response rates and survival and the disease ultimately relapses in a short period of time. This is compounded by toxicity of varying degrees experienced by patients resulting in a low risk–benefit ratio. With emerging therapies that are more target-specific, toxicities are more tolerable, but still present. Aside from one or two examples, these target-specific drugs have yet to fulfil early promise, and response rates and survival benefits remain uncertain. The number of drugs available to treat a cancer patient increases yearly. Increasing early cancer detection and surgery has increased the number of patients who could potentially benefit from **adjuvant** therapies. Choosing the patients that will benefit from these potentially toxic therapies is a difficult but essential goal. Predicting the patients who would not benefit from adjuvant therapy because their disease is unlikely to relapse becomes as important as predicting the patients who would benefit. So the clinical problem remains to select the drug that fits each individual best with the minimum of toxicity and maximum of benefit.

Since the human **genome** was completely sequenced at the turn of the century, there has been an explosion in the amount of genomic information available for each cancer. Currently, over 10 million **single nucleotide** polymorphisms (SNPs) have been discovered in the human genome of 3 billion total bases. Elucidation of **oncogenes, tumour-suppressor genes,** and cellular and subcellular molecular signalling pathways of oncogenesis is moving forward with great momentum, as is evident from this book. With this increase in information, the hope remains of attaining the holy grail of individualised specific therapy based on an individual's genetics (i.e. **pharmacogenomics**).

1.2 Translating it forward

How can one translate this genetic information to full clinical application? There are obstacles that need to be overcome before therapy can be individualised successfully.

1.2.1 A robust phenotype is required

Determining an accurate and reproducible phenotype is a cardinal requirement for a biological marker that is measurable and can be related to an individual's **genotype**. This allows the practising clinician to choose therapy based on a genotype–phenotype correlation that is reliable and accurate. This genotype and phenotype should be easily measurable and reproducible. They should be of adequate positive or negative predictive value of outcome for each tumour sufficient to alter existing practice. The genotype or phenotype should also be of sufficient prevalence in the population at risk to be of any clinical utility. An example lies in dihydropyrimidine dehydrogenase (DPD) gene polymorphisms in predicting DPD activity and toxicity from 5-fluorouracil (5-FU) (Lim & McLeod 2004). DPD is the main catabolic enzyme for 5-FU. DPD deficiency is a reason for severe 5-FU toxicity. There is unfortunately no clinical phenotype that identifies deficiency. There are two recognised ways of determining the deficient phenotype but neither is a great test. The most direct method is to determine absolute DPD activity in tissue. The liver contains the highest concentration of DPD but accessing it for tissue carries considerable morbidity (Lu *et al.* 1995). Efforts to measure DPD levels in peripheral lymphocytes have inconsistent results (Fleming *et al.* 1993; Etienne *et al.* 1994; Di Paolo *et al.* 2001). The assay for DPD activity is also not routinely available. An indirect method is to identify genetic polymorphisms in the DPD gene that encode for low DPD activity. The problems with this approach include: the most common genetic polymorphism that is associated with toxicity (DPD*2A) is of low prevalence (<1% of general Caucasian population) (Raida *et al.* 2001); severe toxicity can be only partially accounted for by DPD*2A (Raida *et al.* 2001; Van Kuilenburg *et al.* 2002); not all genetic polymorphisms are associated with reduced levels of DPD activity

(Collie-Duguid *et al.* 2000); low levels of DPD activity exist even in the absence of coding sequence variants of DPD and could be accounted for by decreased activity of downstream enzymes like dihydropyrimidinase (Van Kuilenbrg *et al.* 2003). Therefore no patient who requires 5-FU today should be denied therapy based on a DPD test in the absence of a clear definable phenotype.

1.2.2 Selecting the right patient

Selecting the patient who will benefit from therapy is difficult. Traditional methods have used gross tumour information, performance status, and demographics to associate with response or toxicity. This was somewhat superseded by simple biological markers in the last decade. A predictive biological marker is one that predicts for response or toxicity to a specific therapy. A prognostic biological marker is one that predicts for outcome independent of therapy. Several terms of reference that are commonly used for deciding the clinical utility of such biomarkers are specificity, sensitivity, positive predictive value, and negative predictive value (Altman & Bland 1994a, b). These are useful tools to help decide how applicable a biomarker as a screening test for toxicity or response will be in clinical practice. Using DPD*2A to illustrate this, while the test is specific for the mutation, its clinical utility is diminished because it has low specificity for the phenotype (60% of patients who carry DPD*2A do not manifest grade 3–4 toxicity with 5-FU therapy implying a high false positive rate), and it has a currently unknown true negative rate for DPD deficiency because of the myriad of other possible reasons for DPD deficiency in the presence of a negative test for the mutation.

There is significant interpatient heterogeneity even within the same tumour type. Gene expression differences account for different phenotypes and different outcomes in several tumour types. This has been validated for several tumours. Diffuse large B-cell lymphomas can now be divided into two distinct groups based on their genetic signature. The initial division into 'germinal centre' like cells and 'activated peripheral' type cells (Alizadeh *et al.* 2000; Huang *et al.* 2002) has been further refined into a predictive set of six genes (Lossos *et al.* 2004) that adds to the clinical International Prognostic Index (Shipp *et al.* 2002). Among other tumours, one of the best characterised is breast cancer (Perou *et al.* 2000; Sorlie *et al.* 2001). Adenocarcinoma of the breast can be reproducibly divided based on their gene expression profiles into 5 subtypes: luminal subtype A, luminal subtype B, basal epithelial origin, ER negative and her2 positive, and normal breast origin. Luminal type A is indolent, while luminal type B is aggressive. Luminal type B overexpresses genes associated with proliferation, has a high rate of **p53** mutation, and is associated with much worse prognosis. Duke B colon cancer has a historical recurrence rate of between 25% and 30% despite adequate surgery. The majority of these patients receive no adjuvant therapy because randomised phase III trials have failed to demonstrate a survival advantage, excepting specific subsets who manifest with obstruction or perforation. These patients can now be divided into two different prognostic subgroups based on a 23-gene signature derived from gene-expression studies (Wang *et al.* 2004). The poor prognostic subgroup has a 13-fold risk of recurrence compared to the good prognosis subset. These approaches argue for a risk-adjusted approach to therapy. The subsets with the best prognosis can be treated with conventional therapies, while those with poorer prognosis may require novel treatment approaches. Although this goes some way to 'individualising' therapy, it is difficult for the patients and the oncologist assigned to a poor prognosis genetic signature. This is because these patients may still form a substantial subset. What constitutes best therapy for them? Even greater detail of the genetics of these individuals is needed. The individual pathways and genes that make the tumour active need to be elucidated, specific targets need to be understood, and therapies tailored.

1.2.3 Selecting the right drug

The complexity of each tumour migrates from single gene defects [e.g. chronic myeloid leukaemia caused by a **translocation** of **chromosome** 9 to 22 (Cannistra 1990)], to a multistep and multigene adenoma-carcinoma model of colon cancer (Vogelstein *et al.* 1988). This interplay of different processes is summarised succinctly by Hahn and Weinberg (2002). These present single or multiple potential targets. Traditional cytotoxic chemotherapy usually causes cytotoxicity through multiple pathways. However, the pools of candidate genes that determine sensitivity or resistance, as generated by gene expression profiling studies, can run into thousands. One novel approach to select candidate genes that determine sensitivity or resistance to cytotoxics uses a panel of CEPH cell lines (Watters *et al.* 2004). This method demonstrates hereditability of chemotherapy sensitivity, and also leads to discovery of novel genes in sensitive and resistant cells to different chemotherapies that can be tested in clinical trials. The patient who overexpresses the 'sensitivity' gene could then be treated with appropriate therapy to which they are likely to respond. Ensuring toxicity is not worse than the disease itself is an enduring call for investigators and a worthy objective. The same methods used for detecting candidate genes for response can be applied to selecting genes that predict for toxicity.

Increasingly there are target-specific drugs on the market where the gene, **RNA**, or protein is the target. This target should be a cornerstone of the tumourigenic process. Shutting it down should lead to regression or termination of this process. In theory, targeted therapies have a high specificity. While specific, they are not highly effective in most tumours. Possible reasons include low prevalence of mutations of the target that make it more sensitive to therapy and genetic variations in the target leading to protein conformational changes that interfere with drug binding. This can be illustrated with imatinib. Activating mutations in c-kit or PDGFRA are necessary for imatinib to be effective (Heinrich *et al.* 2003). Fortunately these are fairly common in c-kit and bcr-Abl, resulting in a high response rate. Subsequent point mutations in the ABL-kinase binding domain in chronic myelogenous leukaemias (Azam *et al.* 2003) and mutations in the ATP-binding pocket of c-kit in gastrointestinal tumours (Bohmer *et al.* 2003) result in decreased binding affinity to imatinib leading to secondary resistance. A pan-tyrosine kinase inhibitor, SU11248 has been shown to be effective in overcoming secondary imatinib resistance in gastrointestinal stromal tumours arising as a result of secondary mutations in the c-kit or PDGFRA (Demetri *et al.* 2004).

Given the multiple pathways for carcinogenesis and specificity of such targeted therapies, single targets may not suffice, and multiple targets in different pathways may be needed. Additive effects have been described in pre-clinical studies combining inhibition of multiple downstream signal **transduction** molecules along the EGFR-MAPK pathway (Bianco *et al.* 2004; Lev *et al.* 2004). Different drugs hitting different parts of the same target may also allow additive gain. Both cetuximab and gefitinib used together demonstrated additive effects on cytotoxicity and tumour regression in cell lines and **xenografts** (Huang *et al.* 2004).

In targeted therapy unlike cytotoxics, the **maximum tolerated dose (MTD)** needs to be replaced with the biologically effective dose (BED). In fact the BED may be well below or above the MTD for any drug. Accurate determination of the BED could improve toxicity profiles and clinical benefits. Phase I studies of gefitinib that incorporated **pharmacokinetic** and **pharmacodynamic** endpoints were used to determine the BED for EGFR TK inhibitor, gefitinib (Wolf *et al.* 2004). From these, it was established that the MTD was observed at doses of 750–1000 mg/day. More importantly, two important observations were made. First, pharmacokinetic data showed that biologically relevant plasma levels were reached at doses >100 mg/day, and second, maximum biological effect was observed at the lowest dose of 150 mg/day (demonstrated by reduction in pMAPK levels) in serial skin biopsies. In order to minimise subtherapeutic exposure due to interpatient variability, a daily dose of at least 250 mg/day was advanced to phase II trials. These trials compared two doses of 250 mg/day and 500 mg/day. The lower dose gave comparable efficacy at lower toxicity, thereby establishing a BED of 250 mg/day. In practice it is difficult to individualise the BED in real-time, and a population-based approach that achieves the BED for the majority of the population at risk as above is still worthwhile.

1.2.4   Validation of current genotype-phenotype correlations

A paradigm shift in how current biomarker and drug discovery studies are carried out is needed. Most drugs do not make it beyond phase II studies because of either overwhelming toxicity or poor efficacy. Subsets of patients however do benefit, and developing markers concurrently to identify these patients would go a long way to individualising therapy and bringing these drugs forward into phase III studies in a more rapid fashion. Academia and pharmaceutical companies will need to cooperate early in the drug development process to ensure logical development so these trials can lead to changes in practice.

1.2.5   Viable alternatives to meet the needs of patients where 'individualisation' fails

Individualised therapy in the adjuvant setting is likely to divide patients into three large groups. Some patients will be predicted to not need therapy, while others are likely to benefit based on their genetic make-up. Lastly there will be a sizeable group of patients who are at risk for disease recurrence and need therapy for when none of the existing agents are predicted to give clinical benefit. The needs of these patients have to be addressed in the context of novel drugs that give at least a chance of anti-tumour activity.

So, in essence, by gradually unravelling the myriad of pathogenic pathways of cancer, we are moving from a blunt approach to more accurate (and hopefully gentler) tailored therapies in the treatment of cancer (Fig. 14.1).

2   Genetic polymorphisms affecting cancer therapy

There exists a myriad of influences that can account for variation of drug effect (Fig. 14.2).

2.1   Pharmacokinetics

Pharmacokinetics describes the effect of the body on drugs. Inter-individual variability in absorption, distribution, metabolism, and elimination of a drug affects plasma and tissue levels. In turn this affects delivery of the drug to the target and toxicity. There are two broad themes that are the focus of investigation now: one is to study how the plasma levels of each drug are affected by dose and scheduling; and secondly how inter-individual variability of these drug levels are dependent on our genetic diversity in drug transport and

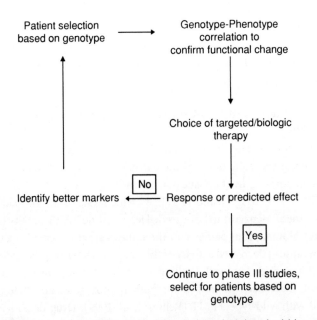

Fig. 14.1 Design of genotype-guided phase I/II studies—bench to bedside and back.

metabolism. The plasma levels of drugs vary with dose and scheduling, even with molecular targeted therapies. So even for the same dose and schedule of drug delivered, inter-individual variation can be very wide (often >10-fold). Part of the reason lies in the genes that govern these pharmacokinetic processes.

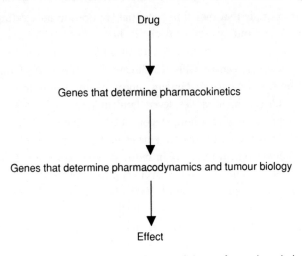

Fig. 14.2 The drug–effect genetic 'sandwich'. Each layer of genetic variation makes individualising cancer therapy complex.

Drug transporters efflux or influx drugs into tumour or normal tissue. Drugs also depend on large families of related drug metabolisers to catabolise them. The product of such catabolism may be an inactive metabolite or an even more toxic metabolite.

2.1.1 (Thiopurine S-methyltransferase) methylates thiopurine (TPMT) drugs

The thiopurines are extensively used in childhood leukaemias and organ transplants. The therapeutic indexes of these drugs are narrow. Therefore accurate dosing is important. In the Caucasian population there are three common alleles, TPMT*2, TPMT*3A, and TPMT*3C, which result in amino acid changes that causes the allo-enzyme to be degraded leaving little TPMT activity (McLeod *et al.* 2002). **Homozygous** patients for these alleles are at increased risk of severe toxicity because of decreased activity of this enzyme. **Heterozygous** patients also tolerate thiopurines less well (Relling *et al.* 1999). Appropriate drug-dose adjustments have been developed for both homozygotes and heterozygotes compared with wild-type TPMT (Relling *et al.* 1999). Drug doses have to be delivered at 1/10 of the dose with careful monitoring in these patients. This is a classic example of individualised therapy where patients at risk of severe toxicity can be identified before treatment. A simple test for a common allelic variant (genotype) is available that has a robust correlation to decreased enzymatic activity (phenotype).

2.1.2 The UGT1A1 (UDP-glucuronosyltransferase 1A1) gene

One similar example that may find potential application in selecting chemotherapy based on avoiding excess toxicity is the UGT1A1 (UDP-glucuronosyltransferase 1A1) gene. Dysfunctional UGT1A1 is responsible for the hyperbilirubinaemia seen in Gilbert's disease. The function of this gene is influenced by the presence of tandem repeats in the **promoter** region. The UGT1A1*28 allele, which carries seven tandem repeats, is common in the Caucasian population with a homozygous allele frequency of 10%, and heterozygous allele frequency of 40% (Bosma *et al.* 1995; Lampe *et al.* 1999). It is a functional polymorphism resulting in reduced gene expression and glucuronidation in both pre-clinical models (Iyer *et al.* 1999; Fisher *et al.* 2000) and in patients (Ando *et al.* 2000; Iyer *et al.* 2002). Irinotecan (CPT-11) is a topoisomerase I inhibitor that is converted in the liver to a highly active metabolite SN38 by UGT family of enzymes (Humerickhouse *et al.* 2000; Xu *et al.* 2002). Toxicity of CPT-11 has been the cause of several fatalities in clinical trials. Both heterozygotes and homozygotes are at risk for toxicity (Ando *et al.* 2000). A recent prospective study demonstrated a positive correlation between unconjugated bilirubin levels and the presence of the homozygous genotype and toxicity (Innocenti *et al.* 2004). The potential impact of this observation is that up to 50% of patients who need irinotecan therapy could be potentially excluded on the basis of the UGT1A1*28 allele (Mcleod & Watters 2004). Prospective clinical trials are now studying the impact of different doses and scheduling of irinotecan in patients with either the 6/6 or 7/7 genotype.

2.2 Pharmacodynamics

Pharmacodynamics studies the drug effects of a drug on the body. This area is increasingly important now with the advent of biological therapy and targeted therapies that are more specific for tumour tissue. Variations in tumour targets and tumour biology are being recognised to determine drug efficacy.

A pertinent recent example is the EGFR tyrosine kinase (TK) inhibitor family of drugs (see Chapter 4). These drugs have high specificity for HER-1 (EGFR) and *in vitro* experiments demonstrated good inhibition of cell growth. When brought to the clinical setting, these drugs in initial phase II mono-therapy trials (Fukuoka *et al.* 2003) showed remarkable effect when they worked (Fig. 14.3) but low response rates. In phase III trials in combination with chemotherapy (Giaccone *et al.* 2004; Herbst *et al.* 2004), EGFR inhibition did not impact an improvement in response. This was explained when activating mutations in the EGFR TK binding domain (Table 14.1) were discovered in a large proportion of responders to gefitinib and absent in tumours of patients who progressed on this therapy (Lynch *et al.* 2004; Paez *et al.* 2004; Pao *et al.* 2004). These mutations were noted to be more frequent in females, adenocarcinoma, non-smokers, and Asians. These mutations made EGFR more sensitive to gefitinib. There are aspects that require further study. Some patients who responded did not carry a mutation in the tyrosine kinase-binding domain on sequencing studies. While mutations are more common in females and adenocarcinomas, there are male patients and patients with squamous cell carcinoma with documented response to such therapy. There is also a significant proportion of patients who develop durable stabilisation of disease not meeting the criteria for a partial response to therapy. The mutation status in these subsets of patients needs to be clarified. The relative contribution of heterodimeric activation of EGFR pathway by other **ligands** such as other members of the HER family, and downstream tumour suppressors that contribute to down-regulation of EGFR signalling, need to be studied. Patients who initially respond also eventually progress on this therapy, and thus it is likely that secondary mutations in the TK binding domain occur similar to c-kit or PDGFR secondary mutations that account for secondary resistance to imatinib. Therefore the true clinical utility of this mutation will only be realised when the sensitivity and specificity of these mutations in predicting for EGFR TK inhibitor response is prospectively studied and validated.

3 Individualised cancer therapy

3.1 Current validated examples

It is revealing that despite such great expansion of our knowledge base in genetics in the last 10 years, the validated examples of individualised cancer therapy are few. In the following section, examples of drugs that have been successfully 'individualised' for therapy and the limitations of current strategies will be discussed.

3.1.1 Trastuzumab and HER-2

Trastuzumab and HER-2 remains one of the best examples of proof of concept in individualising cancer therapy. HER-2 is an oncogene that encodes a 185-kDa transmembrane tyrosine kinase receptor that has partial homology with other members of the epidermal growth factor receptor family. HER-2 is expressed in a small fraction of normal tissue and overexpressed in a range of cancer tissue, from breast to lung cancer. It is an independent prognostic factor for outcome (Slamon *et al.* 1987; Paik *et al.* 1990; Press *et al.* 1997) in breast cancer where it is overexpressed in 25% of patients. For this reason it was evident that development of a **monoclonal antibody** to this oncogene could potentially treat this subgroup of patients. Trastuzumab is a humanised monoclonal antibody to HER-2 receptor. It binds to the extracellular component of HER-2. Its mechanism of action is incompletely understood, however it down-regulates HER-2 expression by receptor **endocytosis** and degradation and induces antibody-dependent cytoxicity in animal models (Roskoski *et al.* 2004). Loss of the extracellular domain is also important for intracellular dimerisation and kinase activation, and trastuzumab may act to prevent this (Molina *et al.* 2001). The pre-clinical efficacy of trastuzumab was demonstrated by down-regulation of oncogene expression by the antibody and cell growth inhibition (Drebin *et al.* 1985, 1986), and efficacy in tumour xenografts (Drebin *et al.* 1988a, b). Synergism with several common chemotherapeutics was subsequently demonstrated in pre-clinical studies (Pegram *et al.* 2000). In phase II monotherapy trials in metastatic disease the objective response rates ranged from 11% to 15% (Baselga *et al.* 1996; Cobleigh *et al.* 1999). In a seminal paper in 2001, Slamon showed that by addition of paclitaxel or anthracyclines to trastuzumab in previously untreated women with HER-2 overexpressing disease (at least 2+ by immunohistochemistry),

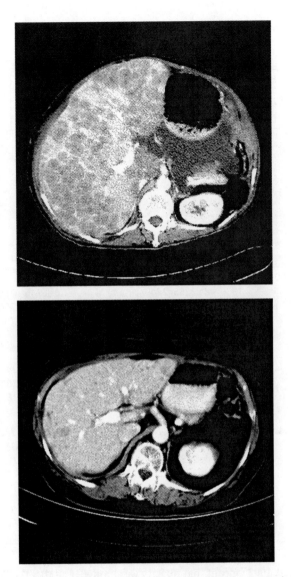

Fig. 14.3 Sequential CT scans of a female Chinese patient with metastatic lung adenocarcinoma treated with gefitinib taken 10 months apart, showing near complete resolution of liver metastases. (Photo courtesy of Dr Wan-Teck Lim, National Cancer Center Singapore.)

these women benefited with a 20% relative reduction in the risk of death at 30 months (Slamon *et al.* 2001). In addition, the paucity of HER-2 expression on normal cells and the presence of HER-2 in both primary and metastatic tumour

Table 14.1 Somatic mutations in EGFR that determine sensitivity to gefitinib.

Exons 25-28	Exons 18-24	Exons 17	Exons 13-16	Exons 8-12	Exons 5-7	Exons 1-4
Regulatory Domain	TK Domain	TM region	Subdomain IV	Subdomain III	Subdomain II	Subdomain I

Study	Exon	Mutation in EGFR gene	Mutation in EGFR protein
Lynch *et al.* (2004)	18	2155 G→T	G719C
	19	del2235–2249	delE746-A750
	19	del2240–2251	delL747-A750,T751S
	19	del2240–2257	delL747–S752,P753S
	21	2573 T→G	L858R
	21	2582 T→A	L861Q
Paez *et al.* (2004)	19	del2239–2247,2248G→C	delL747-E749, A750P
	19	del2240–2257	delL747-S752, P753S
	19	del2238–2255,2237A→T	delL747-S752,E746V
	21	2573 T→G	L858R
Pao *et al.* (2004)	19	del2235–2249	delE746-A750
	19	del2236–2250	delE746-A750
	19	del2239–2256	delL747-S752
	19	del2239–2248,2252–2256	delL747-S752insQ
	19	del2229–2236,2245–2252+T	delE746-T751insl
	20	2326 C→T	R776C
	21	2573 T→G	L858R
	21	2504 A→T	H835L

(Niehans *et al.* 1993) meant that toxicity was limited, and that the therapy was likely to be of use in both the primary and metastatic tumour.

With the development of trastuzumab, the question arose whether all patients who express HER-2 should be offered the drug. The best method to select the patient for therapy remains controversial. The initial studies selected patients for therapy with trastuzumab used over-expression by IHC. Monoclonal antibodies to either the extracellular domain or intracytoplasmic domain were equally effective in selecting patients for treatment in the initial studies. These studies demonstrated that patients who were called 3+ on IHC had a consistently higher response compared to 2+. However because of inter-observer variability, lack of internal standards and a wide variation in response depending on the staining intensity of IHC, some studies utilised fluorescent *in situ* hybridisation (FISH) to detect HER-2 gene amplification in retrospective analyses. Comparative studies of FISH and IHC show fairly high concordance between IHC and FISH in predicting response in patients treated with trastuzumab (Seidman *et al.* 2001; Vogel *et al.* 2002). To date there are no trials that have tested the value of HER-2 testing using FISH alone. This has led to adoption of two methods of selection of patients for therapy with trastuzumab: either treating all patients who express HER-2 3+ using an industry kit and use FISH to confirm HER-2 positivity in patients who were 2+ by IHC; or FISH testing for all patients. Potentially the area where HER-2 overexpression and trastuzumab will find greatest impact in treatment will likely be in adjuvant therapy of breast cancer. In patients with resected breast cancer who overexpress HER-2, and have an overall poorer prognosis, institution of adjuvant chemotherapy with trastuzumab could potentially result in a significant relative reduction in risk of disease relapse and death. This is currently the subject of large phase III trials. In the HERA trial, women with HER-2 positive early breast cancer have been randomised, following adjuvant chemotherapy, to trastuzumab for one year vs. trastuzumab for two years vs. observation. The early results of HERA, those for trastuzumab given every 3 weeks for one year vs. observation, were presented at ASCO 2005 (Piccart 2005). Trastuzumab (T) significantly prolonged disease-free survival (2 years: T 85.8%; observation 77.4%: HR = 0.54, $P < 0.0001$) and relapse-free survival (2 years: T 87.2%; observation 78.6%: HR = 0.50, $P < 0.0001$), significantly reduced the risk of distant metastases and its clinical benefits are independent of the patient's baseline characteristics (including node status and hormone receptor status) and of the type of chemotherapy received. However, more cardiotoxicity was seen in the trastuzumab group. Long-term data will be required before changes can be recommended to clinical practice; the results of the optimal duration, one year vs. two years, will be available by 2008.

Overall, with HER-2 testing, 3 of 10 patients will be selected correctly for treatment with trastuzumab. This still leaves a significant proportion of patients that will fail this pharmacogenetic stratification and this population will require further research to yield viable treatment options.

3.1.2 C-kit/bcr-abl and imatinib

Imatinib is a promiscuous tyrosine kinase inhibitor and inhibits several kinases such as c-kit, bcr-abl, and platelet-derived growth factor receptor alpha (PDGFRa). In this effect, its application now includes chronic myelogenous leukaemias and gastrointestinal stromal tumours (GIST). Bcr-abl is the fusion oncogene created by translocation of the long arm of chromosome 9 and the short arm of chromosome 22 (also known as the **Philadelphia chromosome**) (Nowell 1962; Rowley 1973; Shtivelman *et al.* 1985). It is the genotypic abnormality responsible for leukaemogenesis resulting in chronic myelocytic leukaemia (CML) and selected types of acute lymphocytic leukaemia (ALL). This results in deregulation of Abl tyrosine kinase and phosphorylation and activation of signal transduction pathways that govern cell proliferation, cell survival, and **apoptosis** (Holyoake 2001). Initial *in vitro* studies of imatinib showed that it was a specific agent and inhibited only cells bearing the bcr-abl fusion protein (Druker *et al.* 1996). This observation was subsequently corroborated in clinical studies that showed complete cytogenetic remission in a substantial number of patients (Druker *et al.* 2001a, b). This drug has now been approved for treatment of CML in blast crisis, where the majority of cells are driven by deregulated Abl tyrosine kinase.

Gastrointestinal stromal tumours (GIST) are the most common tumour arising from mesenchymal tissue and there was no effective treatment. It is a relatively slow-growing highly chemotherapy and radiotherapy resistant tumour. It expresses a specific receptor CD117 (also known as c-kit). C-kit is constitutively activated in these tumours and inhibition of activated c-kit tyrosine kinase by imatinib has the effect of reducing cell proliferation, decreasing cell survival and cause apoptosis (Tuveson *et al.* 2001). Identification of this phenotype can be determined by simple immunohistochemistry for c-kit. Around 80% of GIST carry activating c-kit mutations. Imatinib has revolutionised therapy in this disease. Again a robust genotype-phenotype association between activated c-kit mutations and c-kit expression by IHC established a logical pattern for development of imatinib as a targeted therapy. Interest has now turned to the subsets of patients who are c-kit negative by IHC. These patients otherwise have GIST that are clinically, pathologically, and cytogenetically similar. Mutations in PDGFR and c-kit mutation carriers with low or absent concurrent c-kit protein expression have been described (Medeiros *et al.* 2004). Interestingly, treatment with imatinib has been successful in some of these patients (Bauer *et al.* 2003; Heinrich *et al.* 2003; Hirota *et al.* 2003). These mutations in PDGFR appear to an alternate pathway for driving tumour progression aside from or in place of c-kit. Absence of c-kit expression in the presence of c-kit mutations may represent problems with the antibody for IHC, or extremely low expression that cannot be assessed by IHC (Medeiros *et al.* 2004). These findings suggest a need for further evaluation of other biomarkers for this subset in order not to deny therapy to patients who will benefit from imatinib.

3.1.3 CD20 and rituximab

CD20 is a ubiquitous membrane receptor expressed in normal and neoplastic cells of B-cell lineage. The function of CD20 remains largely unknown. There is no known CD20 ligand, and CD20-deficient mice have normal B-cell function (O'Keefe *et al.* 1998). However because of its widespread expression as a cell surface antigen, it is a target of interest. Rituximab is a humanised **chimeric** monoclonal antibody against CD20. It demonstrated synergism with chemotherapy in inducing apoptosis and cell death (Di Gaetano *et al.* 2001; Shan *et al.* 2001). It has shown exciting results in combination with conventional cytotoxic regimens and as monotherapy in large phase III trials of both aggressive and indolent lymphomas of B-cell lineage (Czuczman *et al.* 1999; Coiffier *et al.* 2002). In the process following binding, it has been shown that **complement** activation leading to complement dependent cytotoxicity (CDC) and **antibody-dependent cell-mediated cytotoxicity (ADCC)** results in cell death and apoptosis in B-cell lymphoma cell lines (Cartron *et al.* 2004). Because of the nature of ADCC mediated cytotoxicity, **immunoglobulins** play a major role in affecting cell lysis and cell death. Recent studies show in patients treated with rituximab, response can be better predicted by looking for polymorphisms in the fragment C gamma receptors (FCGR) of immunoglobulin G. A single nucleotide polymorphism in FCGR3A at position 158 that causes a change from valine to phenylalanine increases the affinity of IgG1 for the FCGR3A-158 VV receptor (Koehne *et al.* 1997). This same polymorphism is shown to associate with a higher response rate to rituximab as shown by objective responses and also clearance of the bcl2-JH rearrangement (Cartron *et al.* 2002). The observation that this polymorphism results in differential response has been confirmed in separate studies involving both lymphoma (Weng & Levy 2003) and with inflammatory bowel disease treated with infliximab (another chimerised monoclonal antibody to tumour necrosis factor alpha) (Louis *et al.* 2004). This further suggests that the advantage gained is independent of tumour biology and is dependent on the effects of the monoclonal antibody and ADCC.

4 Current limitations

Progress in translating findings from the bench to the bedside is inexorably slow. There are several reasons.

4.1 Determining functional variants

There is a great degree of genetic diversity. However, not all these variants change the function of the protein. Some of the variants lie in the untranslated or intronic regions of the genomic DNA. While they are less likely to alter function, tandem repeats that occur in the 5′untranslated promoter region can cause changes in gene copy number and function. Sifting out the functional variants is challenging. Considering the number of variants in each gene, overcoming this at both a statistical and clinical level would be a major problem. As such some proponents have suggested using haplotype associations or tag SNPs to reduce the number of variants that need to be associated with outcome. Major consortia are also contributing SNP analyses to a public database (http://hapmap.org) and availability of these SNPs will allow biomarker studies to be pursued more easily.

4.2 Epigenetic phenomenon

There is now increasing evidence that gene expression can be independent of the DNA sequence. This phenomenon called epigenetics is defined as modifications of the genome heritable during cell division that do not involve a change in the DNA sequence (Feinberg 2001). Major epigenetic effects are: DNA methylation; genomic imprinting, where one parental allele compared to the other is silenced by differential methylation of regions near imprinted genes; and transcriptional regulation related to histone modification (Feinberg & Tycko 2004). Epigenetic alterations in cancer were first described in 1983 by Feinberg and Vogelstein (1983). They described hypomethylation in the genes of cancer cells compared to normal ones. Other genes that do not undergo methylation may undergo post-transcriptional changes in RNA or post-translational modification of protein. These may change and influence function in the presence of a constant gene sequence. O^6-methyl guanine DNA methyltransferase (MGMT) is an important DNA repair gene. It is responsible for removing O^6-guanine residue that arises from alkylation. It is silenced by hypermethylation. Tumours with hypermethylated MGMT have greater propensity to induce point mutations in genes because of low activity of MGMT, aberrant pairing of O^6-methyl guanine with thymine, resulting in conversion of guanine–cytosine pairs to adenine–thymine pairs. p53 and k-ras are two important oncogenes where MGMT hypermethylation has resulted in increased mutations. Conversely, MGMT silencing also renders tumours more sensitive to alkylating chemotherapy (Esteller & Herman 2004) such as cyclophosphamide and nitrogen mustard. MGMT inactivation by DNA-damaging agents or guanine analogues has undergone clinical trials in combination with alkylating agents, but its use is likely limited currently because cytotoxicity is not limited to tumour tissue. Myelosuppression is a major problem because of low levels of MGMT in bone marrow.

4.3 Understanding drug and tumour pathways

Our current understanding of pharmacokinetics and pharmacodynamics that determine drug effectiveness is still a piece in evolution. There are large ongoing projects that are attempting to locate and categorise all known SNPs in candidate pharmacokinetic and pharmacodynamic genes, re-sequencing them and correlating them with function. In concert with biostatistics and bioinformatics, they are attempting to separate the genes of highest impact from those of limited utility. They would subsequently be studied in chemotherapeutics and targeted therapies that associate these relevant SNPs with drug toxicity and efficacy. These validation studies need to be done in large datasets of completed prospective trials where there has been uniform tissue and data collection. The markers identified can then be brought into prospectively designed trials that take into account these differences in cancer patients. These clinical studies take time and effort between multidisciplinary groups to complete. They constitute a narrow inlet through which all this generated information is being passed and will slow translation of exciting data from bench to bedside.

4.4 Molecular heterogeneity and clinical trials

There is discordance between drug discovery and ability to translate them to use on human populations. Of 100 drugs in the pipeline that make it to the clinical testing phase, there are only a few that make it to phase II trials in patients that test for toxicity and efficacy. Of these, most are discarded because of either extreme toxicity and/or limited efficacy. Failure of these drugs in phase II trials calls for incorporation of biomarkers that can be used to stratify patients better. An insightful discussion used a hypothetical phase III trial model. Betensky *et al.* determined that if molecular heterogeneity was unaccounted for in the design of such a trial, the trial was likely to be underpowered and fail to detect a truly effective therapy for cancer (Betensky *et al.* 2002). This model was realised soon after with gefitinib and non-small cell lung cancer. Phase II trials showed promising results in a small percentage of patients. Expression by immunohistochemistry of EGFR was not shown to be an effective predictor of outcome. Nevertheless, there were no predictive markers of response planned in the phase III trials in combination with chemotherapy, and molecular heterogeneity was not accounted for in these trials. Not surprisingly the trials showed no differences between either the chemotherapy or chemotherapy and gefitinib arm. It was later that mutations in the tyrosine kinase binding domain were shown to associate with response, showing that indeed molecular heterogeneity accounted for differential responses. Where trials have been designed to stratify for such molecular heterogeneity, e.g. HER-2 in breast cancer, the full benefit of this biomarker and the biotherapy is revealed.

5 Future promise

What can be expected in 5 years time that will be different from today? For one thing the knowledge base will continue to expand. Efforts to integrate more biomarker studies into clinical drug trials in an expeditious and correct manner will continue. Efforts to understand the genome and epigenomic phenomenon will bear fruit. One can hope that in the next 5 years, the current zoo of biomarkers may be distilled down to a single marker or set of markers that can be derived from readily available tissue such as blood or tumour biopsies using an accurate test. Such a biomarker should have a robust genotype-phenotype correlation, and effectively predict for sensitivity/ response or toxicity in individuals undergoing cancer therapy.

References

Alizadeh AA, Eisen MB, Davis RE, Ma C, Lossos IS, Rosenwald A *et al.* (2000) Distinct types of diffuse large B-cell lymphoma identified by gene expression profiling. *Nature*; 403(6769): 503–11.

Altman DG, Bland JM (1994a) Statistics notes: diagnostic tests 2: predictive values. *BMJ*; 309(6947): 102.

Altman DG, Bland JM (1994b) Statistics notes: diagnostic tests 1: sensitivity and specificity. *BMJ* 308(6943): 1552.

Ando Y, Saka H, Ando M, Sawa T, Muro K, Ueoka H *et al.* (2000) Polymorphisms of UDP-glucuronosyltransferase gene and irinotecan toxicity: a pharmacogenetic analysis. *Cancer Res*; 60(24): 6921–6.

Azam M, Latek RR, Daley GQ (2003) Mechanisms of autoinhibition and STI-571/imatinib resistance revealed by mutagenesis of BCR-ABL. *Cell*; 112(6): 831–43.

Baselga J, Tripathy D, Mendelsohn J, Baughman S, Benz CC, Dantis L A *et al.* (1996) Phase II study of weekly intravenous recombinant humanized anti-p185HER2 monoclonal antibody in patients with HER2/neu-overexpressing metastatic breast cancer. *J Clin Oncol*; 14(3): 737–44.

Bauer S, Corless CL, Heinrich MC, Dirsch O, Antoch G, Kanja J *et al.* (2003) Response to imatinib mesylate of a gastrointestinal stromal tumor with very low expression of KIT. *Cancer Chemother Pharmacol*; 51(3): 261–5.

Betensky RA, Louis DN, Cairncross JG (2002) Influence of unrecognized molecular heterogeneity on randomized clinical trials. *J Clin Oncol*; 20(10): 2495–9.

Bianco R, Caputo R, Damiano V, De Placido S, Ficorella C, Agrawal S *et al.* (2004) Combined targeting of epidermal growth factor receptor and MDM2 by gefitinib and antisense MDM2 cooperatively inhibit hormone-independent prostate cancer. *Clin Cancer Res*; 10(14): 4858–64.

Bohmer FD, Karagyozov L, Uecker A, Serve H, Botzki A, Mahboobi S *et al.* (2003) A single amino acid exchange inverts susceptibility of related receptor tyrosine kinases for the ATP site inhibitor STI-571. *J Biol Chem*; 278(7): 5148–55.

Bosma PJ, Chowdhury JR, Bakker C, Gantla S, de Boer A, Oostra BA *et al.* (1995) The genetic basis of the reduced expression of bilirubin UDP-glucuronosyltransferase 1 in Gilbert's syndrome. *N Engl J Med*; 333(18): 1171–5.

Cannistra SA (1990) Chronic myelogenous leukaemia as a model for the genetic basis of cancer. *Hematol Oncol Clin North Am*; 4(2): 337–57.

Cartron G, Dacheux L, Salles G, Solal-Celigny P, Bardos P, Colombat P *et al.* (2002) Therapeutic activity of humanized anti-CD20 monoclonal antibody and polymorphism in IgG Fc receptor FcgammaRIIIa gene. *Blood*; 99(3): 754–8.

Cartron G, Watier H, Golay J, Solal-Celigny P (2004) From the bench to the bedside: ways to improve rituximab efficacy. *Blood*; 104(9): 2635–4.

Cobleigh MA, Vogel CL, Tripathy D, Robert NJ, Scholl S, Fehrenbacher L *et al.* (1999) Multinational study of the efficacy and safety of humanized anti-HER2 monoclonal antibody in women who have HER2-overexpressing metastatic breast cancer that has progressed after chemotherapy for metastatic disease. *J Clin Oncol*; 17(9): 2639–48.

Coiffier B, Lepage E, Briere J, Herbrecht R, Tilly H, Bouabdallah R *et al.* (2002) CHOP chemotherapy plus rituximab compared with CHOP alone in elderly patients with diffuse large-B-cell lymphoma. *N Engl J Med*; 346(4): 235–42.

Collie-Duguid ES, Etienne MC, Milano G, McLeod HL (2000) Known variant DPYD alleles do not explain DPD deficiency in cancer patients. *Pharmacogenetics*; 10(3): 217–23.

Czuczman MS, Grillo-Lopez AJ, White CA, Saleh M, Gordon L, LoBuglio AF *et al.* (1999) Treatment of patients with low-grade B-cell lymphoma with the combination of chimeric anti-CD20 monoclonal antibody and CHOP chemotherapy. *J Clin Oncol*; 17(1): 268–76.

Demetri GD, Desai J, Fletcher JA, Morgan JA, Fletcher CDM, Kazanovicz A *et al.* (2004) SU11248, a multi-targeted tyrosine kinase inhibitor, can overcome imatinib (IM) resistance caused by diverse genomic mechanisms in patients (pts) with metastatic gastrointestinal stromal tumor (GIST). ASCO Annual Meeting Proceedings (Post-Meeting Edition). *J Clin Oncol*; 22(14 Suppl): 3001.

Di Gaetano N, Xiao Y, Erba E, Bassan R, Rambaldi A, Golay J *et al.* (2001) Synergism between fludarabine and rituximab revealed in a follicular lymphoma cell line resistant to the cytotoxic activity of either drug alone. *Br J Haematol*; 114(4): 800–9.

Di Paolo A, Danesi R, Falcone A, Cionini L, Vannozzi F, Masi G *et al.* (2001) Relationship between 5-fluorouracil disposition, toxicity and dihydropyrimidine dehydrogenase activity in cancer patients. *Ann Oncol*; 12(9): 1301–6.

Drebin JA, Link VC, Stern DF, Weinberg RA, Greene MI (1985) Down-modulation of an oncogene protein product and reversion of the transformed phenotype by monoclonal antibodies. *Cell*; 41(3): 697–706.

Drebin JA, Link VC, Weinberg RA, Greene MI (1986) Inhibition of tumor growth by a monoclonal antibody reactive with an oncogene-encoded tumor antigen. *Proc Natl Acad Sci USA*; 83(23): 9129–33.

Drebin JA, Link VC, Greene MI (1988a) Monoclonal antibodies reactive with distinct domains of the neu oncogene-encoded p185 molecule exert synergistic anti-tumor effects *in vivo*. *Oncogene* 2(3): 273–7.

Drebin JA, Link VC, Greene MI (1988b) Monoclonal antibodies specific for the neu oncogene product directly mediate anti-tumor effects *in vivo. Oncogene* 2(4): 387–94.

Druker BJ, Tamura S, Buchdunger E, Ohno S, Segal GM, Fanning S *et al.* (1996) Effects of a selective inhibitor of the Abl tyrosine kinase on the growth of Bcr-Abl positive cells. *Nat Med*; 2(5): 561–6.

Druker BJ, Sawyers CL, Kantarjian H, Resta DJ, Reese SF, Ford JM *et al.* (2001a) Activity of a specific inhibitor of the BCR-ABL tyrosine kinase in the blast crisis of chronic myeloid leukaemia and acute lymphoblastic leukaemia with the Philadelphia chromosome. *N Engl J Med* 344(14): 1038–42.

Druker BJ, Talpaz M, Resta DJ, Peng B, Buchdunger E, Ford JM *et al.* (2001b) Efficacy and safety of a specific inhibitor of the BCR-ABL tyrosine kinase in chronic myeloid leukaemia. *N Engl J Med* 344(14): 1031–7.

Esteller M, Herman JG (2004) Generating mutations but providing chemosensitivity: the role of O6-methylguanine DNA methyltransferase in human cancer. *Oncogene*; 23(1): 1–8.

Etienne MC, Lagrange JL, Dassonville O, Fleming R, Thyss A, Renee N *et al.* (1994) Population study of dihydropyrimidine dehydrogenase in cancer patients. *J Clin Oncol*; 12(11): 2248–53.

Feinberg AP 2001) Cancer epigenetics takes center stage. *Proc Natl Acad Sci USA*; 98(2): 392–4.

Feinberg AP, Tycko B (2004) The history of cancer epigenetics. *Nat Rev Cancer*; 4(2): 143–53.

Feinberg AP, Vogelstein B (983) Hypomethylation distinguishes genes of some human cancers from their normal counterparts. *Natur*; 301(5895): 89–92.

Fisher MB, Vandenbranden M, Findlay K, Burchell B, Thummel KE, Hall SD *et al.* (2000) Tissue distribution and interindividual variation in human UDP-glucuronosyltransferase activity: relationship between UGT1A1 promoter genotype and variability in a liver bank. *Pharmacogenetics*; 10(8): 727–39.

Fleming RA, Milano GA, Gaspard MH, Bargnoux PJ, Thyss A, Plagne R *et al.* (1993) Dihydropyrimidine dehydrogenase activity in cancer patients. *Eur J Cancer*; 29A(5): 740–4.

Fukuoka M, Yano S, Giaccone G, Tamura T, Nakagawa K, Douillard JY *et al.* (2003) Multi-institutional randomized phase II trial of gefitinib for previously treated patients with advanced non-small-cell lung cancer. *J Clin Oncol*; 21(12): 2237–46.

Giaccone G, Herbst RS, Manegold C, Scagliotti G, Rosell R, Miller V *et al.* (2004) Gefitinib in combination with gemcitabine and cisplatin in advanced non-small-cell lung cancer: a phase III trial–INTACT 1. *J Clin Oncol*; 22(5): 777–84.

Hahn WC, Weinberg RA (2002) Rules for making human tumor cells. *N Engl J Med*; 347(20): 1593–603.

Heinrich MC, Corless CL, Demetri GD, Blanke CD, von Mehren M, Joensuu H *et al.* (2003) Kinase mutations and imatinib response in patients with metastatic gastrointestinal stromal tumor. *J Clin Oncol*; 21(23): 4342–9.

Herbst RS, Giaccone G, Schiller JH, Natale RB, Miller V, Manegold C *et al.* (2004) Gefitinib in combination with paclitaxel and carboplatin in advanced non-small-cell lung cancer: a phase III trial–INTACT 2. *J Clin Oncol*; 22(5): 785–94.

Hirota S, Ohashi A, Nishida T, Isozaki K, Kinoshita K, Shinomura Y *et al.* (2003) Gain-of-function mutations of platelet-derived growth factor receptor alpha gene in gastrointestinal stromal tumors. *Gastroenterology*; 125(3): 660–7.

Holyoake DT (2001) Recent advances in the molecular and cellular biology of chronic myeloid leukaemia: lessons to be learned from the laboratory. *Br J Haematol*; 113(1): 11–23.

Huang JZ, Sanger WG, Greiner TC, Staudt LM, Weisenburger DD, Pickering DL *et al.* (2002) The t(14; 18) defines a unique subset of diffuse large B-cell lymphoma with a germinal center B-cell gene expression profile. *Blood*; 99(7): 2285–90.

Huang S, Armstrong EA, Benavente S, Chinnaiyan P, Harari PM (2004) Dual-agent molecular targeting of the epidermal growth factor receptor (EGFR): combining anti-EGFR antibody with tyrosine kinase inhibitor. *Cancer Res*; 64(15): 5355–62.

Humerickhouse R, Lohrbach K, Li L, Bosron WF, Dolan ME (2000) Characterization of CPT-11 hydrolysis by human liver carboxylesterase isoforms hCE-1 and hCE-2. *Cancer Res*; 60(5): 1189–92.

Innocenti F, Undevia SD, Iyer L, Chen PX, Das S, Kocherginsky M *et al.* (2004) Genetic variants in the UDP-glucuronosyltransferase 1A1 gene predict the risk of severe neutropenia of irinotecan. *J Clin Oncol*; 22(8): 1382–8.

Iyer L, Hall D, Das S, Mortell MA, Ramirez J, Kim S *et al.* (1999) Phenotype-genotype correlation of in vitro SN-38 (active metabolite of irinotecan) and bilirubin glucuronidation in human liver tissue with UGT1A1 promoter polymorphism. *Clin Pharmacol Ther*; 65(5): 576–82.

Iyer L, Das S, Janisch L, Wen M, Ramirez J, Karrison T *et al.* (2002) UGT1A1*28 polymorphism as a determinant of irinotecan disposition and toxicity. *Pharmacogenomics J*; 2(1): 43–7.

Koene HR, Kleijer M, Algra J, Roos D, von dem Borne AE, de Haas M (1997) Fc gammaRIIIa-158V/F polymorphism influences the binding of IgG by natural killer cell Fc gammaRIIIa, independently of the Fc gammaRIIIa-48L/R/H phenotype. *Blood*; 90(3): 1109–14.

Lampe JW, Bigler J, Horner NK, Potter JD (1999) UDP-glucuronosyltransferase (UGT1A1*28 and UGT1A6*2) polymorphisms in Caucasians and Asians: relationships to serum bilirubin concentrations. *Pharmacogenetics*; 9(3): 341–9.

Lev DC, Kim LS, Melnikova V, Ruiz M, Ananthaswamy HN, Price JE (2004) Dual blockade of EGFR and ERK1/2 phosphorylation potentiates growth inhibition of breast cancer cells. *Br J Cancer*; 91(4): 795–802.

Lim WT, McLeod HL (2004) Should screening for DPD deficiency be mandatory before 5-FU exposure. *Onkologie*; 27(6): 531–3.

Louis E, El Ghoul Z, Vermeire S, Dall'Ozzo S, Rutgeerts P, Paintaud G *et al.* (2004) Association between polymorphism in IgG Fc receptor IIIa coding gene and biological response to infliximab in Crohn's disease. *Aliment Pharmacol Ther*; 19(5): 511–9.

Lossos IS, Czerwinski DK, Alizadeh AA, Wechser MA, Tibshirani R, Botstein D *et al.* (2004) Prediction of survival in diffuse-large-B-cell lymphoma based on the expression of six genes. *N Engl J Med*; 350(18): 1828–37.

Lu Z, Zhang R, Diasio RB (1995) Population characteristics of hepatic dihydropyrimidine dehydrogenase activity, a key metabolic enzyme in 5-fluorouracil chemotherapy. *Clin Pharmacol Ther*; 58(5): 512–22.

Lynch TJ, Bell DW, Sordella R, Gurubhagavatula S, Okimoto RA, Brannigan BW *et al.* (2004) Activating mutations in the epidermal growth factor receptor underlying responsiveness of non-small-cell lung cancer to gefitinib. *N Engl J Med*; 350(21): 2129–39.

McLeod HL, Siva C (2002) The thiopurine S-methyltransferase gene locus – implications for clinical pharmacogenomics. *Pharmacogenomics*; 3(1): 89–98.

McLeod HL, Watters JW (2004) Irinotecan pharmacogenetics: is it time to intervene? *J Clin Oncol*; 22(8): 1356–9.

Medeiros F, Corless CL, Duensing A, Hornick JL, Oliveira AM, Heinrich MC et al. (2004) KIT-negative gastrointestinal stromal tumors: proof of concept and therapeutic implications. Am J Surg Pathol; 28(7): 889–94.

Molina MA, Codony-Servat J, Albanell J, Rojo F, Arribas J, Baselga J (2001) Trastuzumab (Herceptin), a Humanized Anti-HER2 Receptor Monoclonal Antibody, Inhibits Basal and Activated HER2 Ectodomain Cleavage in Breast Cancer Cells. Cancer Res; 61(12): 4744–9.

Niehans GA, Singleton TP, Dykoski D, Kiang DT (1993) Stability of HER-2/neu expression over time and at multiple metastatic sites. J Natl Cancer Inst; 85(15): 1230–5.

Nowell PC (1962) The minute chromosome (Phl) in chronic granulocytic leukaemia. Blut; 8: 65–6.

O'Keefe TL, Williams GT, Davies SL, Neuberger MS (1998) Mice carrying a CD20 gene disruption. Immunogenetics; 48(2): 125–32.

Paez JG, Janne PA, Lee JC, Tracy S, Greulich H, Gabriel S et al. (2004) EGFR mutations in lung cancer: correlation with clinical response to gefitinib therapy. Science; 304(5676): 1497–500.

Paik S, Hazan R, Fisher ER, Sass RE, Fisher B, Redmond C et al. (1990) Pathologic findings from the National Surgical Adjuvant Breast and Bowel Project: prognostic significance of erbB-2 protein overexpression in primary breast cancer. J Clin Oncol; 8(1): 103–12.

Pao W, Miller V, Zakowski M, Doherty J, Politi K, Sarkaria I et al. (2004) EGF receptor gene mutations are common in lung cancers from 'never smokers' and are associated with sensitivity of tumors to gefitinib and erlotinib. Proc Natl Acad Sci USA; 101(36): 13306–11.

Pegram MD, Lopez A, Konecny G, Slamon DJ (2000) Trastuzumab and chemotherapeutics: drug interactions and synergies. Semin Oncol; 27(6 Suppl 11): 21–5; discussion 92–100.

Perou CM, Sorlie T, Eisen MB, van de Rijn M, Jeffrey SS, Rees CA et al. (2000) Molecular portraits of human breast tumours. Nature; 406(6797): 747–52.

Piccart M. (2005) HERA trial. Available online at http: //www.asco.org/ac/1,1003,_12–002511–00–18–0034–00–19–005816–00–21–001, 00.asp (last accessed 7 July 2005).

Press MF, Bernstein L, Thomas PA, Meisner LF, Zhou JY, Ma Y et al. (1997) HER-2/neu gene amplification characterized by fluorescence in situ hybridization: poor prognosis in node-negative breast carcinomas. J Clin Oncol; 15(8): 2894–904.

Raida M, Schwabe W, Hausler P, Van Kuilenburg AB, Van Gennip AH, Behnke D et al. (2001) Prevalence of a common point mutation in the dihydropyrimidine dehydrogenase (DPD) gene within the 5′-splice donor site of intron 14 in patients with severe 5-fluorouracil (5-FU)-related toxicity compared with controls. Clin Cancer Res; 7(9): 2832–9.

Relling MV, Hancock ML, Rivera GK, Sandlund JT, Ribeiro RC, Krynetski EY et al. (1999) Mercaptopurine therapy intolerance and heterozygosity at the thiopurine S-methyltransferase gene locus. J Natl Cancer Inst; 91(23): 2001–8.

Roskoski R, Jr (2004) The ErbB/HER receptor protein-tyrosine kinases and cancer. Biochem Biophys Res Commun; 319(1): 1–11.

Rowley JD (1973) Letter: A new consistent chromosomal abnormality in chronic myelogenous leukaemia identified by quinacrine fluorescence and Giemsa staining. Nature; 243(5405): 290–3.

Seidman AD, Fornier MN, Esteva FJ, Tan L, Kaptain S, Bach A et al. (2001) Weekly trastuzumab and paclitaxel therapy for metastatic breast cancer with analysis of efficacy by HER2 immunophenotype and gene amplification. *J Clin Oncol*; 19(10): 2587–95.

Shan D, Gopal AK, Press OW (2001) Synergistic effects of the fenretinide (4-HPR) and anti-CD20 monoclonal antibodies on apoptosis induction of malignant human B cells. *Clin Cancer Res*; 7(8): 2490–5.

Shipp MA, Ross KN, Tamayo P, Weng AP, Kutok JL, Aguiar RC *et al.* (2002) Diffuse large B-cell lymphoma outcome prediction by gene-expression profiling and supervised machine learning. *Nat Med*; 8(1): 68–74.

Shtivelman E, Lifshitz B, Gale RP, Canaani E (1985) Fused transcript of abl and bcr genes in chronic myelogenous leukaemia. *Nature*; 315(6020): 550–4.

Slamon DJ, Clark GM, Wong SG, Levin WJ, Ullrich A, McGuire WL (1987) Human breast cancer: correlation of relapse and survival with amplification of the HER-2/neu oncogene. *Science*; 235(4785): 177–82.

Slamon DJ, Leyland-Jones B, Shak S, Fuchs H, Paton V *et al.* (2001) Use of chemotherapy plus a monoclonal antibody against HER2 for metastatic breast cancer that overexpresses HER2. *N Engl J Med*; 344(11): 783–92.

Sorlie T, Perou CM, Tibshirani R, Aas T, Geisler S, Johnsen H *et al.* (2001) Gene expression patterns of breast carcinomas distinguish tumor subclasses with clinical implications. *Proc Natl Acad Sci USA*; 98(19): 10869–74.

Tuveson DA, Willis NA, Jacks T, Griffin JD, Singer S, Fletcher CD *et al.* (2001) STI571 inactivation of the gastrointestinal stromal tumor c-KIT oncoprotein: biological and clinical implications. *Oncogene*; 20(36): 5054–8.

Van Kuilenburg AB, Meinsma R, Zoetekouw L, Van Gennip AH (2002) Increased risk of grade IV neutropenia after administration of 5-fluorouracil due to a dihydropyrimidine dehydrogenase deficiency: high prevalence of the IVS14+1g>a mutation. *Int J Cancer*; 101(3): 253–8.

Van Kuilenburg AB, Meinsma R, Zonnenberg BA, Zoetekouw L, Baas F, Matsuda K *et al.* (2003) Dihydropyrimidinase deficiency and severe 5-fluorouracil toxicity. *Clin Cancer Res*; 9(12): 4363–7.

Vogel CL, Cobleigh MA, Tripathy D, Gutheil JC, Harris LN, Fehrenbacher L *et al.* (2002) Efficacy and safety of trastuzumab as a single agent in first-line treatment of HER2-overexpressing metastatic breast cancer. *J Clin Oncol*; 20(3): 719–26.

Vogelstein B, Fearon ER, Hamilton SR, Kern SE, Preisinger AC, Leppert M *et al.* (1988) Genetic alterations during colorectal-tumor development. *N Engl J Med*; 319(9): 525–32.

Wang Y, Jatkoe T, Zhang Y, Mutch MG, Talantov D, Jiang J *et al.* (2004) Gene expression profiles and molecular markers to predict recurrence of Dukes' B colon cancer. *J Clin Oncol*; 22(9): 1564–71.

Watters JW, Kraja A, Meucci MA, Province MA, McLeod HL (2004) Genome-wide discovery of loci influencing chemotherapy cytotoxicity. *Proc Natl Acad Sci USA*; 101(32): 11809–11814.

Weng WK, Levy R (2003) Two immunoglobulin G fragment C receptor polymorphisms independently predict response to rituximab in patients with follicular lymphoma. *J Clin Oncol*; 21(21): 3940–7.

Wolf M, Swaisland H, Averbuch S (2004) Development of the novel biologically targeted anticancer agent gefitinib: determining the optimum dose for clinical efficacy. *Clin Cancer Res*; 10(14): 4607–13.

Xu G, Zhang W, Ma MK, McLeod HL (2002) Human carboxylesterase 2 is commonly expressed in tumor tissue and is correlated with activation of irinotecan. *Clin Cancer Res*; 8(8): 2605–11.

Glossary

Acquired Immune-Deficiency Syndrome (AIDS) A disease of the human immune system caused by the HIV retrovirus that is characterised cytologically especially by a reduction in the numbers of CD4-bearing helper T cells to 20% or less of normal, thereby rendering the subject highly vulnerable to life-threatening conditions.

Adaptive immunity Immunity generated in response to a specific antigen. Hallmarks are memory and specificity.

Adenovirus Any of a family of DNA viruses shaped like a 20-sided polyhedron, originally identified in human adenoid tissue, causing respiratory diseases.

Adjuvant Assisting in the prevention, amelioration, or cure of disease, e.g. adjuvant chemotherapy following surgery; in immunology, an agent that promotes antigenicity.

Adoptive cellular therapy Therapy that involves the transfer of immune cells with anti-tumour activity to the tumour-bearing host.

Agonist A drug capable of combining with receptors to initiate drug actions.

Alleles Variants of a gene that may occur at a given locus.

Allogeneic Involving, derived from, or being individuals of the same species but that are distinct antigenetically.

Angiogenesis The formation and differentiation of new microvessels from parent microvessels.

Anti-angiogenic Inhibition of the development of new blood vessels.

Antibody-dependent cell-mediated cytotoxicity (ADC) A phenomenon in which target cells, coated with antibody, are destroyed by specialised killer cells that bear receptors for the Fc portion of the coating antibody. These receptors allow the killer cells to bind to the antibody-coated target.

Antibody Directed Enzyme Prodrug Therapy (ADEPT) The use of antibodies to express an enzyme capable of converting a non-toxic prodrug into a cytotoxic species.

Antigen processing/presenting cells Non-lymphocyte cells that carry antigen and present it to lymphocytes, resulting in induction of an immune response.

Anti-idiotype An antibody targeted to the idiotype found on antibodies.

Apoptosis Programmed cell death, a genetically controlled normal physiological process to eliminate DNA-damaged, superfluous, or unwanted cells.

ATP Adenosine triphosphate, a phosphorylated nucleoside $C_{10}H_{16}N_5O_{13}P_3$ of adenine that when reversibly converted especially to ADP releases energy in the cell for many metabolic reactions.

Autocrine Related to, promoted by, or being a substance secreted by a cell and acting on surface receptors of the same cell.

Auto-immunity A state in which the body produces an immune response against its own tissue constituents.

Autologous Derived from the same individual, e.g. as both donor and recipient (as of blood).

B lymphocyte (B cell) Lymphocytes derived from the bone marrow that develop into plasma cells and are responsible for the production of antibodies.

Bacillus Calmette-Guérin (BCG) Strain of tubercle bacilli that causes tuberculosis in humans. Attenuated strain is often used as a vaccination against tuberculosis or as a means to non-specifically stimulate the immune system.

Bystander effect Anti-tumour effect, or cell kill, of cancer cells adjacent to those treated. Generally seen with radiation or transduced cells in gene therapy.

Capsid The protein shell of a virus particle that surrounds its nucleic acid.

Caspases A family of intracellular proteases involved in apoptosis, programmed cell death.

CD4 A large glycoprotein that is found especially on the surface of helper T cells, that is the receptor for HIV, and that usually functions to facilitate recognition by helper T-cell receptors of antigens complexed with molecules of a class that are found on the surface of antigen-presenting cells (as B cells and macrophages) and are the product of genes of the major histocompatibility complex.

CD8 A glycoprotein found especially on the surface of cytotoxic T cells that usually functions to facilitate recognition by cytotoxic T-cell receptors of antigens complexed with molecules of a class that are found on the surface of most nucleated cells and are the product of genes of the major histocompatibility complex.

Cell-mediated immunity Immunity mediated by cells, primarily lymphocytes.

Chemokine Chemokines belong to a large family of chemoattractant molecules involved in the directed migration of immune cells.

Chimeric Composed of parts of different origin, e.g. an individual, organ, or part consisting of tissues of diverse genetic constitution.

Chromosome A structural unit within DNA. A chromosome is composed of genes and transmits hereditary information, normally 46 in humans.

Class I MHC Major histocompatability proteins whose role is to display fragments of proteins originating inside the cell.

Class II MHC Major histocompatibility proteins whose role is to display fragments of proteins from digested microorganisms.

Complement A series of serum proteins involved in the mediation of immune reactions. The complement cascade is triggered classically by the interaction of antibody with specific antigen.

Complementarity-determining regions (CDR) The hypervariable region of the antibody that binds to an antigen.

Cyclin-dependent kinase (CDK) A kinase [catalyses the transfer of phosphate groups from a high-energy phosphate-containing molecule (as ATP or ADP) to a substrate] that is dependent on cyclin (a group of proteins active in controlling the cell cycle and in initiating DNA synthesis) to function

CDK inhibitors (CDKIs) Intracellular proteins that act to inhibit the above phosphorylation reaction of CDKs.

Cytokines A generic term for proteins (e.g. interleukin, tumour necrosis factor, and interferon) released by cells on contact with a specific antigen that serve as messengers between cells. Cytokines effect the growth and differentiation of white blood cells and regulate immune and inflammatory responses.

Cytokinesis   The cytoplasmic changes accompanying mitosis.

Cytoplasm   The organised gelatinous complex of inorganic and organic substances external to the nuclear membrane of a cell and including the cytosol and membrane-bound organelles (as mitochondria or chloroplasts).

Cytosol   The fluid portion of the cytoplasm exclusive of organelles and membranes.

Cytostatic   Tending to retard cellular activity and multiplication.

Cytotoxic   Toxic to cells, causing damage or destruction.

Cytotoxic T lymphocyte (CTL)   A T cell that usually bears CD8 molecular markers on its surface and that functions in cell-mediated immunity by destroying a cell, having a specific antigenic molecule on its surface

Deoxyribonucleic acid (DNA)   The type of nucleic acid found principally in the nucleus of animal and vegetable cells. The repository of hereditary characteristics (genetic information). A large, double-helix molecule (held together by hydrogen bonds between purine and pyrimidine bases, which project inward from two chains containing alternate links of deoxyribose and phosphate) that controls protein synthesis within a cell.

Dendritic cell   Antigen-presenting cells with long irregular processes.

Differentiation   The process of cell development and maturation. Results in ability to perform specialised functions for a particular cell type.

Dose-limiting toxicity (DLT)   The dose of an agent, which, if exceeded, causes unacceptable toxicity to the patient.

Endocytosis   Internalisation of substances from the extracellular environment through the formation of vesicles formed from the plasma membrane.

Endoplasmic reticulum   A system of interconnected vesicular and lamellar cytoplasmic membranes that functions especially in the transport of materials within the cell and that is studded with ribosomes in some places.

Epitopes   A molecular region on the surface of an antigen capable of eliciting an immune response and combining with the specific antibody produced by such a response.

Eukaryotic Descriptor for an organism composed of one or more cells containing visibly evident nuclei and organelles.

FAB Fragment of antibody containing the antigen-binding site, one complete light chain, and part of one heavy chain, generated by cleavage of the antibody with the enzyme papain, which cuts at the hinge region.

Fc Fragment of antibody without antigen-binding sites generated by cleavage with papain. The Fc fragment contains the C terminal domains of the heavy immunoglobulin chains.

Fc receptor Protein on the surface of immune cells that recognises the Fc region of an antibody once it has bound an antigen.

Genome Total genetic information carried by a cell or organism.

Genotype The makeup of DNA: the description of an organism at the genetic level.

Golgi apparatus A cytoplasmic organelle that consists of a stack of smooth membranous saccules and associated vesicles and that is active in the modification and transport of proteins.

Graft versus host disease A condition that results when T cells, from a usually allogeneic tissue or organ transplant and especially a bone marrow transplant, react immunologically against the recipient's antigens attacking cells and tissues, that affects especially the skin, gastrointestinal tract, and liver with symptoms including skin rash, fever, diarrhoea, liver dysfunction, abdominal pain, and anorexia, and that may be fatal.

Guanosine triphosphate (GTP) An energy-rich nucleotide analogous to ATP that is composed of guanine linked to ribose and three phosphate groups and is necessary for peptide bond formation during protein synthesis.

Helper/inducer T cell A subset of T lymphocytes (CD4) whose presence is required by B cells for normal antibody production.

Heterozygous Having the two genes at corresponding loci on homologous chromosomes, different for one or more loci.

Homozygous Having the two genes at corresponding loci on homologous chromosomes, identical for one or more loci.

Human anti-chimeric antibody (HACA) The immune response generated by the infusion of a chimeric antibody into an immunocompetent individual. The response is targeted to the mouse portion of the antibody.

Human anti-mouse antibody (HAMA) The immune response generated by the infusion of a murine antibody into an immunocompetent individual.

Human leukocyte antigen (HLA) A complex group of antigens that define human tissue histocompatibility.

Humoral immunity Immunity mediated by the cell-free portion of the blood primarily by antibodies.

Hybridoma A hybrid cell that results from the fusion of an antibody-secreting cell with a malignant cell and used to culture continuously a specific monoclonal antibody.

Iatrogenic Induced inadvertently by medical treatment or diagnostic procedures or by a clinician.

Idiotype The combined antigen determinants (idiotypes) found on antibodies of an individual that are directed at a particular antigen. Such antigenic determinants are found only in the variable region.

Immune surveillance The concept that immunological mechanisms 'recognise' and remove malignant cells as they arise.

Immunisation The creation of immunity usually against a particular disease with the purpose of making the organism immune to subsequent attack by a particular pathogen.

Immunogen A molecule that provokes an immune response.

Immunogenic Relating to or producing an immune response.

Immunogenicity The state or quality of being immunogenic.

Immunoglobulin Protein molecules composed of four polypeptide chains (two heavy chains and two light chains) that function as antibodies. There are five classes of immunoglobulins: IgG, M, A, D, and E.

Immunotherapy The use of therapy that stimulates the immune system as its mechanism of action.

Innate immunity Non-specific immunity that does not involve the specific recognition of antigen.

Integrins Glycoproteins found on cell surfaces that are composed of two dissimilar polypeptide chains, that are receptors for various proteins that typically bind to the tripeptide ligand consisting of arginine, glycine, and aspartic acid, that promote adhesion of cells (e.g. T cells) to other cells (e.g.

endothelial cells) or to extracellular material (as fibronectin or laminin), and that mediate various biological processes (e.g. phagocytosis, wound healing, and embryogenesis).

Interleukin   Literally, 'between leukocytes'. Compounds of low molecular weight produced by lymphocytes, macrophages, and monocytes, and that function especially in regulation of the immune system and especially cell-mediated immunity.

Isotype   Any of the categories of antibodies determined by their phy-sicochemical properties (such as molecular weight) and antigenic characteristics.

Leukapharesis   A procedure by which the white blood cells are removed from a donor's blood, which is then transfused back into the donor.

Ligand   Something that binds, especially molecules that bind to cells or other molecules.

Liposomes   A fatty droplet in the cytoplasm of a cell *or* an artificial vesicle that is composed of one or more phospholipid bilayers and is used to deliver microscopic substances (as DNA or drugs) to body cells.

Lymphokines   Protein molecules (e.g. an interleukin) of low molecular weight that are not antibodies,   secreted by T cells in response to stimula-tion by antigens that serve as messengers between cells of the immune system.

Lymphokine-activated killer (LAK) cells   Peripheral blood lymphocytes cap-able of lysing a variety of tumour cell lines after exposure to IL-2.

Lysis   Disintegration or dissolution of cells, bacteria, and other structures by a specific agent.

Lysosome   A sac-like cellular organelle that contains various hydrolytic enzymes.

Lytic   Relating to lysis.

Macrophage histocompatibility complex (MHC)   The collection of genes coding for cell-surface compatibility antigens.

Matrix metalloproteinases (MMPs)   A family of zinc-dependent endopepti-dases uniquely able to digest various structural components of the extra-cellular matrix.

Mitogen   A molecule that can induce non-specific division and activation of lymphocytes.

Mitochondria   Any of various round or long cellular organelles of most eukaryotes that are found outside the nucleus, produce energy for the cell through cellular respiration, and are rich in fats, proteins and enzymes.

Mitosis   The process of cell division that results in the production of two daughter cells.

Mitotic index   The proportion (number of cells per thousand cells) of cells in a given tissue that are in mitosis at any given time.

Monoclonal antibody   Literally an antibody from a single clone. A clone is the progeny of a single cell. The antibody is homogeneous.

Monogenic   Relating to or controlled by a single gene.

MTD (maximum tolerated dose)   The dose of a drug, above which toxicity is unacceptable to the patient.

Natural killer (NK) cells   Lymphocytes (non-B or T) that kill a range of tumour cell targets without antigen specificity. Sometimes known as 'large granular lymphocytes'.

Nucleotide   Any compound containing a heterocyclic compound bound to a phosphorylated sugar by an N-glycosyl link; the basic structural units of RNA and DNA.

Nucleus   The central structure within a cell that houses the genetic code.

Oncogene   A gene having the potential to cause a normal cell to become cancerous.

Organelles   A specialised cellular part—small organ (e.g. a mitochondrion, lysosome, or ribosome).

p53 gene   A tumour-suppressor gene that controls the cell cycle transition from the G phase to the S phase.

Perforins   Molecules involved in the destruction of cells. They cause doughnut-shaped holes to form in the cell membrane, allowing cellular contents to leak out.

Pharmacodynamics   Defined simply, what the drug does to the body.

Pharmacogenomics   A biotechnological science that combines the techniques of medicine, pharmacology, and genomics and is concerned with developing drug therapies to compensate for genetic differences in patients which cause varied responses to a single therapeutic regimen.

Pharmacokinetics How the body acts on a drug.

Phenotype The observed characteristics of an organism that result from interaction of genes and the environment.

Philadelphia chromosome An abnormally short chromosome 22 that is found in the haematopoietic cells of persons affected with chronic myelogenous leukaemia and lacks the major part of its long arm which has usually undergone translocation to chromosome 9.

Plasmid A genetic particle physically separate from the chromosome of the host cell that can function stably and replicate.

Polyclonal Proteins from more than a single clone of cells.

Prodrug A drug that can be converted to a toxic metabolite.

Promoter A binding site in a DNA chain at which RNA polymerase binds to initiate transcription of messenger RNA by one or more nearby structural genes.

Protein kinase An enzyme that switches other enzymes on or off by attaching a phosphate group to them.

Proteolysis The hydrolysis of proteins or peptides with formation of simpler and soluble products (e.g. in digestion)

Proteosome A complex cellular structure that degrades proteins removing denatured, damaged, or improperly translated proteins from cells and regulates the level of proteins such as cyclins and some transcription factors.

Proto-oncogenes A gene present in the normal genome that appears to have a role in regulation of normal cell growth that is converted into an oncogene through somatic mutation.

Recombinant Genetically engineered; may refer to a whole organism or a single product system, such as a bacterium to produce biologically active proteins such as interferon.

Retrovirus A virus from the family retroviridae. These viruses possess the enzyme RNA dependent DNA polymerase (reverse transcriptase).

Ribonucleic acid (RNA) A large molecule consisting of ribonucleoside residues attached to the 3' hydroxyl of one nucleoside to the 5' hydroxyl of the next nucleoside by phosphates and are associated with the control of cellular chemical activities.

Ribosomes   RNA and protein-rich cytoplasmic organelles that are sites of protein synthesis.

Signal transduction   A process of transmitting information (signal) received on the cell surface to the cell's inner structures and nucleus.

Single nucleotide polymorphism   A variant DNA sequence in which the purine or pyrimidine base (as cytosine) of a single nucleotide has been replaced by another such base (as thymine).

Somatic   Relating to or affecting the body especially as distinguished from the germ plasm.

Th1   A subset of T-helper cells that secrete cytokines that help defend the body against viral or bacterial invasion. Cytokines secreted include IL-2, IFN, and TNF.

Th2   A subset of T-helper cells that secretes cytokines that assist in protection from parasitic and muscosal infections. Cytokines secreted include IL-4 and IL-5.

T-cell receptor (TCR)   Molecule (as a protein) on the cell surface of the T cell that has an affinity for a specific antigen

T cell   Lymphocytes that possess highly specific cell-surface antigen receptors, and include some that control the initiation or suppression of cell-mediated and humoral immunity (as by the regulation of T- and B-cell maturation and proliferation) and others that lyse antigen-bearing cells.

Telomerase   An enzyme that allows a cell to replicate indefinitely by replacing telomere length, particularly active in cancer cells.

Telomere   The natural end of a chromosome. Each time a cell replicates, the telomeres shorten, which leads to cell senescence and cell death.

Tolerance   The capacity of the body to endure or become less responsive to a substance.

Transcription   The first step in protein synthesis. An RNA molecule or copy of the information within DNA is made within the nucleus. Information transfer from DNA to RNA.

Transgene   A gene that is taken from the genome of one organism and introduced into the genome of another organism by artificial techniques.

Translation The second step of protein synthesis. Information from mRNA is used to make the new protein within the cytoplasmic structures.

Translocation Transfer of part of a chromosome to a different position especially on a non-homologous chromosome.

Tumour-associated antigens (TAA) Antigens expressed to a greater degree on tumour cells than on normal cells. There are four basic types: oncofoetal, unique, antigens from unrelated tissue, and antigens from the same tissue.

Tumour-infiltrating lymphocytes (TILs) Lymphocytes obtained from tumour specimens.

Tumour-suppressor gene A gene that inhibits growth. Loss of function can lead to cell transformation and malignancy.

Ubiquitination Attachment of ubiquitin to proteins which targets them for proteolytic degradation by a proteasome.

Virion A complete virus particle that consists of an RNA or DNA core with a protein coat sometimes with external envelopes and that is the extracellular infective form of a virus.

Virus Subcellular parasite with genes of DNA or RNA. Replicates inside the host cell, upon which it relies for energy and protein synthesis. In addition, it has an extracellular form in which the virus genes are contained inside a protective coat but with no semipermeable membrane. Viruses cause various important diseases in humans, animals, and plants.

Wild type A phenotype, genotype, or gene that predominates in a natural population of organisms.

Xenograft A graft transferred from an donor of one species to a recipient of another.

Index